EATING *for* PREGNANCY

EATING *for* PREGNANCY

Your Essential Month-by-Month Nutrition Guide *and* Cookbook

THIRD EDITION
COMPLETELY REVISED *and* UPDATED

Catherine Jones and Rose Ann Hudson, RD, LD

***with* Teresa Knight, MD, OB-GYN**

Da Capo
LIFE
LONG

Da Capo Press
Hachette Book Group
1290 Avenue of the Americas, New York, NY 10104
dacapopress.com
@DaCapoPress

Printed in the United States of America

First edition originally published in paperback and ebook by Marlowe & Company in January 2003.

Third Edition: July 2019

Published by Da Capo Lifelong Books, an imprint of Perseus Books, LLC, a subsidiary of Hachette Book Group, Inc.

The publisher is not responsible for websites (or their content) that are not owned by the publisher.

Illustration credits: page 75, credit: mart_m/iStock; pages 99, 125, 153, 177, 203, 233, 283, credit: setory/iStock; page 257, credit: lamnee/iStock.

Print book interior design by Trish Wilkinson.

Library of Congress Cataloging-in-Publication Data

Names: Jones, Catherine Cheremeteff, author. | Hudson, Rose Ann, author.
Title: Eating for pregnancy: your essential month-by-month nutrition guide and cookbook / Catherine Jones and Rose Ann Hudson, RD, LD; with Teresa Knight, MD, OB-GYN, FACOG.
Description: Third edition, completely revised and updated. | New York: Da Capo Lifelong Books, 2019. | Includes bibliographical references and index.
Identifiers: LCCN 2019017594| ISBN 9780738285108 (pbk.: alk. paper) | ISBN 9780738285122 (e-book)
Subjects: LCSH: Pregnancy—Nutritional aspects. | Prenatal care.
Classification: LCC RG559 .J665 2019 | DDC 618.2—dc23
LC record available at https://lccn.loc.gov/2019017594

ISBNs: 978-0-7382-8510-8 (paperback); 978-0-7382-8512-2 (ebook)

LSC-C

10 9 8 7 6 5 4 3 2 1

For all mothers-to-be,
who hold the future in their beautiful bellies.

Contents

MONTH 2: EMBRYO EVOLVING: ORGANS AND SYSTEMS DEVELOPING

MONTH 3: FETUS FORMING: CONSTRUCTION ZONE AHEAD

Nourishing Recipes for the Second Trimester: Maturing at Full Speed

MONTH 4: BEGINNING TO LOOK LIKE A BABY

Body-Building Recipes for the Third Trimester: Grow, Baby, Grow

Catherine Jones and Rose Ann Hudson, RD, LD

Welcome to the third edition of *Eating for Pregnancy*! We are thrilled and honored to be a trusted source for pregnancy nutrition for the past fifteen years. We understand what pregnant women want and need and we do our best to deliver! While it's hard to compete with intense cravings for pickles or rocky road ice cream, we offer 150 nutritious recipes that will tickle your taste buds and satisfy all your nutritional needs. We've redesigned this edition to track your baby's monthly development and honed in on the specific nutrients to optimize your little one's growth over the next nine months.

We know that creating a baby (or babies) is no easy feat. But with the combined knowledge and wisdom our amazing team has to offer, we hope you will feel comfortable in the hands of experts. With decades of experience, each of our contributors offers professional advice along with empathy and support.

Since we published the first edition of *Eating for Pregnancy* in 2003, we've noticed a powerful cooking movement toward consuming more whole foods and superfoods. We love this trend! We hope our book inspires you to leap toward eating healthy foods (maybe even trying some for the first time) and cooking at home! And, for all you mamas out there with special dietary needs, we've upgraded our recipes and complete meal ideas by adding notes on how to make recipes gluten-free, dairy-free, vegetarian, vegan, and helpful for women with diabetes during pregnancy.

These pages are filled with family-friendly recipes tested and enjoyed over the years by couples and families like yours. Convenience and speed are number one priorities in our hectic world. We get it. You need to eat well, sleep as much as possible, pee every five minutes, walk the dog, take your toddler to daycare, and head to work. We want to make sure breakfast, lunch, dinner, and all snacks in between are as stress-free, delicious, and healthy as they can be.

We hope the smart eating habits and recipes you incorporate into your lifestyle over the next nine months will stay with you and your family for years to come. Thank you for allowing us to be part of your incredible journey!

Big hugs and lots of love,
Catherine and Rose Ann

A SPECIAL WELCOME FROM
Dr. Teresa Knight, OB-GYN

Hello Goddesses,

Although I have been a practicing obstetrician and gynecologist for many years, a baby's first breath never ceases to amaze me. At every birth, I am deeply moved by the wondrous events that have allowed for that moment to occur. Our bodies are amazing! It is incredible to think what huge physiologic changes we go through to grow and sustain a baby. We truly are goddesses.

Throughout my career, my mission has been to empower women with the knowledge and options available to them to have the healthiest pregnancies and babies possible. I have seen many miraculous pregnancies and births. I have also at times felt helpless when the unexpected has happened to those who are expecting. But eating well is one variable that's always within your control.

My patients ask me daily about their diet. Common questions are about organic foods, safe foods, and "superfoods." My recommendation is always the same: Eat a variety of nutrient-dense foods and avoid processed foods as much as possible. This book provides the support to do just that. It includes a delicious collection of recipes for all kinds of dietary needs without getting bogged down by the latest trendy foods of the day. This comprehensive resource offers options for many different palates and nutritional needs, while covering all the recommended dietary intakes for pregnancy and lactation. It presents all of the ingredients we need to "bake our little bun(s) in the oven," offering food sources and substitutions, easy recipe instructions, and meal ideas that are simple enough that you, your husband, your partner, or your helper can make it all happen.

This book is written with a strong foundation in science and a big dose of compassion from moms who understand that the making of a miracle is sometimes a huge challenge. Our bodies change to accommodate our growing child in ways that are beautiful and amazing, but can also be uncomfortable. You might be experiencing morning sickness, extreme fatigue, indigestion, heartburn, and various other hardships of pregnancy. But they will all pass. And you will have a beautiful baby in your arms.

I'd like to leave you with one of my favorite quotes from the author Marion C. Garretty: "Mother love is the fuel that enables a normal human being to do the impossible."

—Dr. Knight

INTRODUCTION
Welcome to Eating for Pregnancy

Eating for Pregnancy was written to inform you of your specific nutritional needs before, during, and after pregnancy, and to give you delicious, easy ways to meet them—whether you are cooking at home, lunching at your desk, or on bed rest. Looking at the nutritional math of pregnancy is admittedly daunting, and meeting all of the daily dietary goals is indeed a challenge. But there is certainly more to a healthy pregnancy than consuming the perfect amounts of calcium and iron. Aim for balance. Combine a healthy eating plan with exercise and relaxation to make your prepregnancy months and pregnancy a healthy and enjoyable time.

FOR OUR MOMS TRYING TO CONCEIVE . . .

Gold star for planning ahead. Even before that magical moment of conception occurs, getting your beautiful body in prime condition is the best path forward for a healthy baby. Considering that more than 50 percent of women don't plan their pregnancies, living a healthy lifestyle during your childbearing years is a fantastic guarantee that if conception occurs, your body is ready.

As you read this, you might be on your first day of actively planning to conceive, or you might have been trying for a few months, a year, or even longer. We know that the waiting game of tracking monthly ovulation with a thermometer and/or a phone app can be tedious and frustrating. But hang in there, because this is an excellent opportunity to get your body in the healthiest shape possible. We've got a whole section on preconception just for you. Please see pages 67 to 72. We're with you every step of the way!

FOR OUR MOMS WHO ARE PREGNANT . . .

Congratulations! There is nothing quite like a positive pregnancy test to focus your attention on your lifestyle and eating habits. You will soon learn to share your body and your life with another human being who is totally dependent on you. Suddenly, you realize that everything you eat and drink and do with your body can directly affect the new life you are carrying. And, if you're like most mothers-to-be, this profound realization makes you want the best for your baby.

If this is your first pregnancy, you're in for an amazing journey. If you've been pregnant before, you know much about what lies ahead, but as you have probably been told, every pregnancy is different. The bottom line is that pregnancy is hard work. Some women have it harder than others, such as those carrying twins (or more!), women with diabetes or other complications during pregnancy, and women struggling with depression and anxiety.

Please remember that countless women have gone before you and countless more will follow; however, at this moment in time—we're focused on you! Your pregnancy is the most important thing in your life right now. We're here to guide you and to cheer you on. To be your companion at the grocery store, in the kitchen, and when you have a question about your nutritional needs.

Inhale. Exhale. And, relax. Think positive thoughts. We believe in you. Learn to trust your body. In the end, whether your pregnancy was meticulously planned, medically coaxed, or happened by surprise, one thing is certain—your life will never be the same. As a new mom, you're about to experience a special kind of love that surpasses all others on this planet. Mom + Baby. There is no stronger bond, and it begins in the womb.

LET YOUR MIRACULOUS PREGNANCY JOURNEY BEGIN . . .

- Consult your doctor or care team if you think you may be pregnant, or if your at-home pregnancy test is positive.
- Quit smoking, stop drinking alcohol, and strictly limit or give up caffeinated beverages, including coffee, tea, and soft drinks.
- Inform your doctor of any prescription, over-the-counter, and/or illicit drugs you are taking.
- Reevaluate your eating habits. Do you skip breakfast? Eat fast food for lunch? Graze on junk food for dinner? Please inform your care team of any dietary

concerns, food allergies, or medical conditions that may affect nutrient absorption. You may need additional supplements or a customized eating plan.

- Get moving. Exercise will help you maintain an appropriate pregnancy weight and can help prevent gestational diabetes[1] and gestational hypertension.[2] Exercise will increase your energy and can help overcome insomnia, stress, anxiety, and depression. It can also help alleviate gas, heartburn, and constipation. Recruit your partner, significant other, family member, friend, or co-worker to keep you motivated.

- Eliminate as much stress as possible from your work and home environment. Carve out time to unload and detox. This will keep you emotionally stable when your hormones play tricks on you. Take a minute or two to think about tools you can use to de-stress. Is it music, meditation, a walk, exercise, yoga, a nap, movie, phone call, date night, or connecting with friends?

- Get plenty of rest. Pregnancy fatigue is in a class of its own. Don't fight it. Your body needs the extra sleep for a reason. Plan a fatigue schedule for added downtime, especially during the first and third trimesters. During the first trimester, the increased level of progesterone causes sleepiness and shortness of breath, and during the third, carrying the extra body weight often increases fatigue. Aim for eight hours of sleep at night and take short naps with your legs elevated during the day.

- Pregnant women should be aware of certain dangerous food-borne illnesses and take precautions to avoid them. These include listeriosis (see page 33), toxoplasmosis (see page 28), *E. coli* (see page 30), and salmonellosis (see page 31).

- Limit your consumption of certain large fish, such as swordfish and shark, which could potentially contain high levels of methylmercury (see page 35).

- Avoid X-rays, hot tubs, saunas, massages (unless they are done by a trained and certified prenatal therapist), inverted yoga poses, contact sports, and any activity that has an increased risk of falls, such as skiing.

- Finally, enjoy every day of your pregnancy as much as possible. As Rose Ann always tells her patients: You may only experience pregnancy once, so enjoy it as best you can.

Your Nutritional Needs, Plus a Whole Lot More

During pregnancy, good eating habits are more important than ever. Although "eating for two" is a common expression, it is a bit misleading. While you are pregnant, you are not really eating for two; you are eating mindfully for one.

It's important to learn about the nutritional value of the foods you're eating and to pick them with care. Selecting a variety of nutrient-rich foods versus calorie-rich foods will help prevent excessive weight gain, which can put you at risk for high blood pressure, gestational diabetes, and obesity postpregnancy. On the other hand, insufficient calorie intake can result in inadequate weight gain and in the breakdown of stored fats (or ketones) in the mother's blood and urine, which can be harmful for the fetus. We know that might sound scary, but you'll find the balance. Listen to your body, make smart choices, and you're 90 percent of the way there.

So, what is the ideal diet for you? Striking a balance between healthy weight gain and nutritional intake is not as daunting as it seems. We promise! You have a lot of wiggle room to eat according to your preferred diet, food allergies, special needs, and taste buds, which you might find change drastically and without warning during pregnancy. Your prenatal vitamin and any supplements you are prescribed act as a safety net. **The real power behind your baby's development and your own health will be the healthy foods you consume every day.**

YOUR DAILY CALORIE NEEDS

In the second and third trimesters, most pregnant women increase their calorie intake by about 300 calories per day, assuming that their prior caloric intake was adequate. Certain factors may increase nutritional requirements above the estimated demands of pregnancy, including poor nutritional status, obesity, young maternal age (teenage pregnancy), carrying multiples, closely spaced births, breastfeeding one or more children while pregnant, continued high level of physical activity, certain disease states (such as diabetes), and use of cigarettes, alcohol, and legal or illegal drugs. Women who fit into any of these categories should consult a registered dietitian for customized nutritional advice.

How many calories do you specifically need? A pregnant woman should generally consume between 1,800 and 3,000 calories per day depending on her prepregnant height and weight (body mass index, or BMI; see page 337), stage of pregnancy, physical activity level (PAL), and age. To determine your specific calorie needs (also called estimated energy requirement, or EER), refer to the following chart. On page 338, you will find a BMI chart and a formula to adjust calorie requirements if you are underweight, overweight, obese, carrying twins, triplets, or if you are a teenager. Your doctor and care team should always have the final word in your nutritional requirements.

ESTIMATED ENERGY REQUIREMENT (EER) FOR WOMEN 30 YEARS OF AGE DURING PREGNANCY[1]

HEIGHT (M) [FT & IN]	PHYSICAL ACTIVITY LEVEL (PAL)	PREPREGNANCY BMI OF 18.5 KG/M2 CALORIES REQUIRED	PREPREGNANCY BMI OF 24.99 KG/M2 CALORIES REQUIRED
FIRST TRIMESTER			
1.50 (59) [4'11"]	Sedentary	1,625	1,762
	Low Active	1,803	1,956
	Active	2,025	2,198
	Very Active	2,291	2,489
1.65 (65) [5'5"]	Sedentary	1,816	1,982
	Low Active	2,016	2,202
	Active	2,267	2,477
	Very Active	2,567	2,807
1.80 (71) [5'11"]	Sedentary	2,015	2,211
	Low Active	2,239	2,459
	Active	2,519	2,769
	Very Active	2,855	3,141
SECOND TRIMESTER			
1.50 (59) [4'11"]	Sedentary	1,965	2,102
	Low Active	2,143	2,296
	Active	2,365	2,538
	Very Active	2,631	2,829
1.65 (65) [5'5"]	Sedentary	2,156	2,322
	Low Active	2,356	2,542
	Active	2,607	2,817
	Very Active	2,907	3,147

(continues)

HEIGHT (M) [FT & IN]	PHYSICAL ACTIVITY LEVEL (PAL)	PREPREGNANCY BMI OF 18.5 KG/M2 CALORIES REQUIRED	PREPREGNANCY BMI OF 24.99 KG/M2 CALORIES REQUIRED
SECOND TRIMESTER *(continued)*			
1.80 (71) [5′11″]	Sedentary	2,355	2,551
	Low Active	2,579	2,799
	Active	2,859	3,109
	Very Active	3,195	3,481
THIRD TRIMESTER			
1.50 (59) [4′11″]	Sedentary	2,075	2,212
	Low Active	2,253	2,406
	Active	2,475	2,648
	Very Active	2,741	2,939
1.65 (65) [5′5″]	Sedentary	2,266	2,432
	Low Active	2,466	2,652
	Active	2,717	2,927
	Very Active	3,017	3,257
1.80 (71) [5′11″]	Sedentary	2,465	2,661
	Low Active	2,689	2,909
	Active	2,969	3,219
	Very Active	3,305	3,591

For each year below 30, add 7 kcals per day; for each year above 30 subtract 7 kcals per day

PAL = physical activity level

Activity Levels:[2]

Sedentary = Typical daily living activities

Low Active = Typical daily living activities plus 30 to 60 minutes of daily moderate activity

Active = Typical daily living activities plus 60 minutes of daily moderate activity

Very Active = Typical daily living activities plus at least 60 minutes of daily moderate activity plus an additional 60 minutes of vigorous activity, or 120 minutes of moderate activity

RATE OF WEIGHT GAIN

Just as important as the total number of pounds gained is the rate at which the weight is gained. Aim for about 2 to 5 pounds in the first trimester and 3.5 pounds per month for the remainder of pregnancy. Ideally, your total weight gain during pregnancy should be between 25 and 35 pounds; however, your prepregnant weight and certain conditions will affect the amount of weight you may be advised to gain.

AVERAGE WEIGHT GAIN DURING PREGNANCY[3]

PREPREGNANT WEIGHT/ CONDITION	DESCRIPTION	WEIGHT GAIN
Average weight	Within ideal body weight range	25 to 35 lbs
Underweight prepregnant weight	10% below ideal body weight	28 to 40 lbs
Overweight prepregnant weight	20% above ideal body weight	15 to 25 lbs
Obese	30% above ideal body weight	11 to 20 lbs
Woman carrying twins		40 to 45 lbs

At the end of the day, please don't become obsessed with your weight gain—in fact, feel free to put away your scale. Your weight will be closely monitored by your doctor during each office visit. A trend of excessive or inadequate weight gain in more than one month—a gain of more than 5 pounds or less than 2—indicates that your dietary intake may need to be evaluated. If your weight gain is excessive and on an upward trend overall, take an inventory of your eating habits to pinpoint problem areas. It may be the foods and beverages you are consuming, or the portion sizes might be an issue. If you are losing weight or experiencing inadequate weight gain, reevaluate your exercise plan, particularly if you work out every day. In addition to increasing calories, you may also need to increase the amount of protein and calcium in your diet.

Where do all those extra pounds come from? The following is the generally accepted breakdown.[4] Keep in mind that it is not unusual to have a large one-month weight gain sometime in the second trimester. This may be attributable to a 25 percent increase in blood and fluid volume for the mother.

NUMBER OF POUNDS	SOURCE OF WEIGHT GAIN
6 to 8	Baby
4 to 6	Maternal stores of fat and nutrients
3 to 4	Increased blood volume
2 to 3	Increased fluid volume
2	Uterus
2	Amniotic fluid
1.5	Placenta
1 to 2	Breast enlargement

YOUR NUTRIENT NEEDS

It's helpful to understand the most important nutrients, their role in your baby's development, and how they nourish and sustain your own body.

We know this is a lot of information to digest all at once. Please read it in small chunks and refer to it throughout your pregnancy. It's meant as a reference guide. The most important thing is to figure out ways to use the information in your daily food choices and cooking. Together we can make it happen!

INTRODUCING THE MACRONUTRIENTS

Energy

We all need energy, especially during pregnancy. Energy comes from protein, carbohydrates, and fats. Calories are the single most important nutritional factor in determining birth weight. Calorie intakes during pregnancy vary from woman to woman depending on a number of factors, such as her metabolism, prepregnancy weight, whether she is carrying multiples, her stage of pregnancy, and physical activity level. It is estimated that, on average, a pregnant woman requires a total of 85,000 additional calories over the course of forty weeks of pregnancy. This breaks down to approximately the 300 extra calories per day.[5] During the first trimester, energy needs are generally low, and 300 additional daily calories are not required. Needs begin to pick up in the fourth month as the uterus, mammary glands, placenta, and fetus grow and blood volume increases. In the later stages of pregnancy, energy needs climb again to support the growing fetus and the mother's extra weight. To be exact, the recommended general daily intake is an increase in daily calories of 340 calories in the second trimester, and 452 calories in the third trimester.[6]

PROTEIN

During pregnancy, extra protein is needed to help with fetal brain development and muscle and tissue formation. Inadequate amounts of dietary protein can impair the development of the placenta and fetus and may result in low birth weight and intra-uterine growth retardation. For moms, protein is essential for the increase in maternal blood volume and for the formation of amniotic fluid, especially in the mid to later

PREGNANCY WISDOM: MAKE YOUR 300 EXTRA CALORIES COUNT

BE wise about your 300-calorie additional intake in the second and third trimesters. Choose to eat a sandwich with a glass of milk instead of less nutrient-dense processed foods. Try to include a protein in your snacks and mini-meals. Some popular ideas include nut butters, hard-boiled eggs, cottage cheese, yogurt, cheese sticks, nuts and seeds, dried fruit, bean dips (pages 81 and 161) with veggies, cooked meats and poultry, bean and/or lentil salads (pages 114 and 249), whole-grain breads, whole-grain salads, smoothies (pages 131, 157, and 207), green drinks (page 129), chia pudding (page 282), and protein bars, just to name a few. Leftovers make great mini-meals the next day. Also, see "Kitchen Wisdom: Healthy Snacks for 100 to 200 Calories," page 240.

months. It is also critical to stabilize blood glucose levels. Think of it this way—your protein needs increase as your pregnancy progresses. During labor, delivery, and lactation, protein storage reserves are tapped, making it vital to have an excess amount. Most women will need to consume between 60 and 75 grams. The daily recommended intake during pregnancy is at least 71 grams of protein per day. Some good sources of protein include poultry, lean meats, seafood, cottage cheese, pasteurized cheeses, milk, yogurt, eggs, tofu, tempeh, soy products, beans and other legumes, nut butters, nuts, and seeds. For a more complete list of protein sources, see page 339.

CARBOHYDRATES

Carbohydrates, also called carbs (and referred to as CARBS in this book), fuel your brain and body. Adequate intake of carbohydrates is necessary to free up protein that would otherwise be tapped for energy to be used for muscle building and tissue formation in the fetus. As much as you can, choose complex carbohydrates, such as whole grains, beans, whole wheat pasta, brown rice, fruits, and vegetables, which contain vitamins (particularly the B-complex vitamins), iron, and fiber. Simple sugars, such as candy, sodas, and desserts, may give you a temporary energy boost, but they are empty calories and should not be substituted for nutrient-rich foods. For more information on carbohydrates and how they impact diabetes during pregnancy, see "Diabetes During Pregnancy," pages 50 to 58.

PREGNANCY WISDOM: SAFE ARTIFICIAL SWEETENERS

WHEN it comes to sweeteners, natural is always best (always!). Think: sugar, honey, and maple syrup. That said, many women worry whether artificial sweeteners, such as those found in diet sodas, yogurt, gum, sugar-free desserts, and packets of sweeteners, are safe. There is a lot of conflicting information. The short answer is some are considered safe, such as stevia, sugar alcohols (including xylitol and erythritol), and Splenda. All of these should be consumed in moderation. Others, such as saccharin, should be completely avoided. Aspartame should be carefully weighed, since the results are still unclear. Some studies of aspartame show little risk, but others point to more serious risks, including weight gain[7] and obesity.[8] Pregnancy is the ideal time to try to wean yourself off artificial sweeteners and to curb your craving for sweet foods and drinks.

FATS

Healthy fats are essential during pregnancy and throughout life. They provide slow-burning, long-lasting energy to fuel your body and to enhance your baby's development, plus they are critical for the absorption of fat-soluble vitamins A, D, E, and K. Fats play a central role in skin health, cell formation, and fetal brain development.

Understanding the different types of fat can be confusing. The two major fat groups are saturated and unsaturated fats. The second group is the healthier, so we will start with those. There are two types of unsaturated fats: monounsaturated and polyunsaturated. Both of these fats come primarily from plants, nuts, seeds, and cold-water fish. They remain liquid at room temperature. Monounsaturated fats, such as olive oil, will become solid when refrigerated. Polyunsaturated fats, such as fish oil, will not.

Saturated fats come mainly from animal sources. Butter, cheese, whole milk, cream, lard, meat, and poultry are examples. Palm kernel and coconut oils are also considered saturated fats, despite their plant origins. Saturated fats are solid at room temperature. They should be consumed in moderation. Trans fats, a category of synthetic saturated fats, should be avoided. They are usually found in processed and fast foods. Their use has decreased dramatically in recent years, which is excellent news. While there is no scientific evidence that trans fats are particularly harmful to pregnant women, studies show that excessive consumption of trans fats can decrease the body's conversion of omega-3 fatty acids.[9]

One important subgroup of the unsaturated fats are the omega-3 fatty acids. They are so vital to fetal development, we give them the most attention, with docosahexaenoic acid (DHA) getting the star role. If you remember nothing else, think of these fats as major nutrients for your baby's brain, eye, and nervous system development in the womb and during infancy.[10] During pregnancy, the daily dietary goal for omega-3 fatty acids is 650 milligrams, *300 milligrams of which come from DHA*. See more information in the "Benefits and Sources of Omega-3 Fatty Acids" chart, below.

A major source of the omega-3s is seafood. Many women ask whether seafood is safe to consume during pregnancy, and if so, how much. The answer is yes—by all means, consume seafood, unless you are vegetarian, vegan, or don't eat it for some reason, but please refer to our "Limitations on Consumption of Certain Fish" on page 35. Seafood is an excellent source of lean protein, vitamins, fats, and minerals. Fish varieties that are high in DHA and eicosapentaenoic acid (EPA) and that are safe to eat include salmon (especially wild), canned light tuna, sardines, anchovies, herring, trout, and catfish.

Not all prenatal vitamins contain DHA, so ask your doctor whether you need to take a DHA supplement. Deficiency of DHA is associated with poor night vision and other visual and spatial interpretation problems.[11] Benefits of adequate DHA intake for pregnant moms and babies include the following:

- prevention of preterm delivery[12]
- increase in head circumference and birth weight[13]
- prevention of depression during pregnancy and postpartum[14]
- improved ability for infants to solve problems at nine months and infant's visual acuity at 4 months of age[15]
- supports healthy immune system development[16]

BENEFITS AND SOURCES OF OMEGA-3 FATTY ACIDS

OMEGA-3S	RECOMMENDED DAILY INTAKE FOR PREGNANCY	ROLE	SOURCES
DHA (docosahexaenoic acid)	300 mg (3 g)	Brain and eye (retina) development: structural roles	Fish and seafood and DHA micro algae supplements, plus DHA-fortified products, including cereal, eggs, orange juice, peanut butter, milk, oils, margarines, pastas, and chocolate
EPA (eicosapentaenoic acid)	Not available	Brain development: cell-signaling role	Fish and seafood and DHA micro algae supplements
ALA (alpha-linolenic acid)	Not available	Converted to DHA and EPA for brain and eye development	Vegetable oils, nuts, seeds (flaxseeds, chia, and hemp seeds), soybeans, and dark green leafy vegetables

ESSENTIAL MINERALS AND VITAMINS

Minerals and vitamins play a star role in your baby's growth and development, as well as meeting all your changing body's needs. The following pages summarize the minerals and vitamins (in alphabetical order with the B vitamins grouped together) and the wonderful benefits they offer. Your prenatal vitamin acts as your safety net, so please don't stress out about trying to count every microgram or milligram of every nutrient listed in the foods you're consuming. Choose a variety of healthy whole foods and enjoy them.

Your Mineral Needs

CALCIUM

Calcium is an essential mineral for bone and teeth construction for the mother and her baby. The ideal amount is 1,000 milligrams during pregnancy, and more for women carrying multiples and for pregnant adolescents. Bones contain 99 percent of your calcium, and the remaining 1 percent is found in your blood. If calcium intake is not adequate enough to meet a baby's needs, especially during the third trimester to accommodate rapid skeletal growth, calcium reserves of the mother's bones are tapped, resulting in calcium depletion. Ask your doctor or care team about calcium supplements and dosage. Calcium supplements from some natural sources, such as oyster shell or bone meal, may be high in lead. Synthetic supplements made from calcium carbonate, such as TUMS, have much lower levels of lead (1 milligram per tablet), about the same amount of lead found in one serving of cow's milk.

Calcium in the bloodstream is very important, particularly during labor, when it is needed to maintain proper heartbeat, muscle contractions, nerve transmissions, and for blood clotting. Consuming calcium through proper diet and supplements is only one phase of building and maintaining healthy bones. For the body to absorb calcium, the calcium must be combined with vitamin D (see page 19). To prevent interference with iron absorption, calcium supplements should not be taken with a prenatal vitamin and preferably should be taken between meals. See page 25 for information on lactose intolerance, and page 344 for nondairy calcium sources.

CHROMIUM

Chromium enhances insulin and helps with carbohydrate, fat, and protein metabolism. Pork chops, chicken, broccoli, romaine lettuce, potatoes, spinach, tomatoes, whole wheat bread, whole grains, peanuts, and apples are good sources for the 30-microgram recommended daily intake.

COPPER

Copper assists with iron utilization and other metabolic functions. Greens, mushrooms, squash, asparagus, kidney beans, soybeans, tofu, lentils, brown rice, potatoes, whole wheat bread, seeds, nuts, and pineapple juice are all good sources for the daily recommended intake of 1,000 micrograms.

IODINE

Iodine is critical for thyroid functioning and metabolism regulation. A daily recommended intake of 220 micrograms can be obtained from iodized salt, seaweed, cow's milk (by way of iodine-containing products used to disinfect milk-collection vessels), eggs, fish, shellfish, and pork. Iodine deficiency (unlikely in most developed nations) can result in enlargement of the thyroid gland, goiter, or hypothyroidism, which could have detrimental effects on the fetus.

IRON

Iron is essential for the formation of hemoglobin, which carries oxygen in the blood. A daily iron intake of 27 milligrams is recommended for most healthy pregnancies. Women carrying multiples or women suffering from iron-deficiency anemia (see page 46) may need more. Because it is impossible to meet your daily iron requirements through food sources alone, particularly if you started your pregnancy with low iron stores, a prenatal vitamin that contains iron is recommended for all pregnant women. Additional intermittent iron supplementation (1 to 3 times per week) appears to be as effective as daily supplementation for women who have issues tolerating large doses to treat anemia.

Why is iron so important? For moms, iron is essential to keep up with the increase in blood volume during pregnancy and in the case of complications due to blood loss during pregnancy. During the last trimester, a three- to four-month supply of iron is stored in the liver of the fetus for use after birth, before food stores of iron are added to an infant's diet.

Heme iron from animal sources is more easily absorbed by the body than nonheme iron from plant sources. One easy way to increase iron absorption is to eat high-iron foods with a source of vitamin C. While it is true that some of the highest sources of iron (such as beef and eggs) are also high in cholesterol and fat, a low-cholesterol, low-fat diet is not recommended during a normal pregnancy without complications. Cholesterol levels may rise slightly during the second half of pregnancy, but they usually resume to normal levels within six months postpartum. See page 342 for sources of iron.

MAGNESIUM

Magnesium is critical for bone building, muscle function, heart health, immunity, regulation of blood glucose levels, promoting normal blood pressure, and energy metabolism synthesis. Studies show that magnesium may play a role in preventing preeclampsia, but the evidence is not conclusive.[17] The following foods can help meet the daily recommended intake of 350 milligrams: seafood, nuts (Brazil nuts, almonds), seeds (pumpkin, sunflower, chia, flax, and hemp), soybeans, tofu, tempeh, oatmeal, wheat bran, whole grains, beans, brown rice, lentils, potatoes with skin, avocados, spinach, okra, bananas, orange juice, pineapple juice, molasses, and all dairy products.

MANGANESE

Manganese is imperative for bone development, maintaining normal blood glucose levels, nerve cell health, thyroid functioning, and the metabolism of protein, fats, and carbohydrates. The adequate daily intake is 2 milligrams. Some good sources include nuts, seeds (chia), soybeans, beans, oats, lentils, brown rice, whole wheat bread, romaine lettuce, spinach, kale, baked potatoes, raspberries, bananas, pineapple, and molasses.

MOLYBDENUM

Molybdenum is an important trace element in the metabolism of protein and fat. Spinach, whole grains, milk, and lentils can help supply the 50 micrograms recommended daily.

PHOSPHORUS

Phosphorus helps build strong bones and teeth. It is involved in the metabolism of fats, protein, and carbohydrates for energy, and in the formation of genetic material, cell membranes, and enzymes. Pregnant women should aim to consume 700 milligrams daily. Some good sources include meats, poultry, fish and shellfish, sardines in oil, eggs, whole grains, wheat germ, quinoa, all types of beans, all soy products, lentils, chickpeas, nuts and nut butters (Brazil nuts, almonds, cashews), seeds (pumpkin, sunflower, and chia), baked potatoes with skin, goat's milk, and all dairy products.

POTASSIUM

Potassium is necessary for optimal kidney, heart, digestive, and muscle function. Adequate dietary intake helps prevent osteoporosis. Low intake can lead to high blood pressure. The adequate intake of 4,700 milligrams per day can come from salmon, potatoes, dried apricots, bananas, orange juice, dairy products, and seeds.

SELENIUM

Selenium protects cells from free-radical damage, promotes proper thyroid functioning, and boosts the immune system. Pregnant women should aim for 60 micrograms daily. Some good sources include nuts (Brazil nuts), seeds (chia), oatmeal, pork chops, fish (especially canned light tuna), shellfish (crab and shrimp), poultry, eggs, tofu, soy yogurt, peanuts, mushrooms, milk, yogurt, cheese, cottage cheese, and whole grains (couscous and brown rice).

SODIUM

Sodium is necessary for regulation of blood and bodily fluids, communication among nerves, heart activity, and certain metabolic functions. The adequate intake is 2,300 milligrams of sodium per day. Generally, there are no sodium restrictions for pregnant women. Please consult with your doctor if you have questions or concerns about your sodium intake.

ZINC

Zinc is essential for cell growth, maintaining immunity, wound healing, fat metabolism, gene expression, and sexual function. Zinc deficiency can cause poor fetal growth. Dietary sources of zinc include seafood, meat, eggs, dairy products, zinc-fortified cereals, legumes, seeds, cashews, and whole grains. Pregnant women should consume 11 milligrams of zinc daily.

PREGNANCY WISDOM:
THE DANGERS OF ALCOHOL DURING PREGNANCY

AVOID all alcohol during pregnancy. Alcohol in a mother's bloodstream quickly crosses the placenta to her fetus. Drinking alcohol regularly can cause miscarriage, mental and physical deficiencies, learning disabilities, and numerous other behavioral problems for the child. Heavy consumption, four to five drinks per day, may lead to fetal alcohol exposure (FAE) and fetal alcohol syndrome (FAS), resulting in physical defects to the heart, limbs, and facial structure, in addition to other health issues.[18]

Your Vitamin Needs

VITAMIN A

Vitamin A is vital for promoting cell, bone, and tooth formation; normal vision; and healthy skin in the fetus. Pregnant women require 770 micrograms (about 2,300 IU) of vitamin A daily. Excessive intake of vitamin A (more than 10,000 IU in the form of retinol, not beta-carotene) can increase the risk of birth defects, such as malformation of the head, brain, heart, or spinal cord.[19] Fruit and vegetable sources of vitamin A, such as mangoes, cantaloupe, tangerines, sweet potatoes, carrots, broccoli, and asparagus contain beta-carotene, which the body converts to vitamin A based on need. They are not toxic in large doses. There is some concern about consuming too much liver, which is extremely rich in vitamin A. Pregnant women should minimize their consumption of liver.[20] Other good sources of vitamin A include egg yolks, pasteurized cheese, fortified dairy products, and butter (see page 345 for more sources of vitamin A).

VITAMIN C

Vitamin C (also known as ascorbic acid) is essential for iron absorption, wound healing, healthy teeth and gums, and maintaining resistance to infection. A daily increase to 85 milligrams is recommended during pregnancy; however, don't overdo it with supplements. Excessive intake of vitamin C supplements could cause the newborn to have increased requirements for vitamin C, possibly leading to a deficiency syndrome called rebound scurvy. Pregnant women can fulfill their daily requirements of vitamin C by eating citrus fruits, berries, cantaloupe, tomatoes, broccoli, Brussels sprouts, and red bell peppers (see page 346 for more sources).

VITAMIN D

Vitamin D is manufactured by the body after exposure to the sun. It is necessary to promote the utilization of calcium and phosphorus by the body. Pregnant women need 15 micrograms (500 IU) of vitamin D per day. A healthy, nonpregnant woman usually gets adequate amounts from two twenty-minute sessions of exposure to sunlight weekly, without UVA-blocking sunscreen. Be aware that vitamin D through supplements can be toxic in doses larger than 1,000 IU. Ideally, supplements should be labeled D_3 as they tend to have a better absorption rate in the body than D_2. Good sources of vitamin D include egg yolks, butter, fortified milk products, fortified cereals, fortified plant-based milks, canned fish (sardines, salmon, herring, and mackerel), and seafood.

VITAMIN E

Vitamin E protects cells from damage, boosts immune function, assists with DNA repair, and supports metabolic processes. A daily intake of 15 milligrams (28.5 IU) can be obtained from wheat germ, vegetable oils, avocados, nuts (almonds), and seeds (sunflower).

VITAMIN K

Vitamin K ensures normal blood clotting and bone mineralization. The adequate intake is 90 micrograms, which is easily met by the following sources: all greens (especially romaine lettuce and spinach), Brussels sprouts, avocados, broccoli, cabbage, asparagus, and kelp.

THE B VITAMINS

Folic acid (also called folacin and folate; folate is the natural form) is essential for cell division and manufacturing DNA and RNA, the molecules that transfer genetic information and translate it into tissue production. Increased amounts of folic acid help prevent neural tube defects, such as spina bifida and anencephaly. Spina bifida is caused by an incomplete closing of the bony casing around the spinal cord, which results in partial paralysis. Anencephaly is a fatal defect in which a major part of the brain never develops. Research shows that adequate amounts of folic acid can also help prevent oral and facial birth defects, such as cleft palate.[21]

Pregnant women should consume 600 micrograms of folic acid daily. Women carrying multiples and obese pregnant women may be prescribed additional folic acid. Available evidence suggests that synthetic folic acid, found in supplements and fortified foods, is more effective at preventing neural tube defects than is folate from food; *both*, however, are recommended.[22] Some natural sources of folate include lentils, romaine lettuce, asparagus, chickpeas, beans, green leafy vegetables, citrus fruits, wheat germ, brewer's yeast, enriched breads and grain products, and fortified breakfast cereals (see page 347 for more folate sources).

It is important to note that approximately 15 percent of the population is a carrier for a gene called methylene tetrahydrofolate reductace (MTHFR).[23] Most patients do not have symptoms if they are a carrier with one abnormal gene. If they have inherited two abnormal genes, it can affect the metabolism of folate and B vitamins.[24] The subsequent lack of absorption of folate and B vitamins may cause such symptoms as extreme fatigue, but may also increase the risk of blood clotting and the risk of miscarriage. Fortunately, MTHFR is easy to detect by a blood test and easy to treat by adding methyl folate supplements and eating a diet rich in B vitamins. Talk with your health-care provider about testing for MTHFR, especially if there is a family history or you have had recurrent miscarriages.

VITAMIN B$_{12}$

Vitamin B$_{12}$ is essential in the formation of red blood cells and a healthy nervous system. It is found only in animal products (eggs, dairy, meat, poultry, and seafood), vitamin B$_{12}$–fortified cereals and plant-based products (almond or rice milks), and nutritional yeast. The recommended dose of 2.6 milligrams of vitamin B$_{12}$ during pregnancy is usually met through food sources; therefore, supplements are not needed, except perhaps for strict vegetarians or vegans (see page 28 for more information on B_{12} for vegetarians and vegans). Women with Crohn's disease or those who have undergone bariatric surgery might be prescribed intramuscular shots of B_{12}, which increase the ability for absorption.

VITAMIN B_6

Vitamin B_6 assists in the formation of red blood cells and the metabolism of protein and fats. An intake of 1.9 milligrams per day is recommended. Research shows that B_6 may help combat morning sickness.[25] Good natural sources of vitamin B_6 include poultry, fish (salmon and tuna), pork, eggs, whole wheat products, oats, beans, soy products, peanuts, bananas, baked potato, nuts (especially pistachios and walnuts), and seeds (sunflower).

THIAMINE (B_1)

Thiamine helps the body convert carbohydrates into energy. It is also necessary for healthy functioning of the heart and brain, and for healthy nerve cells. Pregnant women should consume 1.4 milligrams of thiamine per day. Some good sources include unrefined cereal, nutritional yeast, pork, legumes, nuts, and seeds.

RIBOFLAVIN (B_2)

Riboflavin is important for body growth and cell reproduction. It is necessary for breaking down amino acids and releasing energy from fats, proteins, and carbohydrates. Pregnant women should consume 1.4 milligrams of riboflavin per day. Some good sources include meat, eggs, poultry, dairy products, whole grains, and green vegetables, such as broccoli, turnip greens, collard greens, asparagus, and spinach.

NIACIN (B_3)

Niacin assists with cell production. Pregnant women should consume 18 milligrams of niacin per day. Some good sources include poultry, meat, tuna, eggs, whole grains, nuts, legumes, and enriched breads and cereals.

PANTOTHENIC ACID (B$_5$)

Pantothenic acid is a major player in the metabolism of fats, carbohydrates, and protein. It helps regulate the body's adrenal activity and is involved with the production of antibodies for wound healing. The adequate intake of 6 milligrams can come from meats, milk, eggs, salmon, and seeds.

CHOLINE

Choline is essential for neural tube development, fetal brain development, and the formation of cell membranes throughout the body. Research studies on the safety and effectiveness of taking choline supplements during pregnancy for improving brain development are under way. Stay tuned for results as they become available. The adequate daily intake of 450 milligrams can be supplied by egg yolks, milk, nuts, fish, and meat.

AT-A-GLANCE DAILY NUTRIENTS FOR PREGNANCY AND LACTATION[26]

NUTRIENT	PREPREGNANCY	PREGNANCY	LACTATION
Biotin (mcg)	30	30	35
Calcium (mg)	1,000	1,000	1,000
Carbohydrates (g)	130	175	210
Choline (mg)	425	450	550
Chromium (mcg)	25	30	45
Copper (mcg)	900	1,000	1,300
Fiber (g)	25	28	29
Fluoride (mg)	3	3	3
Folate (mcg)	400	600	500
Iodine (mcg)	150	220	290
Iron (mg)	18	27	9
Magnesium (mg)	320	350	310
Manganese (mg)	1.8	2.0	2.6
Molybdenum (mcg)	45	50	50
Niacin (mg)	14	18	17
Omega-3 DHA	N/A	300	300

(continues)

NUTRIENT	PREPREGNANCY	PREGNANCY	LACTATION
Pantothenic acid (mg)	5	6	7
Phosphorus (mg)	700	700	700
Potassium (mg)	4,700	4,700	5,100
Protein (g)	46	71	60
Riboflavin (mg)	1.1	1.4	1.6
Selenium (mcg)	55	60	70
Sodium (mg)	2,300	2,300	2,300
Thiamin (mg)	1.1	1.4	1.4
Vitamin A (mcg)	700	770	1,300
Vitamin B_{12} (mcg)	2.4	2.6	2.8
Vitamin B_6 (mg)	1.3	1.9	2.0
Vitamin C (mg)	75	85	120
Vitamin D_3 (IU)	200	500	200
Vitamin E (mg)	15	15	19
Vitamin K (mcg)	90	90	90
Zinc (mg)	9	11	12

PREGNANCY WISDOM: HYDRATE WITH LOTS OF WATER

WHY is water so important? Fluid intake is vital throughout pregnancy for the reasons listed below. During pregnancy, adequate fluid intake from consumption of beverages (water and other liquids) is estimated to be approximately 2.3 liters per day (76 fluid ounces, or about 10 cups), according to the National Academy of Medicine. Additional water is consumed in foods other than beverages to meet the total adequate intake of 3 liters per day. Numerous factors (such as hot climates, humidity, physical activity, and exertion) also influence total water needs.[27] Juice is fine in moderation; ideally, water it down with (you guessed it) water! Skip all sodas, both regular and diet. If water gets boring, jazz it up with a lemon, lime, or orange wedge; or mint sprigs; or add a little juice for flavor. See Ginger-Mint Soother for Morning Sickness (page 103), and Omega-Charged Chia Juice (page 261).

Why water is so important:

- To aid digestion
- To avoid constipation
- To avoid hemorrhoids

(continues)

- To prevent dehydration that may cause contractions in the last trimester
- To reduce the risk of urinary tract infections (bladder infections)
- To eliminate toxins and keep your system clean
- To regulate your body temperature
- To prevent dry and itchy skin
- It can also help relieve swollen ankles and feet. If swelling is excessive, or appears suddenly, contact your caregiver right away, as this may be a sign of preeclampsia.

PREGNANCY WISDOM: CHOOSING THE BEST OVER-THE-COUNTER PRENATAL VITAMINS

PRENATAL vitamins and supplements act as a safety net during pregnancy. Keep in mind that they do not replace real food. You need both to grow a healthy baby. During the first trimester, morning sickness can be exacerbated by certain prenatal vitamins. If you suspect this, try taking your vitamin with food, before bedtime, or ask your doctor to switch brands. Buying a prenatal vitamin over the counter can be very confusing. Different brands contain different ingredients in different amounts. Here are some basics to look for, but please ask your doctor or care team for your specific needs.

- 600 micrograms (mcg) of folic acid
- 200 to 600 IU of vitamin D_3
- 200 to 300 milligrams (mg) of calcium
- At least 75 mg of vitamin C
- 3 mg of thiamine
- 2 mg of riboflavin
- 20 mg of niacin
- 6 mcg of vitamin B_1
- 27 mg of iron

SPECIAL DIETS AND FOOD ALLERGIES DURING PREGNANCY

Women who are on special diets or who have food allergies during pregnancy may need to make certain accommodations to their daily eating habits and may need to modify their nutrition supplements. If you fit into this category, you will want to talk to a registered dietitian who is familiar with your diet, to get personalized recommendations for pregnancy. Inquire about vegetarian and vegan prenatal vitamins and supplements and gluten-free prenatal vitamins. There are many varieties on the market to fit your needs.

Gluten-Free Diets and Celiac Disease

Being gluten-free, whether by choice or if you have celiac disease, should not place any extra burdens on your pregnant health as long as you get adequate amounts of folic acid and other essential nutrients from gluten-free sources. Make sure your prenatal vitamin is gluten-free as well. The following nutrient-dense gluten-free starchy foods will help you maintain a healthy intake of nutrient-dense carbohydrates: quinoa, rice, millet, amaranth, teff, buckwheat, corn, potatoes, sweet potatoes, chia, flaxseeds, and beans, lentils, and other legumes. More and more mainstream gluten-free foods, from bagels and frozen waffles to crackers and boxed cookie mixes, appear on the market every day. Also, gluten-free flour choices are numerous and include almond, coconut, rice, buckwheat, chickpea (garbanzo), teff, oat, and gluten-free all-purpose enriched flour. (See pages 112 and 113 for more information on whole grains and how to use them.)

Lactose Intolerance

Lactose intolerance, or the inability to digest milk sugar contained in dairy products due to a deficiency of the enzyme lactase, is one of the major reasons that women cannot meet their calcium goal during pregnancy. Look for lactose-free milk, or nondairy, fortified beverages, such as soy, almond, rice, and oat milks. Another option is yogurt made with live or active cultures whose bacteria releases lactose-digesting enzymes, making it easier to digest. Or you might consider Lactaid drops or pills. Some good news is that pregnant women may be better able to tolerate lactose in the third trimester. See sources for nondairy calcium on page 344.

Vegetarian and Vegan Pregnancy Nutrition and Meal Plans

For starters, please don't let anyone tell you that a vegetarian or vegan cannot have a perfectly healthy pregnancy and a healthy baby. Most pregnant vegetarians and vegans do not need to drastically change their lifestyle or eating habits unless they were unhealthy to begin with. Getting in top shape before conception is ideal for all women. To optimize nutritional benefits, all women should eat balanced meals that include a variety of foods (see page 357 for "Menus for Vegetarians and Vegan Pregnancies"). Eating a mix of healthy foods maximizes the body's ability to absorb nutrients, particularly calcium, iron, and zinc. Depending on one's eating habits and any special situations, some vegetarians and vegans may find it challenging to meet the requirements for protein, calcium, vitamin D, iron, vitamin B_{12}, zinc, and iodine.[28] We offer some advice here.

Macronutrient, Mineral, and Vitamin Needs for Vegetarians and Vegans

PROTEIN

Meeting the protein requirements of pregnancy is usually not a problem for most vegetarians, although vegans, who do not eat any dairy products, might be a bit challenged. Some vegetarian sources of protein include pasteurized cheese, cottage cheese, fortified milk, yogurt, tofu, tempeh, eggs, enriched soy beverages, cooked beans, peanuts, soybeans, nuts, and nut butters. Vegans may have additional challenges with their protein needs, but with some meal planning, it is absolutely possible to reach your goals (see page 340 for vegan protein sources).

CALCIUM

Vegetarians who eat dairy products can fulfill their calcium and vitamin D requirements from milk, yogurt, and pasteurized cheeses. If your vegetarian or vegan diet excludes all dairy products, a calcium and vitamin D supplement will likely be advised. To ensure vitamin D production, vegans should try to get at least twenty minutes of direct sunlight on their hands and faces two to three times a week. Some good news is that vegetarians and vegans tend to absorb and retain more calcium from foods than do nonvegetarians. However, calcium bioavailability, or the body's ability to absorb calcium, may be reduced by oxalic acid (oxalates) and phytic acid (phytates), found in certain plants and vegetables (such as dark leafy greens, like kale), and unrefined cereals.[29] This information is important to note because some vegetarian diets rely on large amounts of leafy greens and green vegetables for calcium intake. One way to optimize calcium bioavailability is to try to avoid consuming calcium- and iron-rich foods in the same meal.

IRON

The Institute of Medicine has established a higher daily iron requirement for vegetarians and vegans—48.6 milligrams per day, an increase from 27 milligrams per day for nonvegetarians. This is admittedly difficult (impossible) to achieve without supplements.[30] The reason for this increase is because consuming nonheme iron from plant sources is not as easily absorbed by the body as is heme iron from meat. Some good iron sources for plant-based diets include blackstrap molasses, iron-fortified cereals, cooked beans (especially lima beans and soybeans), green leafy vegetables (such as spinach, Swiss chard, kale, and beet greens), lentils, whole and enriched grains, baked potatoes (with skin on), tempeh, meat analogues, seeds, prune juice, and dried fruit (see page 342 for more iron sources). Ask your doctor or care team about a line of plant-based iron supplements called Floradix.

Please note that the tannins in leaf tea, coffee, calcium supplements, and certain foods high in phytic acid can limit iron absorption. To maximize iron absorption, vegetarians and vegans should try to consume iron-rich foods with foods high in vitamin C. Also, they should opt for iron- and zinc-fortified soy products to minimize the inhibitory effect of phytic acid contained in certain soy products, such as soy flour, soy protein isolate, and tofu processed with calcium sulfate. And, ideally, drink tea and coffee at times other than mealtime.

IODINE

Plant-based diets tend to be low in iodine, which can put some vegetarian women at risk for iodine deficiency. Using iodized salt in cooking and on the table is the answer for most diets. Just ¾ teaspoon used in cooking and at the table will provide enough iodine to meet the 220 micrograms per day. Seaweed, such as nori and hiziki, is also high in iodine.

ZINC

While the Institute of Medicine has not specified a zinc RDA for vegetarians, it suggests that the requirement should be as much as 50 percent higher than 11 milligrams per day for omnivores. This would increase the vegetarian zinc recommendation to about 17 milligrams per day.[31] Dairy products are among the best dietary sources of zinc for vegetarians. Vegans can obtain zinc from other sources such as whole grains, legumes, brown rice, spinach, nuts, seeds, tofu, tempeh, fortified cereals, and wheat germ. As with iron, your body's ability to absorb zinc may be reduced by the presence of phytates, oxalates, fiber, calcium supplements, and soy proteins containing phytic acid.

VITAMIN B$_{12}$

Because plants do not contain vitamin B$_{12}$, vegans may need to supplement their diets to ensure an adequate intake of B$_{12}$. Vegetarians who include eggs and dairy products in their diet are seldom at risk for a vitamin B$_{12}$ deficiency. Some good sources of vitamin B$_{12}$ include fortified plant-based milk products (such as soy milk and yogurt), fortified tofu, fortified soy-based products (such as veggie burgers), meat analogues (such as vegan sausages), enriched breakfast cereals, and nutritional yeast. Vegans should discuss the need for increasing B$_{12}$ supplements with their care teams.

FOOD SAFETY TIPS

You have undoubtedly heard from your doctor or care team that certain foods should be consumed in moderation during conception and pregnancy, and some entirely avoided. Before you read on, we want to assure you that very few pregnant women get food-borne illnesses or mercury poisoning, but we would be remiss if we did not thoroughly outline the precautions.

Why spotlight these precautions during pregnancy? During pregnancy, your immune system lets down its guard in some ways to accommodate your baby's "invasion of your body" as he or she makes it a home for the next nine months. The end result is that you become slightly more susceptible to infections, and sometimes these infections can be serious. Keep abreast of news alerts posted on the FDA and CDC websites, and your local news.[32] To make life easy, here is a laundry list of food safety tips. Be assured that we're here to guide you. We want you to eat well, but we also want you to enjoy your pregnancy. You're amazing! You're beautiful! We know pregnancy is not always easy.

Toxoplasmosis and How to Avoid It

Let's start with the nasty Toxoplasmosis, an infection caused by the parasite *Toxoplasma gondii*, which can be transmitted by eating undercooked infected meat, or by handling soil or cat feces that contain the parasite. Other sources of infection may be raw goat's milk and raw eggs. Insects, such as flies and cockroaches, that have been in contact with cat feces can contaminate food as well. Just to be clear, contact with cats themselves does not cause the illness. The toxoplasmosis parasite lives in the ground. Cats may become infected with the parasite, especially if they eat rodents and birds. An indoor cat that has *never* been outside is generally not a threat.

PREGNANCY WISDOM: VEGAN STAPLES TO HAVE ON HAND

- Almond and other fortified plant-based milks and yogurts
- Blackstrap molasses
- Breakfast cereals fortified with iron, B_{12}, omega-3, and folic acid (plus any other essential nutrients)
- Calcium-fortified orange juice and various other fortified beverages
- Canned beans (pinto beans, kidney beans, lentils, soybeans, and chickpeas)
- Chia seeds
- Dried fruits (apricots, raisins, and cranberries)
- Enriched whole wheat pastas and brown rice
- Ground flaxseeds and flaxseed oil
- Hemp seeds
- Legume, seed, and nut spreads (including peanut butter, sunflower seed butter, and almond butter)
- Marmite
- Natto (fermented soybeans)
- Nutritional yeast
- Nuts, all kinds
- Packaged vegan soups
- Seaweed
- Seeds (unsalted pumpkin and sunflower)
- Soybeans (edamame and soy nuts)
- Tofu and tempeh, and tofu-based spreads
- V8 juice, tomato juice, or other vegetable juices
- Vegan frozen meals
- Vegan protein powders
- Vegan whole wheat crackers
- Wheat germ
- Wheatgrass
- Whole grains (such as barley, brown rice, bulgur wheat, and quinoa)

Swelling of the lymph nodes or flu-like symptoms (fever, fatigue, and sore throat) may be present, although most adults have no symptoms. If a woman contracts toxoplasmosis for the first time during her pregnancy (active infection only occurs once in a lifetime; however, the parasite remains in the body indefinitely), there is a 40 percent chance that her unborn child will also become infected. The risk and severity of the baby's infection depend partly on the timing of the mother's infection. Unborn children infected in early pregnancy are the most likely to suffer severe effects, which may include blindness, deafness, hydrocephalus (water on the brain), seizures, and mental retardation. Tests can determine whether an unborn child is infected, and medications can prevent or reduce severity of effects in unborn children. Toxoplasmosis can also result in miscarriage or stillbirth.

Pregnant women should take the following precautions to prevent toxoplasmosis.[33]

- Don't empty your cat's litter box; have someone else do this.
- Don't feed your cat raw or undercooked meat.
- Keep your cat indoors as much as possible to prevent it from hunting birds or rodents.
- Don't eat raw or undercooked meat, especially lamb or pork. Meat should be cooked to an internal temperature of 160° to 165°F throughout (see "Well-Done Temperature Guide" on page 38).
- If you handle raw meat, wash your hands immediately with soap. Never touch your eyes, nose, or mouth with potentially contaminated hands.
- Wash all raw fruits and vegetables before you eat them.
- Wear gloves when gardening, since soil may contain the parasites. Keep your hands away from your mouth and eyes and wash your hands thoroughly when finished. Keep gardening gloves away from food products.
- Avoid children's sandboxes, as cats may use them as a litter box.

E. coli and How to Avoid It

You've probably heard of E. coli, whose formal name is *Escherichia coli* O157:H7 (or Shiga toxin-producing *E. coli* [STEC]), a bacterium usually found in undercooked contaminated ground beef that causes food-borne illness. Other known means of infection are drinking unpasteurized milk and juice, swimming in or drinking sewage-contaminated water, and consuming tainted sprouts, lettuce, and salami. The poor hygiene of infected persons (or caretakers of those persons) suffering from diarrhea can also spread the bacteria.

Escherichia coli O157:H7 can be found on a small number of cattle farms and can live in the intestines of healthy cattle. Meat can become contaminated during slaughter, and organisms can be mixed into the beef when it is ground. Contaminated meat looks and smells normal. Bacteria present on the cow's udders or on equipment may get into raw milk, causing contamination. The symptoms of infection are usually severe bloody diarrhea and abdominal cramps, but symptoms are not always present. Fever is uncommon, and the illness usually runs its course in five to ten days.

Here are a few tips to prevent infection.[34]

- Cook all ground beef and hamburger thoroughly. Because beef can turn brown before disease-causing bacteria are killed, use an instant-read thermometer to check that ground beef has reached the well-done stage of 160°F. Wash the thermometer in between each test of the meat.
- Keep raw meat separate from uncooked foods. Wash hands, counters, and utensils with hot, soapy water after touching raw meat.
- Never put cooked hamburgers or ground beef back on the plate that held the raw patties.
- Drink only pasteurized milk, juice, and cider.
- Wash fruits and vegetables thoroughly, especially those that will not be cooked.
- Avoid alfalfa sprouts.
- Drink municipal water that has been treated with chlorine and other disinfectants or drink bottled water.
- Avoid swallowing lake or pool water while swimming.
- Make sure that persons with diarrhea, especially children, wash their hands, to reduce the risk of spreading infection, and that anyone washes his or her hands after changing soiled diapers.

Salmonella and How to Avoid It

Salmonellosis is a food-borne illness caused by the bacteria *Salmonella*, which can be acquired from infected animals (usually poultry, swine, and cattle), raw milk and raw milk products, undercooked or raw eggs and egg products (see "*Salmonella enteritidis* and How to Avoid It," page 32), and contaminated water. Fecal-oral transmission from person to person, especially in infants, is another cause of *Salmonella* poisoning. Certain pets, such as turtles, tortoises, iguanas, chicks, dogs, cats, and rodents, can also carry the bacteria in their intestines.

The symptoms of gastrointestinal infection usually include fever, nausea and vomiting, abdominal cramping, and diarrhea, which may be bloody. Other complications, such as enteric (typhoid) fever or extra-intestinal infections (infections that have spread outside the intestines), may occur. Following are a few tips to help prevent infection.[35]

- Avoid raw eggs and food that contains raw or partially cooked eggs.
- Avoid raw (unpasteurized) milk and any food that contains raw milk or raw milk products.
- Thoroughly cook all poultry and meat (see "Well-Done Temperature Guide," page 38). Wash instant-read thermometers in between tests of foods that require further cooking.
- Keep raw meat separate from uncooked foods. Wash hands, counters, and utensils with hot, soapy water after touching raw meat.
- Consume only safe drinking water or bottled water, especially when traveling to developing countries.
- Wash hands thoroughly after touching any of the pets mentioned above.
- Make sure that persons with diarrhea, especially children, wash their hands to reduce the risk of spreading infection, and that anyone washes his or her hands after changing soiled diapers.
- Avoid swallowing lake or pool water while swimming.

Salmonella enteriditis *and How to Avoid It*

While *Salmonella* can be contracted a number of different ways, contaminated raw eggs are of particular concern for pregnant women. Unbroken fresh eggs in their shells that appear perfectly normal may contain bacteria called *Salmonella enteritidis* (SE), which can cause food-borne illness. SE silently infects the ovaries of healthy-appearing hens and contaminates the eggs before the shells are formed. SE bacteria are usually in the yolk, but it's possible that the bacteria are in the whites as well.

People with health problems, the very young, seniors, and pregnant women (the risk is to the unborn child) are particularly vulnerable to SE infections. The symptoms include fever, abdominal cramps, and diarrhea. Proper refrigeration, cooking, and handling of raw eggs should prevent most contamination problems. People can and should enjoy eggs and egg dishes, provided they follow these safe handling guidelines:[36]

- Don't eat raw eggs—including raw eggs contained in milk shakes, Caesar salad dressing, hollandaise sauce, homemade mayonnaise, ice cream, or eggnog. Also, avoid tasting any batters (such as cake and cookie batters) that contain raw egg.
- Choose Grade A or AA eggs with clean, uncracked shells. Don't wash eggs.
- Buy only refrigerated eggs and keep them refrigerated in their original egg carton in the coldest part of the refrigerator, and not in the door.
- Don't keep eggs out of the refrigerator for more than 2 hours. Bacteria grow rapidly at room temperature.
- Use raw eggs within 3 to 5 weeks of purchase. Use any leftover yolks or whites within 4 days.
- Hard-cooked eggs can be kept in the refrigerator for 1 week.
- Handle eggs safely. Wash hands, utensils, equipment, and work areas with warm soapy water before and after contact with raw eggs and dishes containing raw eggs.
- Keep raw eggs separate from other foods that will be cooked.
- Cook eggs thoroughly until the yolk and whites are firm. Scrambled eggs should not be runny and there should be no visible liquid egg. Casseroles, soups (such as egg drop), and other egg-based dishes should be cooked to 160°F on an instant-read thermometer.
- Eat eggs promptly after cooking. Refrigerate any leftovers and consume within three to four days.
- Commercially manufactured ice cream and eggnog made with pasteurized eggs have not been linked to SE infections. Dry meringue shells and cookies are safe to eat. It is advisable to avoid meringue-topped pies, chiffon and fruit pies made with raw whipped egg whites, and any custard-based desserts in which the eggs might not have reached a safe internal temperature of 160°F.

Listeriosis and How to Avoid It

Here's the last food-borne illness to be aware of—listeriosis is caused by a bacterium called *Listeria monocytogenes*, found in soil and water. The bacteria are very resistant to common food preservation agents, such as heat, nitrites, nitrates, and acids, and they can continue to multiply in refrigerated foods. *Listeria* is often present in the intestines of seemingly healthy animals. The bacteria can contaminate milk and meat products from infected animals and can also contaminate vegetables fertilized with tainted manure. It is important to note that contaminated food may not look, smell, or taste different from uncontaminated food.

Healthy people are generally resistant to listeriosis, but pregnant women are about twenty times more likely than other healthy adults to get listeriosis. About one third of listeriosis cases happen during pregnancy. Infected pregnant women may experience only a mild, flu-like illness, including fever or a stiff neck. Infections during pregnancy can lead to premature delivery, infection of the newborn, or even stillbirth. Because the symptoms of listeriosis can take a few days or even weeks to appear and can be mild, you may not even know you have it. That is why it is important to take appropriate food safety precautions during pregnancy. Following is a list of guidelines to prevent listeriosis infection provided by the USDA's Food Safety and Inspection Service and the US Food and Drug Administration:[37]

- Do not eat hot dogs, luncheon meats, or deli meats unless they are reheated until steaming hot.
- Do not eat soft cheeses, such as unpasteurized feta or unpasteurized fresh mozzarella, Brie, Camembert, blue-veined cheeses, and Mexican-style cheeses, such as queso fresco (also called queso blanco) and asadero. Pasteurized hard cheeses, semisoft cheeses (such as part-skim low-moisture mozzarella and feta), processed cheese slices and spreads, cream cheese, and cottage cheese can be consumed safely.
- Do not eat refrigerated pâté or meat spreads. Canned or shelf-stable pâté and meat spreads can be eaten.
- Do not eat refrigerated smoked seafood unless it is an ingredient in a cooked dish, such as a casserole. Examples of refrigerated smoked seafood include salmon, trout, whitefish, cod, tuna, and mackerel, which are most often labeled as "nova-style," "lox," "kippered," "smoked," or "jerky." Canned fish, such as salmon and light tuna or shelf-stable smoked seafood, may be eaten safely.
- Do not drink raw (unpasteurized) milk or eat foods that contain unpasteurized milk.
- Use all perishable items that are precooked or ready-to-eat as soon as possible.
- Observe all expiration dates.
- Wash the insides of refrigerators regularly, and be sure to thoroughly clean liquid spills, such as spills from hot dog and luncheon meat packages.
- Use a refrigerator thermometer to make sure that your refrigerator always stays at 40°F or below.
- Wash all fruits and vegetables with water.

- After handling raw foods, wash your hands with warm, soapy water, and wash the utensils, cutting boards, and dishes you used with hot, soapy water before using them again.
- Cook foods to well-done temperatures.

PREGNANCY WISDOM: IS ORGANIC REALLY BETTER?

IS the organic label really worth the extra dollars? Yes, absolutely, if it doesn't break your budget. In a perfect world, we would all be consuming organic, non-GMO whole foods, minimally processed to retain their nutrients. It's better for the environment, farmers, and the health of consumers. The reality is most of us can't and don't eat organic for any number of reasons, from cost, to a lack of time to eat and cook at home every day. When pondering what to buy organic, keep in mind that switching to even a few organic foods during pregnancy might be worthwhile. Here are some good options:

- Buy organic meat, poultry, and eggs that are hormone- and antibiotic-free as much as possible.
- Buy organic fruits and vegetables in the "dirty dozen" group. These include foods with the highest levels of pesticides according to the Environmental Working Group.[38] Think: peaches, apples, sweet bell peppers, celery, nectarines, strawberries, cherries, pears, imported grapes, spinach, lettuce, and potatoes. Foods considered part of the "clean fifteen"[39] category have less chemical exposure and absorption and are not as important to buy organic. They include: avocados, sweet corn, pineapples, cabbage, sweet peas (frozen), onions, asparagus, mangoes, papaya, kiwifruit, eggplant, honeydew melon, grapefruit, cantaloupe, and cauliflower. All fruits and vegetables, regardless of whether they are organic or not, should be washed carefully before eaten or prepared.
- Buy wild-caught fish that contains fewer PCBs (polychlorinated biphenyls) and dioxins than farm-raised fish. See below for more information on mercury and fish.
- Buy organic coffee, if you drink it.[40]

Methylmercury and Limitations on Consumption of Certain Fish

Fish and shellfish are part of a healthy diet and should *not* be excluded, especially during pregnancy. However, certain types of fish can be contaminated with high levels of mercury that may harm an unborn baby or young child's developing nervous system. The risks from mercury in fish and shellfish depend on the amount of fish and shellfish eaten and the levels of mercury in the fish and shellfish. The US Food and Drug Administration and Environmental Protection Agency are advising women who may become pregnant, pregnant women, nursing mothers, and young children to follow these recommendations.

- Do not eat shark, swordfish, king mackerel, or tilefish because they contain high levels of mercury.
- Eat up to 12 ounces (2 average meals) a week of a variety of fish and shellfish that are lower in mercury. Five of the most commonly eaten fish that are low in mercury are shrimp, canned light tuna, salmon, pollock, and catfish.
- Check local advisories about the safety of fish caught by family and friends in your local lakes, rivers, and coastal areas. If no advice is available, eat up to 6 ounces per week of fish from local waters, but don't consume any other fish during that week.
- Pregnant women should also avoid raw fish, especially shellfish (such as oysters and clams), which can be polluted with raw sewage and can contain harmful microorganisms that can lead to severe gastrointestinal illness. All fish and shellfish should be *thoroughly* cooked.

For further information on seafood safety, visit https://www.epa.gov/choose -fish-and-shellfish-wisely/should-i-be-concerned-about-eating-fish-and-shellfish.

QUESTIONS AND ANSWERS ON MERCURY IN FISH AND SHELLFISH AND FISH OIL SUPPLEMENTS[41]

What are mercury and methylmercury?

Mercury occurs naturally in the environment, and it can also be released into the air through industrial pollution. Mercury falls from the sky, accumulating in streams and oceans, where it turns into methylmercury in the water. Fish absorb methylmercury as they feed. High amounts of methylmercury in certain types of fish can potentially be harmful to the neurological development of an unborn baby and young child.

Does all fish and shellfish contain methylmercury?

Nearly all fish and shellfish contain traces of methylmercury. Large fish (such as shark, swordfish, king mackerel, and tilefish) with long life spans have the highest levels of methylmercury, mainly because they've had more time to accumulate it. These fish pose the greatest risk. Other types of fish should be eaten in amounts recommended by the FDA and EPA.

What about fish sticks and fish sandwiches?

Fish sticks and fast-food fish sandwiches are usually made from fish that are low in mercury, so they are safe to eat.

What about tuna steaks?

Because tuna steaks generally contain higher levels of mercury than canned light tuna, you may eat up to 6 ounces (two average meals) of tuna steak per week.

What if I eat more than the recommended amount of fish and shellfish in a week?

One week's consumption of fish does not change the level of methylmercury in your body much at all.

If I'm trying to conceive, should I be concerned about methylmercury?

If you regularly eat fish high in methylmercury, it can accumulate in your bloodstream over time. Methylmercury is excreted from the body naturally, but it may take over a year for high levels to drop significantly. Therefore, it may be present in a woman before she becomes pregnant. For this reason, women who are trying to conceive should also try to avoid eating high-mercury fish, but they certainly should eat other fish.

Are fish oil supplements safe?

The short answer is some brands are of higher quality than others. Reputable manufacturers will provide documentation of third-party lab results that demonstrate the quality and purity of their fish oil. These standards guarantee high-quality fish oil by setting maximum allowances for toxins, heavy metals, and oxidation, so be sure to buy from a manufacturer that can document that their products meet or surpass these standards. In addition, check to see if any of the company's products are backed by independent clinical research studies.

And how much should a pregnant woman consume daily?

If advised by her doctor or care team, a pregnant woman should take a daily supplement that provides a minimum of 300 mg of DHA.

What are the best supplements for vegetarians and vegans?

An omega-3 algae oil supplement can be an excellent vegetarian alternative to fish oil. Be sure to read labels. Make sure you choose a product that supplies enough of both EPA and DHA.

PREGNANCY WISDOM: WELL-DONE TEMPERATURE GUIDE

DURING pregnancy, it's really important to cook all of your meat, poultry, and stuffing to the "well-done" stage, which is different temperatures for different foods. An instant-read thermometer will help you figure out when things are done. Also, cutting into the food is good way to gauge if something is fully cooked.[42]

FOOD	TEMPERATURE °F
Beef	160
Pork	160
Chicken and turkey	
Whole	165
Breast	165
Thigh	165
Ground	165
Stuffing (cooked alone or in the bird)	165
Ground meat and poultry	160
Casseroles	165

SAFE PLASTICS FOR YOU AND YOUR FAMILY

WHILE plastics are getting safer, they still need to be examined before use. Those numbers at the bottom of the bottle do mean something, and not all of the numbers are good. Most clear plastic bottles are labeled #1, which is a safe plastic that should be used only once and then recycled. The safest plastics are #1 PET or PETE (polyethylene), #2 HDPE (high-density polyethylene), #4 LDPE (low-density polyethylene), and #5 PP (polypropylene). Some numbers to avoid whenever possible include #3 PVC (polyvinyl chloride or vinyl), #6 PS (polystyrene, such as Styrofoam), and #7 (polycarbonate or Lexan). In summary, the good numbers are 1, 2, 4, and 5 and the bad numbers are 3, 6, and 7.

Why should certain plastics be avoided? Because studies show that chemicals from those plastics can leach into foods or beverages. Some chemicals, such as BPA (bisphenol-A), have been associated with disruption of the estrogen hormone (though this has not been proven).[43] In 2006, the European Union banned all products with BPA that were made for children under the age of three, including bottles and sippy cups. In 2012, the FDA banned BPA from baby bottles and sippy cups nationwide. In 2013, they were banned from infant formula packaging. For more information, visit the Environmental Working Group website. To be on the safe side, follow these three guidelines when using any plastic products.

- Do not heat foods in plastic containers; use glass or a regular plate in the microwave oven.
- Do not use plastic wrap to cover foods that will be reheated in a microwave oven (use a paper towel instead).
- Thoroughly wash any plastic bottles that you plan to reuse by hand. Do not run them through the dishwasher, where they are exposed to very high heat. Glass bottles are a good option.

COMMON ANNOYANCES DURING PREGNANCY

If this is not your first pregnancy, you will already be familiar with most (maybe all!) of these common annoyances. We hope we can offer you at least one new tip for coping with any of these inconveniences. All first-time moms should remember one thing: This, too, shall pass!

Morning Sickness

Some degree of nausea and vomiting occurs in about 50 percent of all pregnancies. It usually starts around the second month of pregnancy and lasts until about the fourth.

It is called morning sickness because it commonly occurs in the morning, but it can occur anytime and can last all day. It is generally believed that pregnancy hormones are the culprits of morning sickness. Why some women are affected by the increased hormonal levels and others are not remains a medical mystery.

There is no cure for morning sickness. Listen to your body and figure out what works best for you. If you are nauseated and vomiting occasionally, the following tips may help. A severe form of morning sickness, referred to as hyperemesis gravidarum, may require medications prescribed by your doctor and sometimes IV fluids to rehydrate. Keep track of your symptoms and bring any concerns to the attention of your care team. Note: Always talk to your physician before initiating any supplements or medications.

- Take your prenatal vitamins at night or space them throughout the day (if you take more than 1 per day). Consult your doctor to change brands if your vitamin makes you nauseous. Continue taking a folic acid supplement even if you stop taking a prenatal vitamin.
- Vitamin B_6 has been shown to improve morning sickness. Ask your doctor whether B_6 supplements might help you.[44] Food sources of B_6 include avocados, bananas, pistachios, sunflower seeds, meat, seafood, and poultry.
- Talk to your doctor about taking a ginger supplement (please note, this is not the powdered spice). A common dosage is 1 to 1.5 grams orally divided over 24 hours; or 250 milligrams 4 times per day. Some women have reported relief from nausea, not vomiting, with ginger supplements daily.[45] Check out our amazing Ginger-Mint Soother for Morning Sickness (page 103). Other forms of ginger include ginger tea, candies, lollipops, and crystalized ginger.
- Eat small, evenly spaced meals instead of 3 large meals. Don't let yourself get too hungry. Eat slowly and thoroughly chew all foods. Some women tolerate cold foods better than hot foods. Salty foods are sometimes preferred.
- Do not eat and drink at the same time. Drink your fluids between your meals and snacks. Also, do not drink more than 1 cup (8 ounces) of fluid at a time. Avoid caffeinated beverages. Try drinking sips of pure fruit juice, lemonade, coconut water, or ginger ale.
- Eat ice pops, fruit ice, or sherbet between meals. Chew ice or suck on an ice cube.
- Avoid strongly spiced or highly aromatic foods. Avoid greasy or fatty fried foods, especially fast food.

- Strong vegetables, such as cabbage, broccoli, cauliflower, garlic, and onions, can spark nausea. When you cook, open windows to eliminate cooking odors.
- Move slowly upon waking, even from a nap. Allow yourself a few extra minutes when getting out of bed to balance your body and brain. Before you get out of bed in the morning, eat dry toast, crackers, yogurt smoothies, nuts, or whatever works best for you.
- Try to include protein in your meals, especially dinner. Protein helps stabilize your blood glucose levels. You can add protein to a smoothie or green drink.
- Consider eating a small snack before bed. This may reduce morning nausea.
- Get plenty of rest. Physical and emotional fatigue can exacerbate nausea.
- Get plenty of fresh air. Go for a walk in the middle of the day. Make sure your workspace is well ventilated and not too hot. Take deep breaths of fresh air from time to time.
- Try a wristband for motion sickness; some women find acupressure or acupuncture helpful.
- Some women find aromatherapy helpful. Lavender, lemon, and peppermint are some commonly used essential oils that can be used in a diffuser.

Indigestion and Heartburn

Indigestion, heartburn, and reflux are very common complaints during pregnancy, especially during the first and third trimesters. During the first trimester, heartburn is caused by increased hormone levels and smooth muscle relaxation, which allow acids to reflux (come back up) more easily. During the third trimester, decreased stomach capacity limits the space for food and stomach juices, resulting in indigestion and heartburn. Usually, these annoying issues can be controlled by modifying what you eat, when you eat, and other tips. If they become severe, consult with your doctor or health-care provider.

- Avoid greasy, fatty, spicy, or fried foods.
- Avoid gas-forming foods, such as cabbage and beans.
- Avoid caffeinated beverages and chocolate.
- Avoid citrus fruits and juices.
- Sit down when you eat and try to relax.
- Eat slowly and chew thoroughly.
- Don't eat and drink at the same time. Wait 30 to 60 minutes after eating to drink a beverage.

- Don't lie down after eating. Take a walk instead.
- Try not to eat 3 hours prior to bedtime, unless you need a high-protein snack before bed to regulate your blood glucose levels.
- Eat frequent, evenly spaced, smaller meals instead of 3 large ones. Try to eat an early dinner.
- Sip a cup of plain hot water after meals; add a slice of lemon or a mint sprig for flavor.
- If indigestion keeps you awake at night, try to sleep propped up with pillows.
- Wear loose-fitting clothing, especially around the abdomen and waist.
- Avoid bending over at the waist. Bend at the knees. Squat to lift things. Maintain good posture as much as possible.
- Never take any medication for heartburn or an antacid without consulting your doctor or healthcare provider.
- Avoid preparations containing sodium or sodium bicarbonate.

PREGNANCY WISDOM: GAS AND TIPS FOR COPING

EXCESS gas is a normal part of almost all pregnancies. It can be uncomfortable, and even embarrassing. Get used to it, mama. Here are a few tips to help reduce gas.

- Eliminate gas-producing foods in your diet as much as possible. Some common culprits include beans, raw cucumber, raw peppers, raw cabbage, raw onion, cauliflower, and dried fruit.
- Get your body moving! Go for a walk after meals, or whenever you can. This will help keep your digestive tract functioning smoothly.
- Eat smaller meals more frequently.
- Chew foods well.
- Eat slowly.
- Don't eat and drink at the same time. Drink first or wait until after you eat.
- Try to avoid constipation, which can cause gas.
- Ask your doctor before you take any medications or supplements.

WHAT? All of a sudden, you've lost your taste for vegetables? Fruits? Fish? Chicken? But you used to love a good steak with a baked potato smothered in sour cream! Fear not. Food aversions are just as common as food cravings during pregnancy. And, like cravings, they can last for an hour, a day, weeks, or even months. Also, don't be surprised if your food aversion on Monday becomes your craving on Friday, or the other way around.

Why do we get food aversions? Pregnancy is a time when we instinctively become hyperconcerned about what we put into our body. One of the very first physiologic changes that many women will notice in early pregnancy is a strong aversion to certain smells. This is one of the defense mechanisms our body has to keep us away from potentially unsafe environments, chemicals, and foods. Avoiding foods is not usually a problem, but some food aversions may require effort to replace lost nutrients. For example, if you have an aversion to fruit, increase your intake of vegetables—and vice versa. If chicken or beef turn you off, increase your intake of peanut butter, eggs, cheese, dried beans and peas, or tofu. If a food aversion lasts longer than one month, or the appropriate substitutions are not meeting your daily nutrient requirements, discuss the situation with your doctor or a dietitian.

And speaking of cravings, pica is not as common as it once was, thanks in large part to adequate nutrient intakes with prenatal vitamins readily available on the market and by prescription. But the condition still needs to be mentioned because some women do experience it. It has been suggested that pica, the craving for inappropriate substances with little or no nutritional value, may be associated with iron-deficiency anemia. The most common nonfood substances that pregnant women crave are dirt, clay, laundry starch, and ice. Other less common cravings include chalk, air fresheners, charcoal, and mothballs. Whether pica is the cause or effect of anemia remains unknown, but the condition usually clears when the anemia is treated. Consult your doctor or health-care provider if you experience the desire to consume non-food substances.

Constipation and Hemorrhoids

Constipation is a common problem for pregnant women. And hemorrhoids (swollen veins in lower rectum or anus) can happen at any time during pregnancy, but usually in the final stretch. During the first trimester, increased hormonal levels tend to cause constipation, whereas during the third trimester, smooth-muscle relaxation and a cramped and compressed abdominal space slow down waste elimination. Iron and other supplements can also cause constipation. Do not take any form of laxative, bulk-forming supplemental fiber (such as psyllium and methylcellulose), or mineral oil without the consent of your doctor.

- Increase high-fiber foods in your diet, such as whole-grain cereals and breads, beans, lentils, peas, raw fruits and vegetables, and dried fruit. A good fiber intake is about 25 to 30 g per day.
- Consume more chia seeds every day; try our Omega-Charged Chia Juice (page 261). Toss chia on top of smoothies, yogurt, salads, soups, breakfast cereals (hot and cold), or just about anything.
- Increase fluids—drink at least 8 glasses of water per day, and ideally a total of 12 cups of fluid per day.
- With permission from your doctor, get regular exercise, which helps get your intestines moving.
- Go for walks after meals.
- Try a glass of prune juice or some prunes in the morning.
- Iron supplements cause constipation in some women. Try taking your supplement at different times of the day. Ask your doctor about Floradix iron supplements for vegetarians, as they may be less constipating.
- While sitting on the toilet, massage the sides of your back, starting at the base of your ribs, in a downward motion.
- Check out a device called the Squatty Potty as a means to facilitate your bowel movement.

SPECIAL CONDITIONS DURING PREGNANCY

Certain preexisting conditions or pregnancy-related complications require extra care and attention. For these high-risk pregnancies, women usually require a closely monitored, customized medical care plan. Some conditions may call for special nutrition guidelines as well. Following are some of the most common health concerns and high-risk conditions. We've got you covered, mama. You're a super mom. You will prevail!

Obesity During Pregnancy

Obesity in the United States and many other countries has reached epidemic proportions. Currently, obesity prevalence in pregnant women are estimated to be as high as 30 percent.[46] This is of great concern because obesity in pregnancy is associated with numerous maternal and neonatal complications, some of which include difficulty conceiving, increased risk of miscarriage, fetal defects and mortality, increased risk of gestational hypertension, preeclampsia, gestational diabetes, and blood clots.[47]

The best way to prevent these potential complications is to lose as much weight as possible, through diet and exercise, before conception. If you've had bariatric surgery, a special assessment of your nutrient absorption should be done before conception.[48] The latest statistics show that more than 80 percent of bariatric procedures are performed on women, and approximately half of these are performed in reproductive-aged women. It has become increasingly common for women with Crohn's disease or those who have undergone bariatric surgery or gastric bypass to seek preconceptional counseling and/or prenatal care. Ideally, your doctor will advise you to wait at least eighteen months after your surgery to become pregnant.

Obese pregnant women need to maintain their weight, or to gain a minimal amount of weight during pregnancy, usually not more than 15 pounds. This number is likely to change in the near future—it is likely to go down—as more studies are done to figure out the optimal weight gain for overweight and obese mothers. No matter how overweight a woman is, dieting is not recommended during pregnancy because it will deprive the fetus of essential nutrients. This said, a woman might find that due to the metabolic needs of her fetus, she may lose weight naturally in pregnancy. A doctor will want to monitor closely and assign a registered dietitian who will create an individualized meal plan. Increased amounts of folic acid and/or other supplements prior to conception may be prescribed.

High Blood Pressure and Preeclampsia

Contrary to popular belief, when high blood pressure develops during pregnancy (particularly in women with no previous history of high blood pressure), following a strict low-sodium diet is usually not recommended.[49] Instead, increasing protein and calcium seems to be most beneficial. For early detection of elevated blood pressure, blood pressure checks should be done on a regular basis (at least once a month) throughout pregnancy. The following are some of the most common warning symptoms of hypertension. Call your doctor right away if you notice any of them.

- Severe or constant headaches
- Swelling, especially in the face
- Blurred vision and/or sensitivity to light
- Pain in the upper right part of the abdomen

- Sudden weight gain of more than 1 pound per day, or 10 to 12 pounds in 5 days
- Excessive weight gain in the third trimester accompanied by swelling

Sometimes gestational hypertension can lead to a condition called preeclampsia— diagnosed as a combination of high blood pressure and protein in the urine at 20 weeks of gestation. When preeclampsia causes seizures, the condition becomes eclampsia, which can result in fetal complications, low birth weight, premature birth, stillbirth, and serious health risks for the mother.[50] At greatest risk for preeclampsia are:[51]

- Women with chronic hypertension or high blood pressure levels before becoming pregnant
- Women who developed high blood pressure or preeclampsia during a previous pregnancy, especially if these conditions occurred early
- Women who are obese prior to pregnancy
- Pregnant women under the age of 20 or over the age of 40
- Pregnant women carrying multiples
- Pregnant women with diabetes, kidney disease, rheumatoid arthritis, lupus, or scleroderma

No one knows what causes preeclampsia or eclampsia or how to prevent it. Randomized trials have evaluated the role of diet in prevention of preeclampsia; however, no conclusive results have been demonstrated from interventions, which include nutritional advice and supplementation, protein and energy supplements, protein and energy restriction (in obese women), magnesium supplementation, and salt restriction.[52] The important thing is that studies on preeclampsia are ongoing and could potentially bear good news one day.

Iron-Deficiency Anemia

Iron-deficiency anemia is most commonly caused by low iron stores prior to pregnancy, or from blood loss during pregnancy. Certain preexisting or inherited medical conditions can increase the risk of iron deficiency during pregnancy. The most common are sickle cell anemia, an inherited form of anemia occurring primarily in African Americans and women from South and Central America, and a condition called thalassemia, an inherited form of anemia occurring mostly in people of Mediterranean origin and some women of Asian origin.

PREGNANCY WISDOM: ORAL HYGIENE

ORAL hygiene is extremely important during pregnancy. Brushing your teeth multiple times and day and flossing daily is ideal. Why? Because pregnancy causes hormonal changes that increase the risk of developing gum disease (a condition called pregnancy gingivitis), which can affect the health of your developing baby. Pay particular attention to any changes in your gums, such as tenderness, bleeding, or swelling. Should these occur, reach out to your doctor and dentist.

Ideally, try to see your dentist before conception for a routine cleaning and check-up. Inform your dentist if you are pregnant, as sometimes special precautions and/or instructions are given to pregnant women. Routine dental care and any urgent care can be done any time during pregnancy (don't skip your routine appointment because you're pregnant). Dental X-rays are also safe during pregnancy. Your dentist will use extreme caution to protect you and your baby, such as shielding your abdomen and thyroid. A special note to moms experiencing vomiting during pregnancy. If nausea is keeping you from brushing your teeth, try a different toothpaste brand; some are more palatable than others. Rinse your mouth out with water or a mouth rinse after bouts of vomiting. And try to avoid sugary snacks that can increase the risk of decay.

Pregnant women suffering from iron deficiency anemia can experience fatigue, shortness of breath, paleness, dizziness, lightheadedness, or heart palpitations. Anemia can lead to infection, premature labor, low birth weight, and a decreased ability to tolerate blood loss during childbirth. Increased iron supplementation and a high-iron diet may be prescribed by a doctor. Be sure to take all iron supplements with a high–vitamin C food or beverage (such as citrus juice), not milk, as calcium can interfere with iron absorption. Leaf tea, coffee, and high-phytate foods also limit iron absorption.

Pregnant Teens

Pregnant teenagers, aged eighteen years or younger, have more nutritional requirements than do pregnant adults. Teens have to meet their own increased nutritional needs for growth as well as the needs of the developing fetus. Generally, in addition to all of the standard nutrient intake requirements for pregnant women, a pregnant teenager requires 75 to 85 grams of protein, 1,300 milligrams of calcium, 1,250 milligrams of phosphorus, and approximately 400 to 500 additional calories (younger teens will need more calories). A pregnant adolescent should be counseled by her doctor, nurse, and registered dietitian for a meal plan that addresses all her needs. Meal frequency should be evaluated, as teens occasionally skip meals due to school and other activities. Also, the importance of adequate weight gain should be stressed to pregnant teens who may be hesitant to gain weight for fear of becoming fat.

Like all pregnant women, teens should be strongly encouraged to give up alcohol, drugs, smoking, and vaping. Anemia, gestational hypertension, premature deliveries, depression, and babies with low birth weight can be associated with teen pregnancies. Getting prenatal care as early as possible will lead to a healthier baby and a healthier teen mother. Emotional support is a key to positive outcomes. If you are a teen in need of help and support, please reach out to your doctor or care team, or any adult involved with your pregnancy. You're juggling a lot.

PREGNANCY WISDOM:
3 EXCELLENT REASONS TO QUIT SMOKING AND VAPING[53]

- Increased risk for miscarriage, premature birth, babies with a low birth weight, and still-birth. Smoking deprives the fetus and placenta of oxygen, causing extreme harm to the developing baby.
- Increased risk for intellectual deficiencies, learning disabilities, and behavior problems later in childhood.
- Increased risk for breathing problems and other health problems, including SIDS (sudden infant death syndrome).

Pregnancy After 35

Pregnancy after age thirty-five is common today. In fact, more and more women are following this trend. The good news is that pregnancies at this age are generally healthy, although it is good to know what possible risks are involved. Mothers who are over age thirty-five are more likely than younger women to experience gestational diabetes, placental abnormalities, high blood pressure, preeclampsia, miscarriage, premature labor, and stillbirth. Also, babies born to older mothers are more prone to genetic disorders, premature birth, and low birth weight. All this said, older pregnant women are closely monitored by their physicians to try to prevent these problems from arising and to keep them, and their babies, as healthy as possible. Unless a condition pops up, pregnancy dietary recommendations are the same as for younger women. Exercise plans should be discussed with your health-care provider, especially if regular exercise was not a part of your prepregnancy lifestyle.

PREGNANCY WISDOM: BED REST TIPS FOR SPECIAL MOMS

EVERY woman's dream of an uneventful and joyous pregnancy doesn't always come true. Some conditions in pregnancy lead to activity restrictions, which can be as simple as elevating your legs or as strict as conservative bed rest with no bathroom privileges. Bed-rest restrictions cause added stress for the entire family and can make meal planning and food preparation difficult. Often the husband or partner, other family members, and friends will need to help with the cooking, household chores, and care of small children. We hope these tips will help. Hang in. If you're on bed rest, we're sending extra love your way!

- Keep a cooler at your bedside stocked with milk, cheese, cheese sticks, cottage cheese, hummus and bean dips, gazpacho, hard-boiled eggs, cut-up fresh fruit and vegetables (that need to be cool, such as salads and edamame), fruit and vegetable juices, chia juices (for extra fiber), yogurt, smoothies, green drinks, and your other favorite foods. Make sure that your cooler is properly chilled and remains cold throughout the day.
- Keep fresh fruits and vegetables (already cut), raisins and dried fruit, peanut and nut butters, granola bars, protein bars, instant oatmeal packets (with added protein, if available), instant soup (look for low-sodium), whole-grain bread, whole wheat crackers, rice cakes, popcorn, nuts, seeds, individual fruit cups in natural juices, fruit juices, and other snack items within easy reach.
- Keep two or three large sport bottles filled with water within reach. Most bed rest situations also mean an increase in fluid requirements.
- If possible, set up a microwave oven or toaster oven at your bedside to reheat precooked, frozen, or semiprepared meals and to reheat vegetables and other simple dishes.
- Keep a thermos of soup, pasta, or any other food that can be kept warm for a few hours at your bedside.
- Keep plastic utensils, napkins, paper cups, and wipes by your bedside.
- Discuss your prenatal meal plan with your caretaker (your husband or partner, mother, friend, or hired help) and share recipes with family and friends who may be bringing meals to you.

Pregnancy with Multiples

Pregnant women carrying twins, triplets, or more have a particular challenge meeting increased nutritional needs. Generally, on top of the normal pregnancy requirements, a woman carrying twins needs an additional 300 calories per day, and a woman carrying triplets needs an additional 600 calories per day. Because of this increased number of calories, a woman might prefer to eat frequent small meals during the day, which will also help control indigestion and heartburn. The total weight gain for a woman with twins is about 35 to 45 pounds, and 45 to 55 pounds for triplets. Protein, calcium, iron, magnesium, and folic acid requirements increase as well, and a doctor should be consulted for specific recommendations. A woman pregnant with multiples needs to consult a registered dietitian for a customized meal plan appropriate for her situation.

Diabetes During Pregnancy

More and more women are entering pregnancy with existing diabetes or prediabetes, or they are developing diabetes during pregnancy, a condition called gestational diabetes mellitus (GDM). This advice comes from Elna Narula, RN, CDE, who specializes in teaching women who develop GDM. Elna and Rose Ann frequently counsel women with diabetes during pregnancy. They know how stressful this diagnosis can be for patients and how hard some women need to work to manage their blood glucose levels (also called blood sugar levels, or simply sugars). If you passed your glucose screening test, please feel free to skip this section. If you have been diagnosed with GDM, or you have preexisting type 2 or type 1 diabetes, we hope this information is helpful.

WHEN WOMEN ARE DIAGNOSED WITH GDM ONE OF THE FIRST QUESTIONS THEY ASK IS: WHY ME?

Blame it on your hormones! That's right. Stop feeling guilty. It's not your fault. You did not do anything wrong. The same hormones that help your baby develop and grow, increase your blood glucose levels, and make it more difficult for your body to use its insulin. As your pregnancy progresses and placental hormones rise, your insulin resistance may increase, especially during the third trimester. Of course, there are some risk factors for developing GDM that you can't necessarily control; family history and having prediabetes (but not knowing it until pregnancy) are just two, but hormones play a big part.

THE NEXT QUESTION MANY WOMEN ASK IS, WHAT IS GDM AND IS IT HARMFUL TO MY BABY?

GDM is, by definition, any diabetes first diagnosed during pregnancy. The term *pregestational diabetes* refers to women who have existing diabetes (type 1 or type 2) before pregnancy. Diabetes is a condition that occurs when your body can't use glucose (a type of sugar) normally. Glucose is the main source of energy for your body's cells. The levels of glucose in your blood are controlled by a hormone called insulin, which is made by your pancreas. That's the short and sweet definition.

Having high blood sugar levels is not good for a baby in the womb because when blood sugars are high, that extra glucose reaches the baby and causes his or her developing pancreas to work in overdrive to produce more insulin. In addition to transporting glucose into cells for energy, insulin has one more function, which is to promote fat storage. This is why babies born to GDM mothers can end up with more fat pads, which is not only unhealthy, but can lead to neonatal problems at delivery, such as shoulder dystocia and hypoglycemia (low blood sugar), and for moms, an increased chance of C-sections. It can also cause metabolic problems and a greater chance of obesity and type 2 diabetes for the child later in life, as well as possible developmental delays.[54] Moms who maintain good blood sugar control throughout their pregnancies lessen these risks.

Because of these potential side effects, controlling your blood sugars during pregnancy is a top priority for your doctor and care team. The first line of defense is usually a focus on a healthy meal plan and daily exercise. If that does not work, oral medications or insulin may be prescribed. Your GDM meal plan is not meant to be restrictive, but rather a healthy way of eating for pregnancy that incorporates the right combination of healthy carbohydrates, proteins, and fats, eaten at regular intervals. Most women are advised to start the day with a small, nutritious breakfast, followed by a midmorning snack, lunch, a midafternoon snack, dinner, and a bedtime snack. This helps you utilize your insulin and promotes better blood sugar control throughout the day.

- Breakfast is important; don't skip it. Because pregnancy hormones are highest in the morning and decrease as the day continues, it is important to have a small, low-carb breakfast with protein. Most women will be advised to hold off on fruit, especially fruit juice, first thing in the morning. The best way to see what foods work for you (in other words, what foods and beverages don't spike your blood glucose), is to test your blood glucose with a finger prick 1 or 2 hours after breakfast, as prescribed by your doctor. Once you find a good breakfast, try to stick with it.

- Your lunch and dinner meal should ideally be divided up as follows:

  Half a plate of nonstarchy vegetables and greens

  One-quarter plate of whole grains or starches

  One-quarter plate of protein

  Reduced-fat milk or unsweetened reduced-fat yogurt (or fortified unsweet- ened plant-based milk products)

  A small portion of fresh fruit

- Choose high-fiber foods as often as possible. Fiber helps slow down the blood sugar-raising effect of carbs, as do fats and protein. For instance, eating a small fresh orange that contains 15 grams of carbs and 3 grams of fiber is better than drinking ½ cup of orange juice that contains 15 grams of carbs and 0 grams fiber.

- Include a good source of protein at every meal and snack; see protein sources on page 339 for ideas. Protein helps balance your blood sugar levels throughout the day.

- Eat nuts, seeds, and natural unsweetened nut, legume, and seed butters (such as almond, cashew, sunflower, tahini, or peanut), which all add nutrients and protein to your diet. For a great snack, try 2 tablespoons of nut butter with a plain rice cake.

- Eat healthy fats, such as avocados, nuts, seeds, olive oil, and omega-3s.

- Avoid processed sugar and concentrated sweets. Opt for fresh fruit if you feel like having dessert. Once you become comfortable with carb counting, you will be able to substitute a special treat for dessert or special occasions.

- Try to "eat all the colors of the rainbow." Think of the vibrant colors you find in tomatoes, red cabbage, carrots, beets, apples, raspberries, strawberries, apricots, bananas, melons, papaya, mangoes, bell peppers, butternut squash, pumpkin, sweet potatoes, Swiss chard, kale, spinach, broccoli, asparagus, avocados, and artichokes. These all contain phytonutrients, which are important to your baby development, and provide you with protective compounds that are immunity-boosting as well.

QUESTIONS AND ANSWERS ABOUT DIABETES DURING PREGNANCY

Are certain women at more risk than others for developing GDM?

Yes. Pregnant women that fall into the following seven categories are generally at higher risk. Although most women are commonly screened for GDM around the 24th to 28th week of pregnancy (since that is when placental hormones are increasing and insulin resistance tends to go up), if risk factors are present, screening may be done earlier. Risk factors for developing GDM include:

- Previous pregnancy with gestational diabetes
- A strong family history of diabetes
- Obesity or excessive weight gain during pregnancy[55]
- A previous delivery of a 9.5-pound or heavier baby
- Polycystic ovarian syndrome, which increases insulin resistance
- Certain ethnic origins
- Above the age of 35

Do I need to see a diabetes specialist to help me with my diet?

Yes. An appointment with a good dietician who has experience with diabetes in pregnancy can help you and should be a part of your pregnancy plan. Most OB doctors will direct you to a certified diabetes educator or registered dietician who is knowledgeable about GDM. If they don't, then ask for a referral, or find one on your own. What you need to know is:

- How to count carbohydrates to create healthy meals and snacks
- How to read a nutrition label to identify the carbohydrate, fiber, and protein content of the foods and beverages you consume based on serving sizes
- How to follow a healthy pregnancy meal plan that includes all the necessary nutrients for mom and baby
- How to exercise safely
- How to get help with your medications and/or dosing insulin, if needed

Do I need to worry about excessive weight gain during pregnancy?

Your doctor and care team will be tracking your weight gain very carefully throughout pregnancy. They will work with you to determine the ideal amount of weight gain per month or week. During pregnancy, it is advisable for all women to avoid excessive weight gain, and if possible, to maintain a healthy weight before becoming pregnant.

How do I test my blood glucose level?

The first thing you need is an accurate new glucose meter (glucometer). Don't use an old meter from a previous pregnancy or one that belongs to a family member. You also need fresh (unexpired) test strips, a good lancing device with lancets, and a control solution for the glucometers that require it. Consult the manufacturer's manual or the phone number on the glucometer or test strip box if you have any problems setting up or using your meter. Generally, this equipment should be covered by insurance. Medical trends suggest that in the future, more women will be using continuous glucose monitors, which will decrease the need for pricking. Stay tuned.

What are my blood glucose targets?

Most women who develop GDM are advised to check their blood sugars four times a day: fasting, one hour or two hours after breakfast, lunch, and dinner. The following table illustrates the target ranges for specific checks. We learned from a large landmark clinical trial, called the Hyperglycemia and Adverse Pregnancy Outcomes study (HAPO), that even mildly elevated blood sugars can cause macrosomia (large babies) and higher insulin levels in these babies can predispose them to metabolic problems later in life.[56] This has brought about tighter blood glucose targets for GDM.

BLOOD GLUCOSE TARGET LEVELS FOR DIABETES DURING PREGNANCY[57]

Fasting/upon rising before breakfast	Less than 95 mg/dL
1 hour after each meal	Less than 140 mg/dL
2 hours after each meal	Less than 120 mg/dL
Before meals/bedtime*	60-100 mg/dL
2:00 am-6:00 am*	60-100mg/dL

*Generally, for pregestational (pre-existing diabetes before pregnancy) insulin-dependent or insulin-adjusting patients

How can I keep my blood glucose levels in a good target range?

This is a great question. There are some factors you can control and some you cannot. Let's start with what you *cannot* control, such as your pregnancy hormones. Your placental hormones continue to rise as you advance in your pregnancy, which is why it is often the last trimester when some women have a tougher time keeping their blood sugars under control. You may be able to eat the same thing for breakfast or lunch for many weeks, and then, poof! at 35 or 36 weeks, you may notice more insulin resistance. If this requires medication and/or insulin to keep your numbers in control, then so be it. Second, being ill can increase your blood glucose levels. Certain medications, such as steroids and progesterone, do the same. And, bed rest or any condition that limits your physical activity can add to the challenge of keeping your blood glucose levels stable. The things you *can* control that will keep you in a good range include the following.

- Walking after breakfast, lunch, and dinner, or whenever time allows.
- Exercising as often as possible. Exercise is the most potent insulin sensitizer there is, which is why it is also the key ingredient in keeping one healthy throughout life. In fact, exercise is increasingly promoted as an intervention to reduce the risk of gestational diabetes or as part of the therapeutic regimen for nonpregnant individuals with diabetes. In addition to its cardiovascular benefits, exercise can also improve glycemic control.[58]
- Logging your blood sugar readings, foods, exercise, and stress levels every day. Seeing how these factors interact can be a powerful teacher and motivator.
- Keeping your doctor and care team appointments. And reaching out when you don't feel well or if you have questions.
- Taking oral medications and/or insulin, if needed, to keep your blood sugars in control.
- Reducing your stress level and focusing on your general well-being through deep breathing, yoga and other means of relaxing. Try not to sweat the small stuff!

Is it safe for me to exercise during pregnancy if I have GDM or existing diabetes?

Yes. For gestational diabetes, moderate activity is recommended, such as two 30-minute walks per day, within one to two hours after eating. Swimming is a great form of exercise since it makes you feel buoyant. Prenatal yoga is excellent, too. Stretching daily keeps you flexible and in shape for delivery. What's important is to find what works for you, and to stick with it. It's important to check with your doctor or health-care provider before beginning any routine, and please don't overdo it (see page 59 for exercise guidelines and warnings).

PREGNANCY WISDOM: SMART EATING WHILE TRAVELING

WHETHER you are traveling near or far, it is important to use common sense and advance planning during pregnancy. Be sure to inform your doctor of your travel plans and get clearance for your journey. Ask your doctor whether you should take a copy of your medical records with you. Ask about immunizations as well. Although traveling in an airplane is almost always safe during pregnancy, it is not recommended for women who have obstetrical medical conditions that could result in an emergency. Check your airline for its policies. Some require a medical letter or certificate from doctor or midwife confirming your delivery date and no complications if you are beyond 28 weeks. Travel is generally allowed up to the 36th week for single pregnancies and 32 weeks for multiples. Eating on the road can be tricky. Here are some tips to guide you.

- Most important rule: When in doubt, don't eat it!
- Make sure you can identify everything you eat and that it is cooked well-done. Do not eat any raw meat (such as beef carpaccio or salmon gravlax) or raw fish (such as sushi or sashimi).
- If you are traveling to a less-developed country, choose fruits or vegetables with a peel. Wash all fruits and vegetables in water with bleach, and dry your produce before you peel it. About 1 tablespoon (½ fluid ounce) of typical chlorine bleach per gallon of water is the maximum that should be used.
- Be sure to stay well hydrated, especially if you're flying. If the water is unsafe, drink only bottled water. If safe water is unavailable, drink canned or bottled fruit juice or other beverages. Do not drink sodas, beer, or any other beverages from a tap or machine.
- Do not use ice cubes if the drinking water is unsafe.
- Brush your teeth with bottled water if the drinking water is unsafe.
- Explain your dietary needs to your waiter. Most restaurants will fix a special dish following your dietary restrictions.
- Take along your favorite foods if they may be hard to find. Peanut butter, protein bars, instant oatmeal, crackers, nuts, and seeds are all good standby foods.
- Carry all medications, supplements, and important items in your carry-on luggage.
- If you think you may have food poisoning (severe vomiting or diarrhea), seek medical help immediately. Do not wait until you are dehydrated.

How can I reduce the pain of finger pricking?

Developing a good technique for pricking your fingers so they don't hurt is key. First, have all of your equipment ready and within reach before you start. Wash your hands with warm soapy water and dry them. Shake them to get the blood flowing. Choose a finger. Imagine a line down the middle of that fingertip pad. Take your thumb and gently press it below the imaginary line on the *opposite* side from the one you plan to prick. Position the lancing device in the area next to the imaginary line on your finger pad and prick. Tips: Don't poke directly on the top of the finger pad, an area filled with nerve endings. And don't poke too far on either side. Every time you prick, rotate to the different sides of your fingers, and always use a fresh lancet for every prick.

Why did my doctor put me on oral medication and/or insulin?

When your blood glucose levels cannot be controlled with diet and exercise, oral medication and/or insulin are prescribed. This does not mean failure. It just means you need additional help to control your blood sugars. You will be closely monitored to keep doses at the ideal levels. Whatever it takes to have a healthy baby—that is your goal.

If I have type 1 or type 2 diabetes can I have a healthy baby?

Absolutely! It just takes more work. Women with type 1 or 2 diabetes need to start pre-conceptual planning as early as possible, ideally three to six months before conception to get their blood glucose in good control. Consistently high or poorly controlled blood sugars can damage fetal organs in the first 8 weeks of pregnancy and lead to other possible complications. Managing type 1 or type 2 diabetes during pregnancy often requires a team of specialists, including one's obstetrician, endocrinologist, internist or nurse practitioner, and a certified diabetes educator, to ensure an optimal pregnancy.

What is hypoglycemia and how should I treat it?

A blood sugar of 60 mg/dL or below is considered low and of concern for most people. If one has type 1 or 2 diabetes, the base number may be different, depending on their set level for highs and lows. Hypoglycemia (low blood sugar) may cause one to feel weak, shaky, irritable, and hungry. For those who are insulin dependent (such as type 1 autoimmune diabetes), hypoglycemia can progress to confusion, loss of consciousness, seizures, and insulin shock. These women should always carry some form of glucagon with them for emergencies.

It is easy to treat an episode of hypoglycemia, if you remember the *Rule of Fifteens*:

- If you feel low, test your blood sugar.
- If it is below 60 mg/dL, then treat with *15 grams of carbs* of fast-acting glucose (this could be three 5-gram glucose tabs, ½ cup of juice, or 1 tablespoon of honey).
- Retest your blood sugar *15 minutes* later.
- If it is still low, you will need to consume a carb-and-protein snack (such as peanut butter with crackers or a slice of whole-grain bread with cheese).
- Test it again after *15 minutes*. If it is not in a good range, call your doctor immediately. If you feel faint, dizzy, or "not right," call 911.

If I have GDM will I get type 2 diabetes? How can I prevent it?

Type 2 diabetes is the most common form of diabetes. It is a progressive disease of insulin resistance. Your body produces insulin, but it does not work efficiently, causing high blood sugar levels that, if left untreated, may eventually lead to serious complications over time. While there is no cure for diabetes, it is possible to prevent, and in some cases, to reverse type 2 diabetes. For women with GDM, the chances of developing type 2 diabetes later in life is high, some estimates are as high as 50 percent.[59] The good news is that the risk goes down if you lose the weight you gained during that pregnancy. Breastfeeding is a great way to lose pounds naturally, in addition to all the other amazing benefits it offers your baby. The important lessons you learned from managing your diabetes during your pregnancy will ideally help you and your family to live a healthier life in the years ahead.

SAFE EXERCISE DURING PREGNANCY

One last but very important thing to cover before we get to the month-by-month nutrition and recipes—exercise! It's critical for so many reasons during pregnancy and postpartum (see "Exercise Is Key," page 335). New studies are emerging that show that being sedentary during pregnancy is not ideal at all, unless you are on bed rest or have been told to limit your exercise by your doctor or care team. That should be enough to get you moving, but in case you need more reasons, here you go.

Exercise helps . . .

- Keep your muscles strong to carry your extra pregnancy weight and to be in top shape for labor and delivery
- Optimize your weight gain during pregnancy and your weight loss postpartum
- Reduce stress, anxiety, and depression
- Boost your energy level
- Stabilize your blood glucose levels, especially if you walk after meals
- Enhance your circulation, an important factor given your increase in blood and fluid volume
- Prevent lower back pain, shoulder pain, and other aches and pains
- Reduce the risk of gestational diabetes and pregnancy induced hypertension
- With sleep—something all mamas, new and seasoned, need more of

So, exercise, mama, exercise! With your doctor's permission, keep moving as much as possible during pregnancy. If you did not exercise before pregnancy, start slow and work up to ideally thirty minutes of exercise per day; this can be in the form of a long walk or shorter walks. You can break up your exercise time and the type of exercise you do. Strength and resistance is excellent combined with something more aerobic, such as brisk walking. Remember good posture is key. Check your alignment frequently to make sure your chin is in, your shoulders are back, and your chest is open.

There are a couple of important things to keep in mind when you exercise. First, it is more difficult for you to breathe when exercising because oxygen must be supplied to your additional body mass (including your baby) and to your increased volume of red blood cells. Second, as your belly gets bigger, breathing becomes even more difficult, because your uterus increasingly crowds your diaphragm, the large muscle between your chest and abdomen. Third, your increased hormone levels soften your connective tissues, making your joints more susceptible to injury. And fourth, your balance shifts as your abdomen and chest enlarge, which can cause clumsiness and possibly falls.

Two of the best exercises for pregnant women are brisk walking and swimming (but not diving). Swimming is particularly good because it uses many muscle groups while the water supports your extra weight. Another option might be to join a prenatal exercise class. Many prenatal classes offer support group discussions on a range of pregnancy-related topics, including how to stretch your pregnancy wardrobe, how to choose a name for the baby, and tips for breastfeeding.

Following are some exercise guidelines recommended by the American College of Obstetricians and Gynecologists (ACOG).[60] **Warning signs to stop exercising include:** chest pain, dizziness, shortness of breath, palpitations (pounding, racing, or irregular heartbeat), faintness, tachycardia (rapid heartbeat), pubic pain, Braxton Hicks (uterine) contractions, vaginal bleeding/amniotic fluid leakage, absence of fetal movement, muscle weakness, calf pain or swelling, and headaches. Once again, if you have any concerns, please check with your doctor.

- Regular exercise (3 to 4 days per week) is preferable to occasional activity.
- Swimming, stationary cycling, and brisk walking are highly recommended.
- Exercises that require jumping, jarring motions, or rapid changes in direction should be avoided. These can cause damage to connective tissue.
- Exercises done lying flat on the back or right side should be avoided. These positions can allow a woman's expanding uterus to compress the vein that carries blood to the heart, which could interfere with blood flow to the uterus.
- Exercise sessions should be preceded by a 5-minute period of muscle warm-up (for example, slow walking or stationary cycling at low resistance).
- Exercise should be done on a safe surface, such as a wooden floor or a tightly carpeted or outdoor surface, to reduce the risk of injury. Wear comfortable shoes for support.
- Strenuous exercise should not be performed in hot, humid weather or during illness accompanied by fever.
- Moderate or intense aerobic activities should be limited to periods of 15 to 20 minutes. Lower-intensity activities may be conducted continuously over a longer period of time, but should not exceed 45 minutes.
- Heart rate should be measured at times of peak activity and should not exceed 140 beats per minute.
- A pregnant woman's temperature should not exceed 100.4°F while exercising.
- Be sure to drink plenty of water before and after exercise to prevent dehydration and hyperthermia and take a break during exercise if more water is needed.
- Care should be taken to rise from the floor gradually to avoid an abrupt drop in blood pressure, and to continue some form of activity involving the legs for a brief period.
- Exercise sessions should be followed by a brief cooldown period of gradually declining activity that includes gentle stationary stretching. Stretches should not be taken to the maximum of resistance.
- A pregnant woman should consume enough calories to meet the needs of her pregnancy as well as her exercise program. Women should not try to lose weight by exercising during pregnancy.

PREGNANCY WISDOM: EASE YOUR LEG CRAMPS

SOME pregnant women experience leg cramps, usually during the last three months of pregnancy. These often occur during sleep, but they can hit anytime. Leg cramps may be caused by the additional weight gain during pregnancy, changes in your circulation, or added pressure from your growing baby may also be placed on the nerves and blood vessels that go to your legs. They can also be the result of deficiencies in calcium, magnesium, and potassium. The following are some tips for relief.

- Stretch your legs (especially your calf muscles) before going to bed.
- Elevate your legs while resting.
- Wear supportive stockings.
- Avoid pointing your toes while stretching or exercising.
- Stay well hydrated—drink plenty of water (you know you're getting enough water if you're urine is light yellow or clear).
- Eat foods with potassium, such as bananas, dried apricots, and orange juice.
- Try to have 3 or 4 servings of calcium-rich food every day.
- Massage or apply heat to your calves.
- Ask your doctor or care team about taking calcium or magnesium supplements.

- Take the talk test to avoid exercising too hard. You should be able to talk in short sentences, as if having a light conversation, without struggling for breath. If you can't catch your breath, slow down, and take it easy until you can. This is really important during the third trimester, when breathing can be a bit of a challenge for some women.
- Women with diabetes during pregnancy or pregnancy-induced hypertension (PIH) should discuss blood glucose levels and any exercise concerns with their doctor and care team. Women taking oral medications or insulin for diabetes will need to get specific blood glucose targets.

One last thing about exercise, do your Kegels (pelvic floor exercises)! They are a critical part of your pregnancy health and postpartum recovery. Ideally, make Kegel exercises part of your fitness routine before, during, and after pregnancy. The job of the pelvic floor muscles is to hold your pelvic organs (bladder, uterus, and bowel) in place. These muscles tend to become stretched or weakened during pregnancy, and if they become too weakened, or damaged, they cannot function properly. Ideally, exercises should be done throughout pregnancy to help support the extra weight of the body and to prepare for labor, and continued post-pregnancy to re-strengthen the muscles.

How to do pelvic floor exercises: While sitting comfortably on the floor, on a ball, or on a chair, contract your pelvis muscles from the outside area to the inner pelvis. Try to imagine that you are stopping your urine in midflow and tightening your anus muscle at the same time. Hold briefly, then release slowly. Keep your stomach relaxed and breathe naturally. Repeat five times. Try to do these exercises five times a day.

9 Months of Baby Talk,
Nutritional Advice,
and Awesome Recipes

From more than three decades of experience working with expecting moms as a perinatal nutritionist, Rose Ann knows that what pregnant women want and need is a collection of family-friendly, easy, delicious recipes that use all the nutritional information beneficial to their pregnancy. Even more, they want to know the optimal time to eat these healthy foods, to have the greatest impact on their baby's development.

The chapters to come follow each month of your pregnancy, highlighting certain nutrients that are beneficial at critical points of your baby's development. Every month throughout pregnancy, starting with preconception, we will give you a list of important nutrients, foods that contain those nutrients, and recipes created from those healthy foods. *That said, please note that all nutrients should be consumed daily, including proteins, carbohydrates, fats, minerals, and vitamins.* This is really important, and we would not be doing our job if we did not emphasize this important fact.

In each recipe, the nutritional highlights for you and your baby are listed at the top. At the bottom of every recipe, the following nutritional information is noted: calories (cals), protein (grams), carbohydrates (grams), fat (grams), fiber (grams), and sodium (milligrams). When a recipe contains vitamins and minerals that satisfy at least 20 percent or more of the FDA's Daily Value per serving based on a 2,000 calorie nonpregnancy diet, they are also included. The major B vitamins—thiamine, riboflavin, and niacin—are viewed as a single group. The B vitamin folate is so important it is listed independently. Our lineup ends with a carb count for women with diabetes during pregnancy. CARB(S), as this is written throughout the book, indicates the number of "carbohydrate counts" in each recipe based on a "one-count portion" being equal to 15 grams of carbohydrates. This is the standard way of carb counting for diabetes.

Our 150 recipes are specifically designed for pregnancy, but they will surely appeal to everyone. Many of our readers over the years have told us that they still make these recipes even after their kids have gone off to college. That makes us really proud and happy. *Regarding the recipes, we encourage you to use all the recipes in the book at any stage of your pregnancy.* In other words, you can use recipes from Month 9 in Month 1 and from Month 4 in Month 7. They are all interchangeable.

Of course, keep in mind that many of these recipes are flexible and can be customized to suit your needs—read the headnotes for ideas. We offer tips to modify them for special diets, food allergies, or diabetes during pregnancy. Look for the following symbols to quickly identify the recipes that are just right for you:

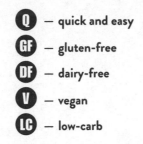

Q — quick and easy

GF — gluten-free

DF — dairy-free

V — vegan

LC — low-carb

Almost all the recipes, except dips, sauces, drinks, dressings, and others like these, come with complete meal ideas. Our readers have found this feature helps them combine foods for maximum nutrient absorption and helps them with menu planning. You'll also see complete meal ideas and tips for diabetes, menus with fewer total carbohydrates. When we suggest certain foods, we've added the word CARB to signal the carb count for the amount that would be ideal to consume. For example, the line "Reduced-fat milk or unsweetened reduced-fat yogurt, 1 CARB" means that you should consume 15 grams or the equivalent of a 1 CARB serving of these foods. These notations apply to grains, starches, baked goods, dairy, and fats. They do not apply to low-carb foods including proteins, green salad, and nonstarchy vegetables. At the back of the book (pages 353 to 364), you'll find menus for pregnancy, menus for vegetarians and vegans during pregnancy, and a collection of menus for diabetes during pregnancy.

PRECONCEPTION

Optimizing Your Body for Pregnancy

We'll say it again—if you're picking up this book before pregnancy, you are brilliant! Now is the time to get your beautiful body in shape. Ideally, give yourself at least three months to make your body the perfect home for your baby. While you're trying to conceive, eating a healthy well-balanced diet, taking a prenatal vitamin or folic acid supplement, and getting exercise are essential. As you probably know, your baby's major organs and systems begin developing at the point of conception and throughout the first eight weeks of pregnancy.

WHAT YOU NEED TO KNOW IF YOU'RE TRYING TO CONCEIVE

- Get prenatal care before you conceive. Inform your health-care provider of your desire to start a family and discuss your general health and any concerns you may have. Inform your doctor of all medications, vitamins, supplements (natural and synthetic), birth control pills, or other substances you are taking, including Accutane or Retin-A.
- Start your prenatal vitamin or folic acid supplement in preparation for conception. Ideally, start taking a folic acid supplement at least one month, and up to three months, before conception. Because half of all pregnancies are unplanned, a daily folic acid supplement of at least 600 micrograms is advisable for all women of childbearing age, especially for women who are trying to conceive.
- Aim to be a healthy weight before pregnancy. Why? One of the biggest reasons is that it will help you control your weight gain during pregnancy. It could also help prevent high blood pressure and gestational diabetes during pregnancy. Plus, a healthy lifestyle will help you lose weight after delivery. Hard to think that far ahead, but you should. On the other hand, if you are underweight and your doctor advises you to gain weight, ask about goals and how best to meet

them. Underweight women can have a harder time conceiving. They are also more at risk for premature delivery and babies with a low birth weight.

- Modify your daily diet to enhance fertility. Prime your body for conception with the proper nutrients. See pages 10 to 23 for information on the nutrients you need and where to get them.

- Make exercise a daily habit. If you needed a push—this is it! Getting physically fit before pregnancy will most likely allow you to exercise throughout your pregnancy, and soon after delivery. Likewise, not being in shape can lead to difficulty when trying to begin an exercise routine during pregnancy, and it can make delivery and postpregnancy weight loss significantly more difficult.

- Stop smoking and vaping, please, please, please. If you need help, don't be shy to ask your care team. Freeing yourself from a nicotine addiction can be very difficult. But there is lots of help out there for you. Although there are no conclusive studies reporting that smoking interferes with conception, quitting smoking will improve your health.

- Stop drinking alcohol. Since you don't know when the magic moment of conception will occur, it is advisable to avoid all alcohol while trying to get pregnant. If you think you may need help, please seek treatment. Heavy drinking can lower your chances of conception and damage your health and the health of your baby.

- Reduce caffeine. Some research shows that caffeine can impair your chances of conception and possibly increase your chances of miscarriage. Studies show that pregnant women who consumed more than 200 milligrams of caffeine a day (about 2 cups of coffee) had twice the risk of miscarriage as women who consumed no caffeine at all.

- If you are entering pregnancy with diabetes or prediabetes, get your blood glucose in good control. *Aim to keep them in an ideal range at least three to six months before conception.* If you are at risk for developing gestational diabetes, work with your doctor to create a plan to reduce or mitigate some of the risk factors that you have control over, such as weight loss, exercise, and diet. Obviously, certain things, such as family history of diabetes, ethnicity, and age, are beyond your control. For lots more information on diabetes during pregnancy, see page 50.

- If you've had bariatric surgery or any other gastrointestinal issues, your doctor will evaluate any nutritional disturbances that should be corrected before conception and into pregnancy (see "Obesity During Pregnancy," page 44).

- If you have an eating disorder or any other condition that could cause infertility or delay conception, please inform your doctors and they will work with you to overcome any foreseeable obstacles.

A quick word about exercise before, during, and after pregnancy. Leading up to pregnancy, there are almost no precautions, unless you fall into any of the following categories, or you are advised not to exercise for any reason. Exercise in moderation is a great thing *during* pregnancy, but consult with your doctor on appropriate exercise for you at different stages of your pregnancy. If in doubt, always ask before beginning a new routine.

- Women with a history of miscarriage
- Women who have experienced preterm labor in this or a previous pregnancy
- Women who have obstetrical complications, including an incompetent cervix, ruptured membranes (broken bag of water), or vaginal bleeding
- Women with diabetes or those who develop gestational diabetes (see page 50)
- Women with preeclampsia or pregnancy-induced high blood pressure
- Women whose fetus is not growing as rapidly as it should be
- Women carrying multiples
- Women with any other pregnancy complication

PREGNANCY WISDOM: MAKE COFFEE WORK FOR YOU

THE amount of caffeine considered safe during pregnancy continues to be a controversial issue. Some studies show that high doses of caffeine may lead to miscarriage. Abstaining from caffeine altogether is the best approach, but some women just need their coffee. If that's you, cut back gradually to avoid some of the unpleasant effects, such as headaches, lethargy, moodiness, and so forth. Try limiting yourself to only one cup of any caffeinated beverage per day. To meet your daily calcium requirements and satisfy your coffee craving at the same time, try increasing the amount of milk (fortified plant-based beverages included) that you add to your coffee. In other words, turn your coffee into a calcium-rich café au lait. One more tidbit of advice regarding coffee is to choose organic brands, especially if you drink it during pregnancy. Conventional coffee is often grown with tons of chemicals, from pesticides to fungicides. How much of this remains after processing is hard to measure.[1]

CAFFEINE CHART[2]

ITEMS	MILLIGRAMS OF CAFFEINE
COFFEE (8 OUNCES)	
Brewed	95–165
Decaffeinated, brewed	2–5
Instant	63
Decaffeinated, instant	2
Espresso (single)	47–64
Latte or mocha	63–123
TEA (8 OUNCES)	
Brewed, black	25–48
Brewed, green	25–29
Decaffeinated, black	2–5
Ready-to-drink bottle (8 ounces)	5–40
Energy drink (8 ounces)	27–164
Energy shot (1 ounce)	40–100
Soda, cola (8 ounces)	24–46
Hershey's chocolate reduced-fat milk	2
Hershey's cocoa powder (1 tablespoon)	8
Hershey's milk chocolate (1.6-oz piece)	9
Dannon coffee yogurt (6 ounces)	30

MAKING THIS THE HEALTHIEST TIME FOR YOU

Getting your body prepped for pregnancy is just plain smart. The fantastic news is that all of the foods that are good for you are also perfect for your partner and the rest of your family. Adding them into your daily meal plan is a win for everyone!

Ideal Nutrition

During preconception, your nutritional focus is on cell structure and genetic material, just as it will be in the first months of your pregnancy. These nutrients are your best friends for supporting your baby's cell, brain, and nervous system development.

- B vitamins: cell division, brain formation, nervous system development, and morning sickness
- Folate: neural tube development
- Phosphorus: genetic material
- Selenium: cell structure
- Vitamin A: cell structure
- Vitamin E: cell structure and genetic material
- Zinc: cell structure and genetic material

OPTIMAL FOODS FOR PRECONCEPTION

PROTEIN	DAIRY	GRAINS/ LEGUMES	VEGETABLES	FRUITS	FATS/OTHER
Eggs	Cheese: goat and ricotta	All-bran cereal and other fortified breakfast cereals	Artichokes	Bananas	Brewer's or nutritional yeast
Meats	Enriched plant-based milks (rice soy, and almond)	Beans: black, navy, pinto, kidney, white, great northern, black-eyed, pink, cranberry, and cannellini	Asparagus	Cantaloupe	Olive oil
Nuts: almonds, cashews, pistachios, Brazil nuts, walnuts and nut butters	Fortified dairy milk	Chickpeas	Avocados	Citrus fruits: oranges, tangerines, grapefruit	Omega-3s
Pork	Yogurt	Corn tortillas	Baked potato with skin on	Dried apricots	
Poultry		Edamame	Beets	Mangoes	
Seafood (fish and shellfish): salmon, tuna, sardines in oil		Folic acid–fortified products	Broccoli and broccoli rabe		
Seeds: sunflower, pumpkin, chia, flaxseed		Lentils	Brussels sprouts		
Tofu and tempeh		Oatmeal	Butternut squash		
		Peanuts	Carrots		
		Wheat germ	Dark, leafy greens: kale, collards, mustard, and Swiss chard		
		Whole grains: quinoa, barley, brown rice, bulgur, and whole wheat couscous	Mushrooms		
			Pumpkin		
			Red bell peppers		
			Romaine lettuce		
			Spinach		
			Sweet potatoes		

This preconception chapter does not have its own set of recipes. Use Month 1's recipes or any others throughout this book to meet your nutritional needs before you get pregnant. Remember, while we're putting the spotlight on certain nutrients during each month, *all the recipes in this book are appropriate for any stage of preconception, pregnancy, and postpartum.*

PREGNANCY WISDOM: HOW IS YOUR DUE DATE CALCULATED?

YOUR doctor or midwife will give you your due date. Or you can use an app or website to figure it out. Or you can calculate it the old-fashioned way, using a calendar with months. Figure out the day when your last menstrual period (LMP) began (example: March 1). Pinpoint that day and subtract 3 whole months from it (example: December 1). Add 7 days (example: around December 8). Your due date is a magical day, but don't be surprised if it gets moved (hint: it probably will).

Now, to confuse things a bit, there are two ways to calculate your due date during pregnancy. "Gestational age" is used to determine your pregnancy from your LMP (info above). "Fetal age" is the actual age of your growing baby. *Your gestational age will always be two weeks ahead of your baby's fetal age.* For instance, if gestational age is 24 weeks, fetal age is 22 weeks. Most calculations of pregnancy, including this book, are measured in gestational age.

Fortifying Foods and Recipes for the First Trimester

Let the Countdown Begin

MONTH 1

Fertilization and Implantation

Weeks 1 Through 4

Welcome to your first month! Yeah! For most women, a home pregnancy test registers positive at Week 4—a time to celebrate and think about fun ways to share the news. That's why we suggest using Month 1's recipes (or any others) while you're trying to get pregnant. That way, you'll already be eating the right foods when the good news hits.

During these early weeks, your baby's major organs and systems have begun to develop. Imagine a heart taking shape (and beating!), a brain developing new cells every second, a circulatory system forming, kidneys, liver and lungs growing, and a neural tube that will eventually become a spinal cord. These are just some of the totally wonderful things that happen in the first eight weeks. That gorgeous baby of yours is a bunch of microscopic cells developing rapidly into an embryo. By the end of Week 4, he or she is the size of a poppy seed.

YOUR BABY'S DEVELOPMENT

- This is the month when fertilization, the journey down the fallopian tubes, and implantation unfold. The total process takes about three weeks.

- Once implantation occurs, the placenta starts to develop and the amniotic sac forms and starts to fill with fluid. The purpose of the amniotic sac is to cushion the baby from bumps, to regulate temperature, and to enhance lung formation.
- As you approach Week 4, your baby's neural tube starts to form.

CHANGES IN YOUR BODY

Some moms may experience some very early signs and symptoms of pregnancy in the first weeks, including fatigue, nausea, feeling sensitive to hot and cold, acute sense of smell, or light spotting when the egg implants. Breasts may feel full or tender, and areolas may get darker. Some women also experience bloating and gas, constipation, frequent urination and excess saliva. For other women, these symptoms may appear weeks later, and some may avoid them entirely. See page 39 if you need tips for coping with morning sickness.

IDEAL NUTRITION

During Month 1, your nutrition focus is foods to optimize your baby's cell structure and genetic material, and preventing neural tube defects. The following nutrients play major roles.

- B vitamins: cell division, brain formation, nervous system development, morning sickness (B_6 for morning sickness)
- Folate: neural tube development
- Phosphorus: genetic material
- Selenium: cell structure
- Vitamin A: cell structure
- Vitamin E: cell structure and genetic material
- Zinc: cell structure and genetic material

OPTIMAL FOODS FOR MONTH 1

PROTEIN	DAIRY	GRAINS/ LEGUMES	VEGETABLES	FRUITS	FATS/OTHER
Eggs	Cheese: goat and ricotta	All-bran cereal and other fortified breakfast cereals	Artichokes	Bananas	Brewer's or nutritional yeast
Meats	Enriched plant-based milks (rice soy, and almond)	Beans: black, navy, pinto, kidney, white, great northern, black-eyed, pink, cranberry, and cannellini	Asparagus	Cantaloupe	Olive oil
Nuts: almonds, cashews, pistachios, Brazil nuts, walnuts, and nut butters	Fortified dairy milk	Chickpeas	Avocados	Citrus fruits: oranges, tangerines, grapefruit	Omega-3s
Pork	Yogurt	Corn tortillas	Baked potato with skin on	Dried apricots	
Poultry		Edamame	Beets	Mangoes	
Seafood (fish and shellfish): salmon, tuna, sardines in oil		Folic acid–fortified products	Broccoli and broccoli rabe		
Seeds: sunflower, pumpkin, chia, flaxseed		Lentils	Brussels sprouts		
Tofu and tempeh		Oatmeal	Butternut squash		
		Peanuts	Carrots		
		Wheat germ	Dark, leafy greens: kale, collards, mustard, and Swiss chard		
		Whole grains: quinoa, barley, brown rice, bulgur, and whole wheat couscous	Mushrooms		
			Pumpkin		
			Red bell peppers		
			Romaine lettuce		
			Spinach		
			Sweet potatoes		

RECIPES FOR MONTH 1

Gingery Cran-Bran Muffins

B vitamins and folate promote your baby's cell, brain, and neural tube development, and the fiber helps your digestion.

THESE healthy muffins make a great breakfast or snack. The cranberries, ginger, and walnuts are all optional—work with what you have in your pantry and what you like to eat. If you can't find All-Bran cereal, any cereal with a high bran content will work. No buttermilk in the fridge? Make your own by adding 1 tablespoon of cider vinegar to 1 cup of milk. Vegan? Use your favorite nondairy milk made into buttermilk and omit the egg. These muffins will keep in the fridge for five days and they freeze beautifully.

MAKES 15 REGULAR MUFFINS OR 52 MINI MUFFINS

Cooking spray (optional)
Bran or similar cereal
1 cup boiling water
¼ cup canola oil or melted unsalted butter
¾ cup sugar
1 cup buttermilk
1 large egg
1¼ cups all-purpose flour
1¼ teaspoons baking soda
¼ teaspoon salt
½ teaspoon ground ginger
½ cup dried cranberries or chopped dried apricots (optional)
½ cup chopped walnuts (optional)
⅓ cup chopped candied ginger (optional)

- Preheat the oven to 400°F. Spray the muffin wells with cooking spray or line with muffin liners.
- Place the cereal in a small bowl and pour the boiling water over it—do not stir. Set aside.
- Combine the canola oil and sugar in a large bowl and whisk together. Add the buttermilk and egg and whisk again. Add the flour, baking soda, salt, and ground ginger, and whisk just until well combined. Add the cereal mixture and mix with a spoon, then add the dried cranberries, walnuts, and/or candied ginger, if using, and mix just until combined. (The batter will be quite thick.) Let the batter sit at room temperature for 10 minutes.
- Stir the batter, then divide evenly among the prepared muffin wells. Bake until a tester inserted into the center of a muffin comes out clean: about 20 minutes for regular muffins, about 12 minutes for mini muffins. Transfer the muffins to a wire rack to cool.

Meal ideas

- Protein, such as natural nut butter or eggs
- Reduced-fat milk or yogurt (Mango-Chia Smoothie, page 157)
- Fresh fruit

Meal ideas and tips for diabetes

- Opt for making mini muffins or reduce your portion size.
- Protein, such as natural nut butter or eggs
- Reduced-fat milk or unsweetened reduced-fat yogurt, 1 CARB

1 regular bran muffin: Calories: 205 cals; Protein: 5 g; Carbohydrates: 35 g; Fat: 7 g; Fiber: 6 g; Sodium: 60 mg; B_6: 1 mg; B_{12}: 3 mcg; Niacin: 4 mg; Riboflavin: 0.3 mg; Thiamine: 0.3 mg; Folate: 213 mcg; Manganese: 1 mg; 2 CARBS
1 mini bran muffin: Calories: 59 cals; Protein: 1 g; Carbohydrates: 10 g; Fat: 2 g; Fiber: 2 g; Sodium: 17 mg; B_{12}: 0.8 mcg; 1 CARB

Just Plain Yummy Avocado Toast

Protein, vitamin K, B vitamins, folate, iron, and fiber enhance your baby's cell, brain, and neural tube development, plus your digestion and iron stores.

LOVE avocados? Enjoy this toast for breakfast, lunch, snack, or dinner! If you don't have time to mash your avocado, simply slice it and place on top of the bread. Choose the best enriched, bakery-quality bread you can find to suit your dietary needs, whether you are gluten-free, vegan, or dairy-free. It should be dense, moist, and as healthy as possible. For more flavor, you can spread a thin layer of pasteurized goat cheese on the bread before topping it with the avocado. For added protein, top with scrambled eggs.

MAKES 2 SLICES TOAST; 2 SERVINGS

1 ripe avocado
2 tablespoons freshly squeezed lemon or lime juice
1 teaspoon olive oil
Salt and freshly ground black pepper
2 slices bread, toasted
¼ cup pumpkin or sunflower seeds
2 cups baby greens, such as spinach or arugula

OPTIONAL TOPPINGS

Radishes, thinly sliced
Cucumbers, thinly sliced
Sliced chives and/or fresh herbs
Pomegranate seeds
Chia seeds or flaxseeds
Chopped walnuts

- Halve the avocado and remove the pit. Scoop out the flesh into a bowl and mash with the back of a fork to your desired consistency. Add the lemon juice and olive oil and season to taste.

- Spread the avocado mixture on the toasted bread. Top with the seeds, baby greens, and other optional toppings, if desired.

Meal ideas

- Salad or soup (Gazpacho [Without the Gas], page 289)
- Reduced-fat milk or yogurt
- Fresh fruit

Meal ideas and tips for diabetes

- Use a small piece of bread for the toast.
- Protein, such as meat, poultry, seafood, eggs, dairy, or plant-based
- Salad or soup (above)
- Reduced-fat milk or unsweetened reduced-fat yogurt, 1 CARB
- Fresh fruit, 1 CARB

1 avocado toast (without any optional toppings): Calories: 363 cals; Protein: 11 g; Carbohydrates: 33 g; Fat: 24 g; Fiber: 9 g; Sodium: 172 mg; Vitamin K: 66 mcg; Niacin: 4 mg; Thiamine: 0.2 mg; Folate: 138 mcg; Copper: 0.5 mg; Iron: 4 mg; Magnesium: 166 mg; Manganese: 2 mg; Phosphorus: 348 mg; Selenium: 20 mcg; Zinc: 3 mg; 2 CARBS

High-Folate Spinach Bean Dip

Vitamins A and K and folate optimize your baby's cell, brain, and neural tube development.

THIS delicious dip will disappear quickly. Serve with whole wheat crackers, veggies, or corn chips. Or spread on toast and top with nuts and seeds for an awesome snack or lunch. Transform any of the leftover artichoke hearts, beans, feta, or spinach into a salad. Lactose intolerant or vegan? Skip the feta. This dip keeps for four days refrigerated.

SERVES 5; MAKES 2 CUPS

2 cups packed baby spinach
½ cup artichoke hearts,
    in brine or oil, drained
    (5 hearts)
1 cup canned white beans,
    drained and rinsed
½ cup pasteurized feta cheese
3 sprigs parsley, leaves only
1 tablespoon olive oil, or to
    desired consistency
2 tablespoons freshly
    squeezed lemon juice, or
    to taste
Salt and freshly ground black
    pepper

- Place all the ingredients in the bowl of a food processor and process to the desired consistency—make it as creamy or chunky as you wish. Adjust the seasoning and serve.

Generous ⅓ cup spinach dip: Calories: 114 cals; Protein: 7 g; Carbohydrates: 15 g; Fat: 3 g; Fiber: 4 g; Sodium: 367 mg; Vitamin A: 3,381 IU; Vitamin K: 191 mcg; Folate: 103 mcg; Manganese: 0.5 mg; 1 CARB

Lentil Soup with Brown Rice and Spinach

Protein, vitamins A and K, B vitamins, and folate promote your baby's cell, brain, and neural tube development.

THE combination of lentils, brown rice, and spinach bursts with nutrition. The vinegar, added to the soup at the last minute, gives it a wonderful tang—balsamic vinegar is perfect—while the olive oil adds richness. The bay leaves are optional. Slow cooker/Instant Pot instructions follow. This soup keeps refrigerated for three days and can be frozen for up to one month.

SERVES 8; MAKES ABOUT 10 CUPS

2 tablespoons olive oil
1 medium-size onion, chopped
2 garlic cloves, minced
4 carrots, peeled and finely diced, or 2 cups sliced peeled baby carrots
½ cup uncooked brown rice (or any rice except instant)
1 tablespoon dried thyme
2 bay leaves
10 cups stock or water, or more as needed
1 cup dried green lentils, picked over and rinsed
1 (5-ounce) bag baby spinach
Salt and freshly ground black pepper

OPTIONAL FLAVOR ENHANCERS

Vinegar, any kind
Olive oil

- Heat the olive oil in a 6-quart saucepan over medium heat. Add the onion and sauté for 3 minutes.
- Add the garlic, carrots, brown rice, thyme, and bay leaves, and sauté for 3 minutes. Add the stock and lentils, stir, and bring to a boil. Skim off the foam with a spoon, then lower the heat and simmer for about 35 minutes, or until the lentils are cooked.
- After 25 minutes of cooking, remove the bay leaves from the soup, and stir in the spinach. If the finished soup is too thick, add more stock or water ¼ cup at a time.
- Adjust the seasoning, place in bowls, and add a couple of drops of vinegar and olive oil to taste, if using.

Meal ideas

- Whole wheat bread or roll (Best-Ever Bruschetta, page 266)
- Reduced-fat milk or yogurt
- Fresh fruit

Meal ideas and tips for diabetes

- Reduce your portion size, if necessary.
- Protein, such as meat, poultry, seafood, eggs, dairy, or plant-based
- Green salad (Quick Romaine and Avocado Salad, page 109)
- Reduced-fat milk or unsweetened reduced-fat yogurt, 1 CARB

1 cup lentil soup (made with vegetable stock): Calories: 196 cals; Protein: 9 g; Carbohydrates: 32 g; Fat: 4 g; Fiber: 5 g; Sodium: 856 mg; Vitamin A: 7,424 IU; Vitamin K: 94 mcg; Thiamine: 0.3 mg; Folate 162 mcg: Copper: 0.2 mg; Manganese: 0.9 mg; 2 CARBS

(continued)

SLOW COOKER OR INSTANT POT INSTRUCTIONS:

- Use 9 cups of stock instead of ten.
- Using a large skillet instead of a saucepan, or your Instant Pot, sauté the onion as directed in Step 1, then add the garlic, carrots, thyme, and bay leaves and sauté for 3 minutes more.
- Transfer the contents of the skillet to the slow cooker, then add the lentils and stock. Cover and cook on HIGH for 6 hours, or until the carrots and lentils are soft. Add the brown rice and spinach and cook for 30 minutes longer. Thin the soup with stock or water, if desired, and finish the soup as directed in Step 3.

Everyone's Favorite Caesar Salad

Q

Protein, vitamins A and K, B vitamins, folate, and fiber optimize your baby's cell, brain, and neural tube development, plus your digestion.

IT'S hard to turn down a Caesar salad, especially a delicious homemade one! Our readers love this salad. If you want to make it a meal, add cooked chicken or shrimp, or sautéed tofu. Short on time? Use bottled Caesar dressing. Vegan? Use vegan mayonnaise and omit the Parmesan and sprinkle with nutritional yeast. This dressing will keep refrigerated for up to three days. Whisk or shake it to reemulsify before using. If you love the taste of olive oil, use 6 tablespoons of olive oil and skip the canola oil.

SERVES 4

**CAESAR DRESSING
(MAKES ABOUT ½ CUP)**

1 tablespoon mayonnaise

1 small garlic clove, minced, or pinch of garlic powder

2 tablespoons freshly squeezed lemon juice, or to taste

1 tablespoon Dijon mustard

2 teaspoons Worcestershire sauce

¼ cup grated Parmesan cheese

Salt and freshly ground black pepper

¼ cup olive oil

2 tablespoons canola oil

SALAD

About 8 cups romaine lettuce sliced into bite-size pieces, or bagged baby romaine, or a mixture of romaine and baby kale

¼ cup grated Parmesan cheese

1 cup canned chickpeas

⅓ cup sunflower seeds

1 cup croutons

Salt and freshly ground black pepper

- For the Caesar dressing, combine all the ingredients, except the olive oil and canola oil, in a small bowl and whisk until smooth. Gradually add the oils, whisking until emulsified; set aside.

- Combine all the salad ingredients in a large bowl, add half of the dressing to start, and toss gently to mix. If you need more dressing, add 1 tablespoon at a time. Adjust the seasoning and serve promptly.

Meal ideas

- Protein, such as meat, poultry, seafood, eggs, dairy, or plant-based (Easy Black Bean Soup, page 107)
- Whole-grain roll or bread
- Reduced-fat milk or yogurt
- Fresh fruit

Meal ideas and tips for diabetes

- Skip the croutons.
- Protein, such as meat, poultry, seafood, eggs, dairy, or plant-based (above)
- Reduced-fat milk or unsweetened reduced-fat yogurt, 1 CARB
- Fresh fruit, 1 CARB

One quarter of the Caesar salad: Calories: 415 cals; Protein: 10 g; Carbohydrates: 24 g; Fat: 32 g; Fiber: 6 g; Sodium: 294 mg; Vitamin A: 8,305 IU; Vitamin K: 117 mcg; Niacin: 4 mg; Thiamine: 0.3 mg; Folate: 231 mcg; Copper: 0.4 mg; Manganese: 0.8 mg; Selenium: 13 mcg; 2 CARBS

KITCHEN WISDOM: TIPS FOR CLEANING AND STORING GREENS AND FRESH PRODUCE

WHEN washing fresh produce, tap water will do just fine. Liquid solutions for washing fresh produce can be effective in removing more bacteria than water, but exactly how much more is unknown. Disinfecting fruits and vegetables with chlorine or iodine is not necessary unless the drinking water has been deemed unsafe, as in developing countries or after natural disasters.

- Greens: Leafy greens (such as spinach, lettuce, Swiss chard, and collards) and fresh herbs are best washed by plunging them into a sink or large bowl of water. Be sure to lift the greens out of the water, leaving the dirt behind. Do not pour them into a colander to drain, which would throw the dirt back on them. Repeat this procedure until no dirt or sand remains in the sink or bowl. Dry with a salad spinner. Place the greens in a resealable plastic bag and store in the vegetable bin of the refrigerator. Greens washed and stored this way will keep for five days. Prepackaged baby greens and boxed lettuce (including spinach, baby romaine, and kale) tend to deteriorate quickly when they become moist. If they are triple washed, there is no need to rewash them at home. If you do want to rewash, do so just before serving.
- Fruits and veggies: Always wash fruits and vegetables before they are peeled or sliced, as the blade of the knife or peeler can move bacteria from the skin to the interior. Large fruits, such as melons or pineapples, and vegetables, such as winter squash, should also be washed before slicing. Ideally, store cleaned and cut fruit and vegetables in a glass or plastic container or bowl with a lid. Shelf life will depend on the produce.
- Mushrooms: Clean just before using. They require a quick rinse (do not soak them, they are like sponges) followed by drying with paper towels. You can also use a mushroom brush to brush off any dirt. Trim the stems after you wash them.
- Root vegetables: Wash well before using, and ideally scrub fresh produce with a vegetable brush, as it causes friction in the hard-to-reach nooks and crannies. Peel if necessary.

Fusilli Pesto Salad with Mozzarella and Artichokes

Protein, vitamins A, E, and K, B vitamins, and calcium promote your baby's cell and brain development, plus strong bones for you.

SEARCHING for a delicious pasta salad? Here you go! This looks complicated, but there are only two steps. Water is substituted for some of the oil in this pesto recipe, resulting in a superb, reduced-fat pesto that is scrumptious on hot linguine, fish, or poultry. Vegan? Use vegan pasta, pasta made from whole grains, or rice noodles and skip the cheese. This salad keeps for three days refrigerated. The leftover pesto will lose its bright green color, but the taste will remain unaffected.

**SALAD SERVES 6;
MAKES ABOUT 8 CUPS**

**BASIL PESTO
(MAKES ABOUT 1 CUP)**

2 cups tightly packed fresh
    basil leaves
¼ cup plus 1 tablespoon olive
    oil or canola oil
3 tablespoons grated
    Parmesan cheese
⅓ cup pine nuts, toasted
1 large garlic clove, peeled
Salt and freshly ground black
    pepper
2 tablespoons water

- Prepare the pesto: Pulse all the pesto ingredients in a food processor until smooth, scraping down the sides of the bowl as necessary. Adjust the seasoning. Transfer to a bowl and cover the pesto with plastic wrap directly against the surface. Refrigerate until needed.

Meal ideas
- Green salad or green vegetable (see Awesome Homemade Salad Dressings, page 114)
- Reduced-fat milk or yogurt
- Fresh fruit

One sixth (1 heaping cup) of the pasta salad: Calories: 471 cals; Protein: 19 g; Carbohydrates: 44 g; Fat: 25 g; Fiber: 4 g; Sodium: 383 mg; Vitamin A: 1,344 IU, Vitamin K: 77 mcg; Vitamin E: 3 mg; Niacin: 3 mg; Copper: 0.3 mg; Calcium: 373 mg; Phosphorus: 273 mg; Manganese: 1 mg; 3 CARBS

(continued)

PASTA SALAD

4½ to 5 cups cooked fusilli (ideally whole wheat) or your favorite shaped pasta (Note: 2½ cups dry fusilli yields about 4½ cups cooked pasta)

2 tomatoes, diced, or 1 cup cherry or grape tomatoes, halved

1 cup artichoke hearts, drained and cut into wedges

8 ounces pasteurized mozzarella cheese, diced (about 1½ cups)

½ cup pitted olives

½ cup Basil Pesto or store-bought pesto, or to taste

Salt and freshly ground black pepper

- Prepare the salad: Combine all the salad ingredients in a large bowl and toss gently until well mixed. Adjust the seasoning and serve.

Meal ideas and tips for diabetes

- Use less pasta in the salad and add more vegetables and/or protein.
- Use whole wheat pasta or a high-fiber brand.
- Reduce your portion size, if necessary.
- Green salad or nonstarchy vegetable (see Awesome Homemade Salad Dressings, page 114)
- Reduced-fat milk or unsweetened reduced-fat yogurt, 1 CARB

Sweet Potato Rounds

Vitamins A and C and B vitamins foster your baby's cell and brain development, plus your immunity.

THE spices make these potato rounds special. The oven must be hot to get the caramelization going. You can keep the skin on these wedges; just scrub the potatoes really well. Try to choose long sweet potatoes versus the shorter, thicker ones. Please note that these rounds are not crisp like traditional deep-fried French fries.

SERVES 4

1¼ pounds sweet potatoes, cut into circles about ½ inch thick

1½ teaspoons total of your favorite spice(s), such as cayenne pepper, chili powder, red pepper flakes, or ground cinnamon, nutmeg, cloves, ginger, or cumin

Salt

¼ cup light brown sugar

2 tablespoons olive oil or cooking spray

- Center an oven rack and preheat the oven to 425°F. Line a rimmed baking sheet with parchment paper or foil. Place the sweet potato rounds on the baking sheet. Sprinkle with the spices, salt to taste, and brown sugar. Add the olive oil and toss until the potatoes are well coated, or spray them with cooking spray. Spread out the potatoes in a single layer so they are not touching one another. Roast for 15 minutes, then turn the potatoes with a spatula and roast for another 10 minutes, until tender. If they are browning too quickly, lower the oven temperature to 400°F.
- Serve promptly.

Meal ideas

- Protein, such as meat, poultry, seafood, eggs, dairy, or plant-based (Awesome Chicken Burgers, page 94)
- Green salad or vegetable
- Reduced-fat milk or yogurt
- Fresh fruit

Meal ideas and tips for diabetes

- Reduce or omit the brown sugar.
- Reduce your portion size, if necessary.
- Protein, such as meat, poultry, seafood, eggs, dairy, or plant-based (above [omit bun])
- Green salad or nonstarchy vegetable

One fourth of the potatoes: Calories: 222 cals; Protein: 3 g; Carbohydrates: 38 g; Fat: 7 g; Fiber: 5 g; Sodium: 54 mg; Vitamin A: 1,362 mcg; Vitamin C: 28 mg; B$_6$: 0.4 mg; Copper: 0.3 mg; Manganese: 0.7 mg; 2½ CARBS

Easy Rice and Green Lentil Side Dish

GF DF V

Folate optimizes your baby's neural tube development.

COMBING enriched rice with green lentils is an easy way to make rice healthier. You can jazz up the flavor with stock instead of water, and by adding a sprinkle of cumin seeds, a cinnamon stick, bay leaves, and/or cloves in Step 2. If you have a rice cooker, by all means use it. In a hurry? Pick up cooked rice from the prepared foods section of your grocery store and add to it some rinsed and drained canned lentils, or your favorite beans.

MAKES ABOUT 4 CUPS

1 cup long-grain enriched rice
½ cup dried green lentils
3 cups water or stock
½ teaspoon salt, or to taste
A few drops of olive oil

OPTIONAL GARNISHES

Sunflower or pumpkin seeds
Pine nuts, toasted
Pumpkin or sunflower seeds
Chopped fresh herbs, such as
    dill, parsley, or cilantro

- Place the rice and green lentils in a bowl, cover with water, and gently swish with your fingers to remove the excess starch. Drain in a sieve, then return the rice mixture to the bowl, add enough water to cover, and let soak while you bring the fresh water or stock to a boil.

- In a medium-size saucepan, bring the water to a boil. Drain the rice mixture and add to the boiling water, along with the salt and olive oil. Stir, return to a boil, then lower the heat to low, cover, and gently simmer until the rice and lentils are soft, 20 to 25 minutes. Turn off the heat and let sit, covered and undisturbed, for 10 minutes. Then, using a fork, gently lift and separate the grains of rice. Adjust the seasoning, add any of the optional garnishes, and serve.

Meal ideas

- Protein, such as meat, poultry, seafood, eggs, dairy, or plant-based (Baked Salmon and Broccoli Rabe with Scallion-Ginger Sauce, page 275)
- Green salad or vegetable
- Reduced-fat milk or yogurt
- Fresh fruit

Meal ideas and tips for diabetes

- Reduce your portion size, if necessary.
- Use brown rice for more fiber (you may need to increase the cooking time slightly).
- Protein, such as meat, poultry, seafood, eggs, dairy, or plant-based (above)
- Green salad or nonstarchy vegetable

½ cup rice and green lentils: Calories: 127 cals; Protein: 5 g; Carbohydrates: 26 g; Fat: 0 g; Fiber: 2 g; Sodium: 292 mg; Folate: 110 mg; 2 CARBS

Swiss Chard with Soy Sauce

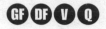

Vitamins A, C, E, and K boost your baby's cell and brain development, plus your immunity.

SWISS chard or spinach, with this garlicky soy sauce dressing, is a tasty side for just about any main course. The sauce can be made up to two days in advance. Sprinkle the finished dish with sunflower, pumpkin, or sesame seeds for even more nutrition.

SERVES 3

SOY SAUCE DRESSING

1 tablespoon light soy sauce or wheat-free tamari (for gluten-free)
¼ teaspoon minced garlic
2 teaspoons light brown sugar, or to taste
1 tablespoon canola oil
A drop or two of toasted sesame oil

SWISS CHARD

1 tablespoon canola oil
12 ounces red or green Swiss chard, or
1 (10-ounce) package baby spinach leaves

- Prepare the dressing: Combine the soy sauce, garlic, and brown sugar in a small bowl. Stir until the sugar dissolves, then add the canola oil and sesame oil, stir, and set aside.
- Prepare the chard: Heat the canola oil in a large skillet over medium-high heat. Add the Swiss chard and sauté just until wilted, about 3 minutes (if it does not fit in the pan all at once, you may need to sauté half of it, then add the rest after it has wilted). Transfer the cooked greens to a serving dish, leaving any watery juices behind in the pan. Add the sauce to the greens and mix gently. Serve hot or at room temperature.

Meal ideas

- Protein, such as meat, poultry, seafood, eggs, dairy, or plant-based (Salmon with Toasted Almonds, Capers, and Herbs, page 144)
- Whole grain or starch
- Reduced-fat milk or yogurt
- Fresh fruit

Meal ideas and tips for diabetes

- Protein, such as meat, poultry, seafood, eggs, dairy, or plant-based (above)
- Whole grain or starch, 1 CARB
- Reduced-fat milk or unsweetened reduced-fat yogurt, 1 CARB

One third of the Swiss chard: Calories: 72 cals; Protein: 3 g; Carbohydrates: 7 g; Fat: 5 g; Fiber: 2 g; Sodium: 577 mg; Vitamin A: 6,935 IU; Vitamin C: 34 mg; Vitamin: E: 3 mg; Vitamin K: 944 mcg; Copper: 0.2 mg; Magnesium: 94 mg; ½ CARB

Three-Bean Chili

Protein, vitamins A and C, B vitamins, folate, iron, and fiber boost your baby's cell, brain, and neural tube development, plus your iron stores and digestion.

AN awesome chili with lots of healthy ingredients and three easy steps. Vegetarians wanting extra protein can add cooked extra-firm tofu or texturized vegetable protein in Step 2. Nonvegetarians might consider adding cooked ground chicken, turkey, or beef. Garnishes to pass at the table include grated Cheddar cheese, sliced romaine lettuce, scallions, black olives, seeds, or cilantro. Slow cooker/Instant Pot instructions follow. This chili keeps for five days refrigerated, and it can be frozen for one month. Freeze in single-meal-size portions in resealable plastic bags or plastic containers for quick and easy lunches or dinners.

SERVES 6; MAKES ABOUT 7 CUPS

2 tablespoons olive oil
1 onion, chopped
1 garlic clove, minced
1 tablespoon chili powder
2 teaspoons ground cumin
1 teaspoon dried oregano
1 red bell pepper, cored, seeded, and diced
8 ounces mushrooms (any kind), washed and sliced
1 (15.5-ounce) can black beans, drained and rinsed
1 (15.5-ounce) can red kidney beans, drained and rinsed
1 (15-ounce) can white beans, drained and rinsed
2 cups diced tomatoes, or 1 (14.5-ounce) can diced tomatoes (do not drain)
1 cup vegetable stock or water
2 tablespoons cornstarch dissolved in ¼ cup water
Balsamic vinegar, for serving (optional)

- Heat the olive oil in a 6-quart saucepan over medium-high heat. Add the onion and sauté for 3 minutes. Add the garlic, chili powder, cumin, and oregano and sauté for 30 seconds. Add the red bell pepper and mushrooms and sauté for 3 minutes.

- Add the black beans, red kidney beans, white beans, diced tomatoes, and vegetable stock and bring to a boil. Lower the heat to a gentle simmer and cook for 30 minutes, or until slightly thickened. Add the cornstarch slurry, stir, and cook for 5 minutes, or until thickened.

- Adjust the seasoning and serve with the balsamic vinegar on the side, if using.

Meal ideas

- Whole-grain or a whole wheat roll
- Green salad or vegetable (Lemony Slaw, page 164)
- Reduced-fat milk or yogurt
- Fresh fruit

Meal ideas and tips for diabetes

- Reduce the amount of beans in the recipe.
- Whole-grain or a whole wheat roll, 1 CARB
- Green salad or vegetable (above)
- Fresh fruit, 1 CARB

(continues)

One sixth (1 heaping cup) of the three-bean chili: Calories: 273 cals; Protein: 15 g; Carbohydrates: 44 g; Fat: 5 g; Fiber: 12 g; Sodium: 444 mg; Vitamin A: 1,371 IU; Vitamin C: 43 mg; Folate: 167 mcg; Niacin: 6 mg; Thiamine: 0.3 mg; Riboflavin: 0.3 mg; Copper: 1 mg; Iron: 4 mg; Magnesium: 103 mg; Phosphorus: 272 mg; Selenium: 12 mcg; Potassium: 1,049 mg; Zinc: 2 mg; 3 CARBS

Three-Bean Chili (continued)

SLOW COOKER OR INSTANT POT INSTRUCTIONS:

- Use 1½ cups of water or vegetable stock instead of 1 cup.

- Follow Step 1, using a skillet instead of a saucepan, or your Instant Pot.

- Transfer the contents of the skillet to the slow cooker and add the black beans, kidney beans, white beans, tomatoes, and water. Cover and cook on HIGH for 5 hours. Add 2 tablespoons of cornstarch dissolved in ¼ cup of water during the last 30 minutes of cooking. Finish the chili as directed in Step 3.

Asian-Style Soba Noodles with Chicken

Protein, vitamins E and K, B vitamins, and folate boost your baby's cell, brain, and neural tube development.

YUMMY and versatile. Feel free to swap out the chicken for sautéed extra-firm tofu or another protein. And use red bell peppers, baby corn, green beans, broccoli, asparagus, or snow peas instead of the vegetables called for. Gluten-free? Use rice noodles and wheat-free tamari. Serve at room temperature. Refrigerate leftovers.

SERVES 5; MAKES ABOUT 5 CUPS

SESAME SAUCE

3 tablespoons toasted sesame oil

2 tablespoons natural peanut butter

3 tablespoons cider vinegar

3 tablespoons light soy sauce or tamari

1½ teaspoons light brown sugar

1 teaspoon minced garlic

2 tablespoons hot water

NOODLES

8 ounces soba or somen noodles

1 tablespoon toasted sesame oil

½ cup grated carrots

1 cup cucumber, cut into matchsticks

1 cup cooked edamame

2 cups cooked chicken breast, shredded or diced

⅓ cup sliced scallion

¼ cup sunflower seeds

- Prepare the sauce: Combine all the sauce ingredients in a small bowl and mix well; set aside.
- Prepare the noodles: Cook the noodles according to the package directions, rinse with cold water, and drain well. Place in a serving bowl and mix with the sesame oil. Arrange the carrots, cucumber, and edamame on top of the noodles, then top with the chicken. Evenly spoon the sesame sauce over the dish and garnish with the scallions and sunflower seeds. Adjust the seasoning. Add more vinegar, soy sauce, or sesame oil as desired.

Meal ideas

- Green salad or vegetable (see Awesome Homemade Dressings, page 214)
- Reduced-fat milk or yogurt
- Fresh fruit

Meal ideas and tips for diabetes

- Use less soba noodles, whole-grain noodles, or swap out for zucchini noodles (see page 169)
- Green salad or nonstarchy vegetable (above)
- Reduced-fat milk or unsweetened reduced-fat yogurt, 1 CARB

1 heaping cup of noodles: Calories: 466 cals; Protein: 31 g; Carbohydrates: 43 g; Fat: 19 g; Fiber: 5 g; Sodium: 1,520 mg; Vitamin E: 4 mg; Vitamin K: 33 mcg; B_6: 0.5 mg; Niacin: 10 mg; Thiamine: 2 mg; Folate: 138 mcg; Copper: 0.3 mg; Magnesium: 94 mg; Manganese: 1 mg; Phosphorus: 313 mg; Selenium: 24 mcg; 3 CARBS

Awesome Chicken Burgers

LC

Protein and B vitamins boost your baby's cell and brain development.

FLAVORFUL and juicy, these burgers are good warm or cold with mustard, ketchup, or your favorite sauce—they may become a weekly go-to meal. Put them in a whole wheat bun or pita pocket or on top of a salad. Top with your favorite relish, slaw (cabbage or broccoli), chutney, jalapeños, cheese, lettuce greens, spinach, or anything you like. The raw burgers can be frozen for up to one month. Thaw before cooking. Gluten-free? Use gluten-free flour. To really rock these burgers, see "How to Check the Flavor of Your Meat Loaf, Burgers, or Meatballs," on page 96.

SERVES 4

1 pound ground chicken
¼ cup crumbled feta cheese
1 tablespoon Worcestershire sauce
2 tablespoons thinly sliced fresh basil leaves
1 tablespoon freshly squeezed lemon juice
1 small garlic clove, crushed, or ½ teaspoon garlic powder
3 tablespoons thinly sliced scallion, green part only
¼ teaspoon salt
About 3 tablespoons all-purpose flour
Cooking spray or canola oil

- Combine all the ingredients, except the all-purpose flour and cooking spray or canola oil, in a large bowl and mix until well blended. Divide the chicken mixture into four equal parts, then form each portion into a patty.
- Place the flour on a large plate. Lightly coat both sides of each patty with the flour, pat off the excess flour, and set aside.
- Preheat an indoor grill to high or heat a large skillet over medium-high heat. Spray the grill with cooking spray or add canola oil to the skillet. Add the burgers and cook on the indoor grill for a total of 5 to 6 minutes, or in the skillet for 2 to 3 minutes on each side. Check for doneness by cutting into a burger; the middle should be fully cooked and the juices should be clear.

Meal ideas

- Green salad or green vegetable (Everyone's Favorite Caesar Salad, page 84)
- Whole wheat bun or cooked whole grain
- Reduced-fat milk or yogurt
- Fresh fruit

Meal ideas and tips for diabetes

- Green salad or nonstarchy vegetable (above)
- ½ whole wheat bun or ⅓ cup cooked whole grain, 1 CARB
- Reduced-fat milk or unsweetened reduced-fat yogurt, 1 CARB

1 chicken burger (without a bun): Calories: 246 cals; Protein: 28 g; Fat: 14 g; Carbohydrates: 2 g; Fiber: 0.2 g; Sodium: 359 mg; B_6: 0.7 mg; B_{12}: 0.7 mcg; Niacin: 12 mg; Riboflavin: 0.4 mg; Phosphorus: 303 mg; Selenium: 18 mcg; Zinc: 2 mg; 0 CARBS

Make It Again Meat Loaf

LC

Protein, vitamin K, B vitamins, and iron enhance your baby's cell and brain development, plus your iron stores.

THE name says it all. Our readers love this recipe. If your kids (or others) object to green things in their meat loaf, leave out the fresh herbs. Serve it hot with traditional mashed potatoes or sweet potatoes, or cold in a sandwich with some good mustard and pickles. The meat loaf can be assembled and refrigerated up to six hours before baking. The baking time may increase by ten to fifteen minutes. The cooked meat loaf keeps for three days refrigerated. Gentle reminder: Be sure to wash your hands thoroughly with warm water and soap for at least twenty seconds after handling the raw meat. Gluten-free? Use gluten-free bread crumbs and ketchup. To really rock this meat loaf, see "How to Check the Flavor of Your Meat Loaf, Burgers, or Meatballs," on page 96.

SERVES 10

Cooking spray or olive oil

GLAZE (OPTIONAL)

⅓ cup ketchup
1 tablespoon molasses
1 teaspoon seasoned
  rice vinegar

- Preheat the oven to 350°F. Line a large baking pan with parchment paper or foil and lightly grease it with cooking spray or olive oil.
- Prepare the glaze, if using: Mix together all the glaze ingredients in a measuring cup or a small bowl; set aside.

> **Meal ideas**
> - Whole grain or starch (Roasted New Potatoes and Bell Peppers, page 139)
> - Green salad or vegetable
> - Reduced-fat milk or yogurt
> - Fresh fruit

(continues)

One tenth of the meat loaf: Calories: 278 cals; Protein: 28 g; Carbohydrates: 13 g; Fat: 12 g; Fiber: 1 g; Sodium: 606 mg; Vitamin K: 64 mcg; B_6: 0.4 mg; B_{12}: 2 mcg; Niacin: 8 mg; Riboflavin: 0.3 mg; Choline: 112 mcg; Iron: 4 mg; Selenium: 26 mcg; Zinc: 7 mg; 1 CARB

MEAT LOAF

2 pounds lean ground beef (preferably chuck) or a meat loaf mix of pork, veal, and beef

2 large eggs, lightly beaten

⅔ cup thinly sliced scallion

¼ cup chopped fresh parsley

¼ cup chopped fresh dill

1 teaspoon dried oregano

1 tablespoon Worcestershire sauce

2 teaspoons Dijon mustard

1 cup plain bread crumbs

1½ teaspoons salt

½ teaspoon freshly ground black pepper, or a couple of drops of Tabasco sauce

½ cup plain reduced-fat yogurt or whole milk

- Prepare the meat loaf: Combine all the meat loaf ingredients in a large bowl and mix with a fork or your hands (wet your hands first, to reduce sticking) until well blended. Form the mixture into a large ball and transfer it to the baking pan. Using your hands, form it into an oval-shaped loaf about 10 inches long and 2½ inches high. Using the back of a spoon, evenly "frost" the meat loaf with the glaze, if using.

- Bake for 1 hour 25 to 30 minutes, or until completely cooked: an instant-read thermometer should read 160°F, and the juices should run clear when the center of the loaf is pierced with a knife or skewer. Remove the meat loaf from the oven and allow it to rest for 15 minutes before slicing.

Meal ideas and tips for diabetes

- Whole grain or starch (Roasted New Potatoes and Bell Peppers, page 139), 1 CARB
- Green salad or nonstarchy vegetable
- Reduced-fat milk or unsweetened reduced-fat yogurt, 1 CARB

KITCHEN WISDOM: HOW TO CHECK THE FLAVOR OF YOUR MEAT LOAF, BURGERS, OR MEATBALLS

IF you have the time, it's always a good idea cook a small "test patty" to check the seasoning and consistency of your meat loaf, meatballs, and burgers (including veggie and tofu) before actually cooking them. To do this, heat a bit of oil in a small skillet and cook 1 or 2 tablespoons of the mixture until well done. Taste the cooked patty and adjust the seasoning or other ingredients in the remaining mixture, if necessary.

No-Bake Nutty Energy Balls

B vitamins and fiber promote your baby's cell and brain development, plus your digestion.

THIS recipe has won the hearts of all our recipe testers. These balls can be stored in the refrigerator for two weeks or frozen for up to three months (if frozen, let thaw before eating). Special note: If your dates are dry and they don't feel sticky and moist, soak them in hot water for ten minutes and drain before processing. This will make the processing easier. Enjoy!

MAKES 50 TEASPOON-SIZE BALLS; 5 BALLS PER SERVING

½ cup unsweetened finely shred coconut

1 cup packed dates, pitted (Medjool are ideal)

1 teaspoon pure vanilla extract

¼ cup pure maple syrup or honey (use maple if vegan)

½ cup creamy unsalted natural peanut butter or almond butter

1 cup chopped raw nuts, such as sliced almonds, walnuts, or pecans

¼ cup whole flaxseeds or chia seeds

1½ cups quick-cooking oats

- Have ready a small bowl or large freezer bag filled with the coconut for coating the balls.
- Place the dates, vanilla, syrup, and peanut butter in the bowl of a food processor and pulse until the mixture comes together, about 2 minutes, scraping down the sides of the bowl as needed.
- Add the nuts and seeds and pulse until incorporated. Add the oats and pulse until the mixture comes together and the ingredients are well blended but still hold their shape for the most part. Transfer to a bowl.
- To form the balls, place a piece of parchment paper, large enough to hold fifty balls, on the counter. Using a teaspoon, scoop out heaping portions of the mixture and place the date mixture on the paper. Repeat this until all the mixture is portioned. Next, roll each portion into a ball.
- Once all the balls are formed, coat them with the coconut, by tossing them in the prepared bowl or bag of coconut. Store them in a sealed container. They can be stacked; they won't stick together. Refrigerate for at least 2 hours before eating.

> **Tips for diabetes**
> - Reduce your portion to 1 or 2 balls.

5 balls: Calories: 313 cals; Protein: 9 g; Carbohydrates: 35 g; Fat: 18 g; Fiber: 6 g; Sodium: 71 mg; Niacin: 3 mg; Magnesium: 104 mg; Copper: 0.3 mg; Manganese: 1 mg; 2 CARBS

TGIF Strawberry-Lime Marga-Chia

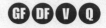

Vitamin C fosters your immunity and iron absorption, while fiber helps with digestion.

YOU made it through the week! Woo-hoo! Time to celebrate with a cool and healthy virgin margarita. Slushy and delicious, you'll have a hard time limiting yourself to just one! For a thicker drink, use less water. If you use fresh strawberries, add three ice cubes to the blender. Sprinkle the chia on top or rim the glass—either way is just plain good!

SERVES 2; MAKES ABOUT 2 CUPS

½ cup orange juice
¼ to ½ cup water, or to desired consistency
3 tablespoons freshly squeezed lime juice, or to taste
2 tablespoons sugar, agave nectar, or your preferred sweetener, or to taste
1 cup frozen strawberries
1 tablespoon chia seeds
Lime wedge (optional)

- Combine everything, except the chia seeds and lime wedge, in your blender and blast on high speed for 30 to 60 seconds, or until smooth. You may need to stop the machine to mix the fruit. Tweak the flavors to taste and adjust the consistency, if necessary. Sprinkle with the chia and enjoy!
- Serving suggestion (optional): Run a lime wedge around the rims of two margarita glasses. Instead of sprinkling on the drinks, pour the chia seeds onto a plate and carefully dip the top rims of the glasses into the mixture.

Tips for diabetes
- Not recommended.

1 cup: Calories: 294 cals; Protein: 4 g; Carbohydrates: 60 g; Fat: 5 g; Fiber: 7 g; Sodium: 4 mg; Vitamin C: 75 mg; 4 CARBS

Embryo Evolving: Organs and Systems Developing

Weeks 5 Through 8

Welcome to your busy second month! Tons (tons!) of development is going on as your baby becomes an embryo. This is a critical phase for organ development. At the beginning of Week 5, your baby is the size of a sesame seed. Over the course of the next four weeks, she or he will transform into a raspberry, about ½ inch in size. That's an amazing amount of growth in just one month!

YOUR BABY'S DEVELOPMENT

- In Week 5, your blastocyst becomes an embryo. Major organs have started to develop. The heart is taking shape, and the circulatory system is operational. In fact, your baby's heart has started beating (incredible, right?), but you won't hear it until Week 10 to 12. The developing umbilical cord will pump oxygen, remove waste, and supply your baby with nutrients to grow and develop.
- In Week 6, dark spots appear where eyes and nostrils are forming. Your baby's jaw, cheeks, chin, nose, ear canals, and eye lenses are under construction.
- In Week 7, your baby's mouth and tongue develop. Leg and arm buds emerge. Your embryo has a tiny tail.
- In Week 8, lungs start to develop. The brain has begun to create about 100 new brain cells every minute. The arm and leg buds start to look more like real arms

and legs, complete with webbed fingers and toes. They begin to twitch, but you won't feel them yet. Your baby's head is quite large compared to his or her body. The neural tube is starting to fuse together.

CHANGES IN YOUR BODY

Some moms will experience a bit of bleeding or spotting; most women will officially miss a period. Breast soreness is common, and breasts may get fuller as your blood volume increases. Montgomery glands can appear. Areolas often darken and veins running to your nipple area become more visible. By Week 7, some weight gain may be noticeable. Fatigue can get intense. Some women may encounter gastrointestinal issues: nausea, bloating and gas, constipation, heartburn, and indigestion. Many also experience an increased sensitivity to smell, along with food aversions and cravings. A white vaginal discharge may occur and continue throughout your pregnancy. Occasional headaches, lightheadedness, or dizziness can be an issue now and throughout pregnancy.

One other thing that might appear at this stage, or any stage: placenta brain! You may experience mood swings, weepiness, irritability, forgetfulness, absentmindedness—all of this is normal. Best thing to do when it hits is to try not to overthink things. Breathe. Relax. Exhale all the way. Everything is going to be great. You're rocking this pregnancy stuff. Tell yourself that you are strong and powerful. Your body is doing miraculous things. And, you're going to be an awesome mom.

IDEAL NUTRITION

Your nutrition focus is foods to optimize your baby's cell, brain, and eye development. The following nutrients will help achieve this.

- B vitamins: cell division, brain formation, nervous system development, and morning sickness
- Folic acid: neural tube defect prevention
- Omega-3s: brain, eye, and nervous system development
- Phosphorus: genetic material
- Potassium: nerve and muscle function
- Selenium: cell structure
- Vitamin A: cell structure, bones, teeth, nervous system
- Vitamin E: cell structure and genetic material
- Zinc: cell structure and genetic material

OPTIMAL FOODS FOR MONTH 2

PROTEIN	DAIRY	GRAINS/ LEGUMES	VEGETABLES	FRUITS	FATS/OTHER
Eggs	Cheese: goat and ricotta	All-bran cereal and other fortified breakfast cereals	Artichokes	Bananas	Brewer's or nutritional yeast
Meats	Enriched plant-based milks (rice soy, and almond)	Beans: soy, black, navy, pinto, kidney, white, great northern, black-eyed, pink, cranberry, and cannellini	Asparagus	Cantaloupe	Olive oil
Nuts: almonds, cashews, pistachios, Brazil nuts, walnuts, and nut butters	Fortified dairy milk		Avocados	Citrus fruits: oranges, tangerines, grapefruit	Omega-3s
Pork	Yogurt		Baked potato with skin on and all other potatoes	Dried apricots	Seaweed
Poultry		Chickpeas	Beets	Mangoes	
Seafood (fish and shellfish): salmon (wild and Atlantic), tuna, mackerel, herring, sardines in oil, halibut, cod, and catfish		Corn tortillas	Broccoli and broccoli rabe		
		Edamame	Brussels sprouts		
		Folic acid–fortified products	Butternut squash		
		Lentils	Carrots		
Seeds: sunflower, pumpkin, chia, hemp seed, and flaxseed		Oatmeal	Dark, leafy greens: kale, collards, mustard, and Swiss chard		
		Peanuts	Mushrooms		
Tahini		Wheat germ	Pumpkin		
Tofu and tempeh		Whole grains: quinoa, barley, brown rice, bulgur, and whole wheat couscous	Red bell peppers		
			Romaine lettuce		
			Spinach		
			Sweet potatoes		

RECIPES FOR MONTH 2

Ginger-Mint Soother for Morning Sickness

GF DF V Q LC

Provides hydration and nausea relief for you.

MOMS tell us this really works for morning sickness! For a boost of vitamin C, feel free to eat the oranges, lemons, or ginger after you drink the tea. Wash the fruit really well before slicing it—try to buy organic ingredients for this recipe. Make a large batch and keep it in the fridge. It's delicious cold, too!

SERVES 1

1 ginger or mint tea bag, with or without caffeine
2 orange slices, cut in half
1 lemon slice
1 sprig mint
3 to 5 thin slices peeled ginger (size is not important)
2 cups boiling water
Honey or sugar, if desired (use sugar if vegan)

- Combine all the ingredients in a large mug or teapot. Let steep for 15 minutes.

1 serving (without added honey or sugar): Calories: 30 cals; Protein: 0 g; Carbohydrates: 0 g; Fat: 0 g; Fiber: 0 g; Sodium: 0 mg; Fiber: 0; 0 CARBS

French Toast Banana Sandwich

Q

B vitamins and folate enhance your baby's cell, brain, and nervous system development.

THIS snappy French toast sandwich is delicious topped with syrup, honey, cinnamon, and sugar, or sliced fresh fruit. We suggest using a calcium-rich bread, such as Roman Meal brand, because two slices have as much calcium as one glass of milk! Of course, you can use any bread you have, including gluten-free. Refrigerate leftovers. To reheat, place the French toast on a plate and microwave for a few seconds.

MAKES 4 SLICES TOAST, FOR 2 SANDWICHES

2 large eggs
½ cup milk
1 tablespoon unsalted butter or canola oil, plus more as needed
4 thick slices calcium-enriched bread, or your favorite whole wheat bread
2 bananas, sliced

OPTIONAL TOPPINGS

Pure maple syrup
Honey
Nuts and/or seeds

- In a bowl, mix together the eggs and milk.
- Melt the butter in a large skillet over medium-high heat. Place a slice of bread in the egg mixture and turn to coat both sides, then add the slice to the skillet and cook for 2 minutes on each side, or until thoroughly cooked and golden brown on both sides. Repeat with the remaining bread.
- As you cook the toast, add some of the sliced bananas to the skillet and cook them, about 2 minutes on each side.
- Place a slice of the French toast on each plate, top with some of the banana slices, cover with another piece of toast, and serve with your favorite topping.

Meal ideas

- Fresh fruit (if not using bananas)
- Reduced-fat milk or yogurt
- Fruit (Supergreen Drink, page 129)

Meal ideas and tips for diabetes

- Reduce your portion size, or skip this recipe.
- Omit the banana or use less.
- Omit any syrups or use a low-sugar jam (such as Polaner All Fruit; 2 teaspoons are FREE).

2 slices French toast with bananas, made from calcium-enriched bread (without optional toppings): Calories: 283 cals; Protein: 9 g; Carbohydrates: 45 g; Fat: 8 g; Fiber: 3 g; Sodium: 234 mg; Niacin: 4 mg; Thiamine: 0.3 mg; Riboflavin: 0.4 mg; Folate: 72 mcg; Selenium: 22 mcg; 3 CARBS

Perfect Homemade Granola

Protein and B vitamins promote your baby's cell, brain, and nervous system development, and fiber helps your digestion.

HOMEMADE granola has always been one of the most popular recipes in this book. And, when you get the hang of it, making your own granola is quick, easy, and fun. Toss in your favorite ingredients, such as sunflower seeds, flaxseeds, pumpkin seeds, coconut flakes, raisins, or dried cherries, apples, mango, apricots, or bananas. And if you're feeling queasy, candied ginger is great, too. For a flavor boost, add 1 teaspoon of ground cinnamon or 1 teaspoon of pure vanilla extract in Step 1. Feel free to add other grains, including rye or wheat flakes (if you aren't gluten-free), or uncooked quinoa. Adding puffed grains to the finished granola is a great option, too. It lightens the granola and cuts some of the calories. Store in an airtight container or resealable plastic bag at room temperature for up to 2 weeks. You can make a large batch and freeze it for up to 3 months.

MAKES ABOUT 5 CUPS

Cooking spray
½ cup pure maple syrup
¼ cup canola oil
3½ cups old-fashioned rolled oats
½ cup chopped walnuts or your favorite nuts
⅓ cup dried cranberries
⅓ cup chopped dried mango, pineapple, apples, or your favorite dried fruit

- Preheat the oven to 275°F. Lightly spray a large, rimmed baking sheet with cooking spray; set aside.
- Combine the maple syrup and canola oil in a Pyrex measuring cup and place in a microwave oven to warm. Mound the rolled oats and walnuts on the prepared baking sheet, then pour the maple syrup mixture over them and toss with two large spoons until well combined. Spread the mixture evenly on the baking sheet.
- Bake for about 20 minutes, then remove from the oven and carefully stir. Bake for another 20 minutes, or until light golden. Note: Do not overbake or the granola may develop a bitter, burnt taste. The oats will still be a bit soft when they come out of the oven, but will harden as they cool.
- Allow the granola to cool completely, then add the dried fruit and mix well.

Meal ideas

- Protein, such as eggs, dairy, or plant-based
- Fresh fruit
- Reduced-fat milk or yogurt (Berry-Peach-Flax Smoothie, page 287)

Meal ideas and tips for diabetes

- Reduce your portion size, or skip this recipe.
- Reduce the amount of maple syrup.
- Omit the dried fruit.
- Protein, such as eggs, dairy, or plant-based

½ cup (made with dried walnuts and mango): Calories: 362 cals; Protein: 10 g; Carbohydrates: 53 g; Fat: 13 g; Fiber: 7 g; Sodium: 3 mg; Thiamine: 0.4 mg; Riboflavin: 0.3 mg; Copper: 0.5 mg; Phosphorus: 308 mg; Magnesium: 110 mg; Manganese: 3 mg; Selenium: 14 mcg; Zinc: 3 mg; 3 CARBS

Vitamin-Rich Butternut Squash Soup   GF DF V

Protein, vitamins A, C, and E, and B vitamins boost your baby's cell, brain, and nervous system development, and vitamin C helps your immunity.

EASY and healthy with only two steps. You can prepare this in a slow cooker or Instant Pot as well. The fresh cilantro, nuts, and seeds add extra flavor and crunch. You can also add diced tomato, cucumber, or radishes to the soup. To save time, use prepeeled and cut-up fresh butternut squash. This soup keeps refrigerated for five days. It can be frozen for up to one month.

**SERVES 6 TO 8;
MAKES ABOUT 8½ CUPS**

2 tablespoons olive oil
1 medium-size onion,
    chopped
2 tablespoons minced fresh
    ginger
1¼ pounds peeled and cut-up
    butternut squash (4 cups)
⅓ cup dried apricots
5 cups stock, any kind
½ teaspoon salt, or to taste
1 teaspoon ground ginger
    (optional)
¼ cup chopped fresh cilantro
¼ cup pumpkin or sunflower
    seeds
½ cup chopped walnuts

- Heat the olive oil in a 6-quart saucepan over medium heat. Add the onion and fresh ginger and sauté for 3 minutes. Add the squash, apricots, stock, salt, and ground ginger, if using. Bring to a boil, then lower the heat and simmer for 10 to 15 minutes, or until the squash and apricots are tender.

- Remove the soup from the heat and allow to cool slightly, then puree in batches. Return the pureed soup to the rinsed-out saucepan and reheat over medium-high heat just until the soup reaches a boil. Adjust the consistency by adding more water, if needed. Adjust the seasoning and garnish with the cilantro, seeds, and nuts.

Meal ideas

- Green salad or vegetable (Quick Romaine and Avocado Salad, page 109)
- Whole wheat bread or roll
- Reduced-fat milk or yogurt
- Fresh fruit

Meal ideas and tips for diabetes

- Green salad or nonstarchy vegetable (above)
- Whole wheat bread or roll, 1 CARB
- Reduced-fat milk or unsweetened reduced-fat yogurt, 1 CARB

1 cup soup: Calories: 293 cals; Protein: 11 g; Carbohydrates: 30 g; Fat: 16 g; Fiber: 6 g; Sodium: 617 mg; Vitamin A: 15,556 IU; Vitamin C: 24 mg; Vitamin E: 3 mg; B_6: 0.4 mg; Niacin: 7 mg; Copper: 0.5 mg; Magnesium: 109 mg; Manganese: 1 mg; 2 CARBS

Easy Black Bean Soup

Protein, vitamins A and C, B vitamins, and folate boost your baby's cell, brain, and nervous system development, and vitamin C helps your immunity and keeps your gums and teeth healthy.

THE key to a really good black bean soup is not only the soup, but the fixin's! Think: Cheddar cheese, avocado, diced tomatoes, scallions, chopped cilantro, and sour cream. Canned beans are a real time-saver. The spices and garnishes add color and a burst of flavor. More stock or water can be substituted for the tomato juice. Need more protein? Add cooked chicken or tofu (if vegetarian or vegan) to the soup. The soup keeps refrigerated for one week, and it can be frozen for up to one month. Slow cooker/Instant Pot instructions follow.

SERVES 7; MAKES 7 CUPS

2 tablespoons olive oil
1 large onion, chopped
2 carrots, sliced
½ red bell pepper, cored, seeded, and chopped (optional)
2 garlic cloves, crushed
2 teaspoons ground cumin
2 teaspoons dried oregano or basil
1 teaspoon chili powder
2 (15-ounce) cans black beans, drained and rinsed
5 cups stock or water, or more as needed
1 cup tomato or V8 juice
Salt and freshly ground black pepper
Fresh cilantro, for garnish

- Heat the olive oil in a 6-quart saucepan over medium-high heat until hot. Add the onion and sauté for 3 minutes. Add the carrots, and the bell pepper, if using, garlic, cumin, oregano, and chili powder and sauté for 3 minutes. Add the beans, stock, and juice and bring to a boil, then lower the heat and simmer, uncovered, for 20 minutes, or until the carrots are tender.
- Allow the soup to cool slightly, then puree 3 cups of it. Return the pureed soup to the saucepan and stir. Add stock or water to thin the soup, if desired. Adjust the seasoning, add the cilantro and your desired fixin's, and serve.

Meal ideas

- Green salad or vegetable
- Whole wheat bread or roll (Easy Cheese-y Toast, page 243)
- Reduced-fat milk or yogurt
- Fresh fruit

Meal ideas and tips for diabetes

- Green salad or nonstarchy vegetable
- Whole wheat bread or roll (above), 1 CARB
- Reduced-fat milk or unsweetened reduced-fat yogurt, 1 CARB

(continues)

1 cup black bean soup (no fixin's): Calories: 237 cals; Protein: 13 g; Carbohydrates: 33 g; Fat: 6 g; Fiber: 10 g; Sodium: 520 mg; Vitamin A: 4,867 IU; Vitamin C: 45 mg; Niacin: 4 mg; Thiamine: 0.3 mg; Riboflavin: 0.4 mg; Folate: 104 mcg; Copper: 0.4 mg; 2 CARBS

Easy Black Bean Soup (continued)

SLOW COOKER OR INSTANT POT INSTRUCTIONS:

- Use 3½ cups of stock instead of 5 cups. Because this recipe calls for canned black beans, the cooking time is short, even in a slow cooker or Instant Pot. When the carrots are soft, the soup is essentially ready, usually after 4 hours on high heat.

- Using a large skillet instead of a saucepan, or your Instant Pot, sauté the onion as directed in Step 1, then add the carrots, bell pepper (if using), garlic, cumin, oregano, and chili powder, and sauté for 3 minutes.

- Transfer the contents of the skillet to the slow cooker, then add the black beans, stock, and tomato juice. Cover and cook on HIGH for 6 hours. Finish the soup as directed in Steps 2 and 3.

Quick Romaine and Avocado Salad

Vitamins A, E, and K, B vitamins, and folate foster your baby's cell, brain, and nervous system development, and fiber helps your digestion.

A salad and dressing made in one bowl. What could be easier? The order in which you add the ingredients is important. Adding the olive oil first coats the leaves so they are not "burned" by the acid of the lemon juice. The seeds are optional, but they are a great way to boost the nutritional value with no effort. Vegan or lactose intolerant? Skip the Parmesan or replace it with a nondairy cheese or nutritional yeast.

SERVES 2

4 cups sliced romaine lettuce, or a mixture of your favorite greens

¼ cup grated Parmesan cheese

1 ripe avocado, peeled, pitted, and sliced

1½ tablespoons olive oil, or to taste

Juice of ½ lemon, or to taste

Salt and freshly ground black pepper

2 tablespoons sunflower or pumpkin seeds

1 tablespoon whole flaxseeds

• Place the romaine lettuce, Parmesan cheese, and avocado in a salad bowl. Drizzle the olive oil evenly over the top, then toss gently. Add the lemon juice and salt and pepper to taste and toss gently again. Adjust the seasoning, sprinkle with the seeds and flaxseeds, and serve promptly.

Meal ideas

- Protein, such as meat, poultry, seafood, eggs, dairy, or plant-based (Pr-Egg-O Salad, page 110)
- Whole grain or starch
- Reduced-fat milk or yogurt
- Fresh fruit

Meal ideas and tips for diabetes

- Protein, such as meat, poultry, seafood, eggs, dairy, or plant-based (above)
- Whole grain, roll, or starch, 1 CARB
- Reduced-fat milk or unsweetened reduced-fat yogurt, 1 CARB

Half of the romaine salad: Calories: 286 cals; Protein: 5 g; Carbohydrates: 12 g; Fat: 26 g; Fiber: 8 g; Sodium: 14 mg; Vitamin A: 8,290 IU; Vitamin E: 6 mg; Vitamin K: 116 mcg; B_6: 0.4 mg; Thiamine: 0.3 mg; Niacin: 3 mg; Folate: 209 mcg; Copper: 0.3 mg; 1 CARB

Pr-Egg-O Salad

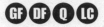

Protein, vitamins A, D, and K, and B vitamins boost your baby's cell, brain, and nervous system development, and vitamin D helps you absorb calcium.

KEEP it simple or doctor up this egg salad with sliced scallions or chives, chopped fresh parsley or dill, paprika, curry powder, or your favorite spice. And, as with many recipes in this book, you can throw in seeds for crunch and added nutrients. Refrigerated leftovers will keep for three days.

MAKES A GENEROUS ½ CUP SALAD; 1 SERVING

2 large eggs, hard-boiled, peeled, and chopped
2 tablespoons diced celery
2 tablespoons light mayonnaise, or to taste
Salt and freshly ground black pepper
½ cup baby greens, such as arugula
2 to 3 slices tomato

• Gently mix the eggs, celery, mayonnaise, and salt and pepper to taste in a small bowl. Adjust the seasoning and serve with the baby greens and tomato. Refrigerate leftovers.

Meal ideas

• Whole-grain bread, roll, or starch
• Salad or vegetable (see Awesome Homemade Salad Dressings, page 214)
• Reduced-fat milk or yogurt
• Fresh fruit

Meal ideas and tips for diabetes

• Whole-grain bread, roll, or starch, 1 CARB
• Salad or vegetable (above)
• Reduced-fat milk or unsweetened reduced-fat yogurt, 1 CARB
• Fresh fruit, 1 CARB

½ cup egg salad: Calories: 270 cals; Protein: 14 g; Carbohydrates: 6 g; Fat: 21 g; Fiber: 1 g; Sodium: 350 mg; Vitamin A: 1,248 IU; Vitamin D: 87 IU; Vitamin K: 72 mcg; B$_{12}$: 1 mcg; Riboflavin: 0.6 mg; Selenium: 31 mcg; ½ CARB

Best-Ever Tabbouleh Salad

Protein, vitamins A, C, and K enhance your baby's cell, brain, and nervous system development, and fiber helps your digestion.

TABBOULEH is a superhealthy Middle Eastern dish made from bulgur wheat and vegetables. Packaged tabbouleh mixes are convenient and tasty, and a good starting point for adding other ingredients. If you can't find bulgur wheat, feel free to swap out for your favorite whole grain or a mix of grains. Serve this salad with hummus (the traditional pair), create a pita pocket with additional veggies and cheese (nondairy if necessary), add it to your salad in a jar (see page 212), or serve it as a side dish (especially good with grilled foods). This salad keeps for two days refrigerated.

SERVES 4 TO 6; MAKES ABOUT 4 CUPS

1 (6-ounce) package tabbouleh, such as Near East Taboule Wheat Salad

2 tablespoons freshly squeezed lemon juice, or to taste

3 tablespoons olive or canola oil

2 tomatoes, diced

⅔ cup seeded and diced red bell pepper (½ pepper)

½ cup canned chickpeas or your favorite beans, drained and rinsed

½ cup pine nuts or other nuts, toasted

¼ cup pumpkin or sunflower seeds

Salt and freshly ground black pepper

¼ cup chopped fresh parsley

- Place the contents of the tabbouleh package in a medium-size bowl and add boiling water (not cold water) in the amount stated on the package. Stir, then cover and let sit for 20 minutes.

- Add the remaining ingredients and mix thoroughly. Adjust the seasoning and serve.

Meal ideas

- Protein, such as meat, poultry, seafood, eggs, dairy, or plant-based
- Green salad or vegetable (Greek-Style Broccoli, page 248)
- Reduced-fat milk or yogurt
- Fruit with vitamin C

Meal ideas and tips for diabetes

- Reduce your portion size, if necessary.
- Protein, such as meat, poultry, seafood, eggs, dairy, or plant-based
- Green salad or nonstarchy vegetable with vitamin C (above)
- Reduced-fat milk or unsweetened reduced-fat yogurt, 1 CARB

¾ cup tabbouleh salad: Calories: 332 cals; Protein: 10 g; Carbohydrates: 36 g; Fat: 20 g; Fiber: 9 g; Sodium: 331 mg; Vitamin A: 1,262 IU; Vitamin C: 36 mg; Vitamin K: 66 mcg; Copper: 0.3 mg; Magnesium: 97 mg; Manganese: 1 mg; 2 CARBS

COOKING grains at home is easy and convenient. You can make them in large batches and freeze them in small portions for a quick side dish or healthy addition to your salads or soups. Quinoa, couscous, brown rice, barley, and bulgur wheat are some common grains used in recipes in this book. Feel free to mix them together. The following tips and cooking instructions will help you incorporate these grains in your everyday meal plans.

Quinoa

Uses: Salads, side dishes, stuffing, patties, mix into oatmeal

Basic cooking instructions: Use 1¾ cups of water to 1 cup of quinoa. Combine the rinsed quinoa and water in a medium-size saucepan and bring to a boil. Reduce the heat and simmer, covered, for 15 to 20 minutes, or until the grains look transparent and the spiral-like germ has separated. Remove from the heat and let stand for 5 minutes, then fluff with a fork. Sautéing cooked quinoa with olive oil or butter, then adding salt, pepper and fresh herbs, makes a lovely side dish or accompaniment to eggs for breakfast.

Tip: The grains of boxed quinoa (such as Ancient Harvest Quinoa) tend to be larger, sweeter, and fluffier when cooked.

Couscous

Uses: Salads, side dishes, stuffing

Basic cooking instructions: Use 1½ cups of water to 1 cup of couscous. Bring the water to a boil in a medium-size saucepan. Add the couscous, stir, return to a boil, simmer for 3 to 5 minutes, cover, and remove from the heat. Let sit, covered, for 7 minutes. Fluff with a fork.

Tips: Whole wheat couscous contains more fiber and iron than regular couscous. Israeli, Mediterranean, or Middle Eastern couscous (all the same thing) are larger rounder grains of toasted pasta that have no fiber or iron, but they make a fun salad.

Brown Rice

Uses: Side dishes, salads, soups, risottos, pilafs, stuffing

Basic cooking instructions: Use 2 cups of water to 1 cup of rice. Stovetop cooking method: Bring the water to a boil in a large saucepan. Add the rice, return to a boil, lower the heat to a simmer, cover, and cook for about 45 minutes, or until the grains are tender and the water has evaporated. Oven method: Preheat the oven to 400°F. Bring the water to a boil and set aside. Place the rice in an 8-inch Pyrex dish, add the water, cover, and bake for 45 minutes, or until the grains are tender.

Tips: Brown rice comes in short, medium, or long grains, or basmati rice. The outer hull, or bran, is left on the brown rice grain, adding twice as much fiber as that of white rice, in addition to vitamin E. Lundberg Family Farms produces fabulous brown rice in an assortment of varieties and mixtures.

Barley

Uses: Soups, casseroles, side dishes, salads, hot cereals, stuffing

Basic cooking instructions: Bring 3 cups of water to a boil in a medium-size saucepan, add ½ cup of barley, and simmer, uncovered, for 45 minutes, or until the grains are soft. Drain, rinse under cold running water, and drain again. Add directly to soups. (Note: One-half cup of raw barley makes about 2 cups of cooked barley.)

Tips: Quick-cooking barley, such as Quaker Oats' Mother's Quick Cooking Barley, cooks in about 10 minutes. Barley flakes, which resemble rolled oats, can be made into hot cereal. Barley grits, a fine grind of the grain, are used for hot cereal.

Bulgur Wheat

Uses: Salads, tabbouleh, pita pocket sandwiches with hummus, stuffing

Basic cooking instructions: Use 1½ cups of water to 1 cup of the grains. (The amount of water will depend on the size of the grain. Drain off any water that is not absorbed after 25 minutes of soaking.). Bring the water to a boil. Place the grains in a heatproof bowl, add the boiling water, stir, cover with plastic wrap, and let sit at room temperature for 20 to 25 minutes, or until the grains are soft and all of the water is absorbed. If not soft by then, add more hot water.

Tips: Boxed tabouleh mixes that contain the spices are quick and easy to prepare. The best brand is Near East Taboule Wheat Salad Mix—it seems to have the perfect balance of spices to grains.

Superhealthy Lentil Salad

Protein, vitamins E and K, B vitamins, and folate enhance your baby's cell, brain, and nervous system development, and iron boosts your iron stores, while fiber helps digestion.

POWER-PACKED with nutrition, salads don't come much healthier than this. If you like cheese, add pasteurized feta cheese or goat cheese for a nice tang. To save time, pick up as many ingredients as you can from a salad bar. This salad keeps refrigerated for three days.

SERVES 4; MAKES ABOUT 3 CUPS

DRESSING

2 tablespoons cider vinegar, or to taste
2 teaspoons Dijon mustard
1 small garlic clove, minced, or ½ teaspoon garlic powder
¼ cup olive oil

SALAD

1 (15-ounce) can lentils, drained and rinsed, or 1½ cups cooked
1 cup cooked quinoa or brown rice
⅓ cup diced celery
⅓ cup sliced red radishes
1 large vine-ripened tomato, diced, or 12 cherry or grape tomatoes, halved
¼ cup chopped fresh parsley
Salt and freshly ground black pepper
¼ cup sunflower seeds

- Prepare the dressing: In a small bowl, whisk together the vinegar, mustard, and garlic. Add the olive oil and continue to whisk until emulsified.
- Prepare the salad: Combine the lentils, quinoa, celery, radishes, tomatoes, and parsley in a serving bowl. Add the dressing and mix gently. Adjust the seasoning, top with the seeds, and serve.

Meal ideas

- Protein, such as meat, poultry, seafood, eggs, dairy, or plant-based
- Green salad or vegetable (Greek-Style Broccoli, page 248)
- Reduced-fat milk or yogurt
- Fruit with vitamin C

Meal ideas and tips for diabetes

- Protein, such as meat, poultry, seafood, eggs, dairy, or plant-based
- Green salad or nonstarchy vegetable with vitamin C (above)
- Reduced-fat milk or unsweetened reduced-fat yogurt, 1 CARB

¾ cup: Calories: 329 cals; Protein: 11 g; Carbohydrates: 29 g; Fat: 19 g; Fiber: 9 g; Sodium: 90 mg; Vitamin E: 6 mg; Vitamin K: 80 mcg; Folate 195 mcg; B$_6$: 0.4 mg; Niacin: 4 mg; Thiamine: 0.3 mg; Copper: 0.5 mg; Iron: 4 mg; Magnesium: 95 mg; Manganese: 1 mg; Phosphorus: 281 mg; 2 CARBS

Kale with Cranberries and Walnuts

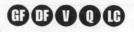

Vitamins A, C, and K and folate optimize your baby's cell, brain, and nervous system development, and vitamin C boosts your immunity.

THIS tasty side dish is filled with good stuff. The sweet cranberries balance the kale and the walnuts give it a nice crunch. Feel free to modify all the ingredients. Any greens will work. For tips on cleaning and storing greens, see page 85.

SERVES 4

2 tablespoons olive oil
1 medium-size onion, chopped
12 ounces kale, stems trimmed, leaves sliced, or baby kale (about 5 cups)
3 tablespoons balsamic vinegar
¼ cup dried cranberries
¼ cup chopped walnuts, toasted
Salt and freshly ground black pepper

- In a large skillet, heat the olive oil over medium-high heat. Add the onion and sauté for 3 minutes.
- Lower the heat to medium, add the kale, and cook, uncovered, stirring frequently, for about 5 minutes, or until wilted. If the kale sticks to the skillet, add a little water, 2 tablespoons at a time. Add the vinegar, cranberries, and walnuts during the last 2 minutes of cooking. Adjust the seasoning and serve.

Meal idea

- Protein, such as meat, poultry, seafood, eggs, dairy, or plant-based (Chili-Rubbed Pork Chops, page 174)
- Whole grain or starch
- Reduced-fat milk or yogurt
- Fruit with vitamin C

Meal ideas and tips for diabetes

- Protein, such as meat, poultry, seafood, eggs, dairy, or plant-based (above)
- Whole grain or starch, 1 CARB
- Reduced-fat milk or unsweetened reduced-fat yogurt, 1 CARB

One quarter of the kale: Calories: 183 cals; Protein: 5 g; Carbohydrates: 17 g; Fat: 12 g; Fiber: 4 g; Sodium: 34 mg; Vitamin A: 8,372 IU; Vitamin C: 102 mg; Vitamin K: 595 mcg; Folate: 129 mcg; Copper: 1 mg; Manganese: 1 mg; 1 CARB

Old Bay Tofu Cakes with Cocktail Sauce

Protein, vitamin C, and B vitamins promote your baby's cell, brain, and nervous system development, and iron keeps your gums and teeth healthy, while calcium keeps your bones strong.

OLD Bay seasoning isn't just for crab cakes anymore! Rose Ann shared this recipe for the first edition of *Eating for Pregnancy*, and it has been a favorite ever since. Pressed for time? Use store-bought cocktail sauce, ketchup, chutney, or your favorite dipping sauce. Gluten-free? Use gluten-free bread crumbs and ketchup. Dairy-free? Omit the Parmesan cheese and sour cream in the sauce. Vegan? Omit all dairy, replace the eggs with 3 tablespoons of flaxseeds, and use vegan mayonnaise. The tofu cakes can be shaped, covered, and refrigerated for up to twenty-four hours. Do not freeze. This sauce can be made up to three days in advance.

SERVES 4

TOFU CAKES (MAKES ABOUT 8 CAKES)

1 (15-ounce) package (drained weight) extra-firm tofu, drained, finely crumbled (use your hands or a fork), and blot well with paper towels

1 cup plain or seasoned bread crumbs or panko

3 large eggs, lightly beaten

2 teaspoons Old Bay seasoning, or to taste

⅓ cup grated Parmesan cheese

⅓ cup chopped fresh cilantro, basil, or dill

¼ cup diced jarred roasted red peppers (optional)

2 tablespoons olive oil

- Prepare the tofu cakes: Combine the tofu, ½ cup of the bread crumbs and the eggs, Old Bay seasoning, Parmesan cheese, cilantro, and bell peppers in a bowl and mix until well blended. Using a ⅓-cup measuring cup, portion out the mixture onto two large plates, then form each portion into a patty.
- Place the remaining ½ cup of bread crumbs on a separate plate. Cover each patty with the bread crumbs before cooking.
- Heat the olive oil in a large skillet over medium-high heat. Add the cakes, in batches, and cook for 3 to 4 minutes on each side, or until golden brown and heated through. If they begin browning too quickly, lower the heat.
- Serve hot with the cocktail sauce.

Meal ideas

- Tossed salad or vegetable (Roasted Brussels Sprouts, page 295)
- Whole wheat bun or whole grain
- Reduced-fat milk or yogurt
- Fresh fruit

2 tofu cakes (no buns): Calories: 335 cals; Protein: 20 g; Carbohydrates: 24 g; Fat: 18 g; Fiber: 2 g; Sodium: 422 mg; Vitamin C: 17 mg; B_{12}: 0.5 mcg; Niacin: 6 mg; Thiamine: 0.3 mg; Riboflavin: 0.4 mg; Choline: 145 mg; Calcium: 344 mg; Copper: 0.3 mg; Iron: 4 mg; Manganese: 0.9 mg; Phosphorus: 289 mg; Selenium: 31 mcg; 2 CARBS

3 tablespoons cocktail sauce: Calories: 48 cals; Protein: 0.4 g; Carbohydrates: 6 g; Fat: 3 g; Fiber: 0 g; Sodium: 196 mg; ½ CARB

(continued)

COCKTAIL SAUCE (MAKES ½ CUP)

⅓ cup ketchup

1 tablespoon prepared horseradish, or to taste

½ teaspoon grated lemon zest

1 tablespoon freshly squeezed lemon juice, or to taste

1 teaspoon Worcestershire sauce

2 tablespoons light mayonnaise

2 tablespoons sour cream or Greek yogurt, or to taste

- Prepare the sauce: Combine all of the ingredients in a bowl and mix until well blended. Adjust the seasoning, cover, and refrigerate until ready to serve.

Meal ideas and tips for diabetes

- Tossed salad or nonstarchy vegetable (Roasted Brussels Sprouts, page 295)
- Whole grain or starch, 1 CARB
- Reduced-fat milk or unsweetened reduced-fat yogurt, 1 CARB

Panfried Chicken with Tzatziki

Protein is for muscle building and the B vitamins boost your baby's cell, brain, and nervous system development.

THIS Greek-style chicken combo is sure to become a go-to recipe. Start marinating the chicken up to twelve hours in advance—the longer the better. You can panfry or grill the chicken. Both taste great. Make the tzatziki a few hours before serving, for the flavors to develop. For extra power, add chopped walnuts or seeds to the tzatziki just before serving.

SERVES 4

CHICKEN

Juice of 1 lemon
3 tablespoons olive oil
1 teaspoon dried oregano
½ teaspoon salt
Freshly ground black pepper
½ teaspoon garlic powder
4 chicken breasts (about
    1 pound), pounded to even
    thickness, pricked with
    a fork
¼ cup chopped fresh parsley,
    for garnish
Lemon wedges, for garnish

- Marinate the chicken: Combine the lemon juice, 2 tablespoons of the olive oil, and the oregano, salt, pepper to taste, and the garlic powder in a shallow bowl or resealable plastic bag. Add the chicken and coat with the marinade. Refrigerate for at least 1 hour, or up to 12. You can also marinate the chicken in a bowl; cover and refrigerate.

- When ready to cook, heat the remaining tablespoon of olive oil in a large grill pan or skillet over medium-high heat until hot. Cook the chicken breasts in batches for 4 to 5 minutes per side, depending on their thickness. Check for doneness by cutting into the thickest part of the breast. The meat should be completely cooked and the juices should run clear. Transfer to a platter and cover for 5 minutes before slicing. Add the chopped parsley and lemon wedges.

Meal ideas

- Whole grain or starch
- Green salad or vegetable (My Big Fat Greek Salad, page 163)
- Reduced-fat milk or yogurt
- Fresh fruit

Meal ideas and tips for diabetes

- Whole grain or starch, 1 CARB
- Green salad or nonstarchy vegetable (above)
- Fresh fruit, 1 CARB

1 chicken breast: Calories: 136 cals; Protein: 26 g; Carbohydrates: 0 g; Fat: 3 g; Fiber: 0 g; Sodium: 51 mg; B₆: 0.9 mg; Niacin: 16 mg; Selenium: 26 mcg; 0 CARBS

5 tablespoons tzatziki: Calories: 86 cals; Protein: 5 g; Carbohydrates: 3 g; Fat: 6 g; Fiber: 0 g; Sodium: 20 mg; 0 CARBS

(continued)

TZATZIKI (MAKES ABOUT 1½ CUPS)

½ cup grated cucumber (gently squeeze out the juice)

1 cup plain Greek yogurt

Pinch of garlic powder, or a tiny bit of minced fresh garlic

1 tablespoon chopped fresh dill (optional)

1 tablespoon olive oil

1 tablespoon cider vinegar

Salt and freshly ground black pepper

- Prepare the tzatziki: Mix together all the tzatziki ingredients in a bowl until well combined. Serve or cover and refrigerate for up to 5 days.

BBQ Chicken Two Ways

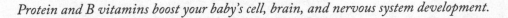

Protein and B vitamins boost your baby's cell, brain, and nervous system development.

ANY cut of chicken can be used with these two delicious barbecue sauces. If you want a break from the traditional red BBQ sauce, our lemon-rosemary sauce will fit the bill. Boneless, skinless breasts cook the quickest, but they are the least juicy. Skinless thighs or breasts on the bone or drumsticks provide a juicier meat. In a hurry? Start cooking the chicken in the oven, then finish it off on the grill. Discard all leftover marinade. Gluten-free? Use gluten-free ketchup and tamari. The barbecued chicken keeps for three days refrigerated.

MAKES ENOUGH MARINADE FOR UP TO 4 POUNDS BONE-IN CHICKEN; SERVES 6

WHITE BBQ SAUCE

¼ cup mayonnaise
Grated zest of 1 lemon
⅓ cup freshly squeezed lemon juice
2 tablespoons finely chopped fresh rosemary (Note: Dried rosemary does not work well.)
2 teaspoons Dijon mustard
2 teaspoons honey or sugar
1½ teaspoons garlic powder
1 teaspoon salt
Freshly ground black pepper

- Prepare either barbecue sauce: Combine all the sauce ingredients of choice in a bowl and mix until well blended.
- Marinate the chicken: Using a fork, pierce the chicken all over to allow the marinade to seep in. Place the chicken in a 1-gallon resealable plastic bag or in a bowl, add the barbecue sauce, seal (or cover the bowl with plastic wrap), and refrigerate for at least 2 hours, or up to 48.
- Before grilling or broiling, have a platter ready for the barbecued chicken. Grill the chicken, turning to cook on all sides, over high heat for about 5 minutes, or until the sauce is caramelized. Or, to broil, remove about half of the sauce from the pan and discard it, then place the chicken under the broiler and cook, turning once, for a couple of minutes on each side.

Meal ideas

- Salad or vegetable
- Whole grain or starch (Mexican-Style Rice and Beans, page 220)
- Reduced-fat milk or yogurt
- Fresh fruit

Meal ideas and tips for diabetes

- Salad or nonstarchy vegetable
- Whole grain or starch (above), 1 CARB
- Reduced-fat milk or unsweetened reduced-fat yogurt, 1 CARB

4 ounces chicken (white meat only, sauce is for marinating only): Calories: 155 cals; Protein: 32 g; Carbohydrates: 0 g; Fat: 3 g; Fiber: 0 g; Sodium: 355 mg; Niacin: 16 mg; Phosphorus: 266 mg; Selenium: 44 mcg; 0 CARBS

(continued)

RED BBQ SAUCE

½ cup ketchup
2 tablespoons molasses
⅓ cup light soy sauce or
    tamari
½ teaspoon ground ginger
¼ teaspoon ground cloves,
    allspice, or cinnamon, or
    a mixture
1 garlic clove, minced
2 tablespoons minced fresh
    ginger

4 pounds chicken parts
    (see headnote)

- To precook the chicken in the oven before grilling, preheat the oven to 400°F. Transfer the chicken with all the sauce to a large baking dish. Bake for 30 minutes, or until an instant-read thermometer inserted into the center (through the side) of the breast meat or thigh reads 165°F, and the juices run clear when the chicken is pierced with a knife. Remove from the oven. Grill for 10 minutes to get the "grill flavor."

Juicy Turkey Burgers

Protein, vitamins C and K, and B vitamins enhance your baby's cell, brain, and nervous system development. The iron boosts your iron stores, fiber aids your digestion, and vitamin C fortifies your immune system and keeps your gums and teeth healthy.

SOME of our readers make these turkey burgers a weekly staple! The ricotta cheese keeps the burgers moist and the fresh herbs add a burst of flavor. Serve with or without buns, accompanied by the usual lineup of burger fixin's and condiments: lettuce, tomatoes, pickles, relish, and so on. You can substitute ground chicken for the turkey; ground lamb works well, too. The burgers can be formed, covered, and refrigerated up to four hours in advance, or frozen for up to one month. Thaw before cooking. These burgers keep refrigerated for three days. To really rock these burgers, see "How to Check the Flavor of Your Meat Loaf, Burgers, or Meatballs," page 96.

MAKES 4 LARGE BURGERS, OR 6 SMALLER ONES

1 pound lean ground turkey
½ cup part-skim ricotta cheese
1 cup shredded zucchini, water squeezed out
¼ cup sun-dried tomatoes in oil, drained and chopped
½ teaspoon salt
2 teaspoons Worcestershire sauce
2 teaspoons Dijon mustard
1 tablespoon freshly squeezed lemon juice
3 tablespoons chopped fresh parsley
1 tablespoon canola oil or cooking spray
4 whole wheat hamburger buns (optional)

- Combine all the ingredients, except the canola oil and buns, in a bowl and mix until well blended. If the mixture is too pasty or sticky, add up to 1 tablespoon of water. The consistency should be softer than a burger made with ground beef, but firm enough to hold its shape.

- Divide the turkey mixture into four portions, form each portion into a patty, and place on a large plate.

- If panfrying, heat the canola oil in a large skillet over medium heat. Add the burgers to the skillet and cook for 6 minutes, or until the underside is dark brown. Flip and cook on the second side for about 6 minutes, or until the center of the burgers is completely opaque and cooked through.

Meal ideas

- Whole grain or starch (if not using a bun)
- Green salad or vegetable (Lemony Slaw, page 164)
- Reduced-fat milk or yogurt
- Fresh fruit

1 turkey burger on a whole wheat bun: Calories: 380 cals; Protein: 32 g; Carbohydrates: 34 g; Fat: 14 g; Fiber: 6 g; Sodium: 512 mg; Vitamin C: 18 mg; Vitamin K: 48 mcg; B_6: 0.5 mg; B_{12}: 1.5 mcg; Niacin: 11 mg; Riboflavin: 0.3 mg; Copper: 0.2 mg; Iron: 4 mg; Phosphorus: 302 mg; Selenium: 27 mcg; Zinc: 3 mg; 2 CARBS

(continued)

- If grilling, before preheating the grill, position a piece of foil over the grill rack and poke holes in it. (This will prevent the burgers from sticking to the grill and falling apart.) Just before cooking the burgers, generously spray the foil with cooking spray. Cook as in step 3.
- Serve with the buns, if desired.

Ricotta Cheesecake with Berries

Protein helps your baby grow and keeps you strong, too.

THIS cheesecake is crammed with protein and it's a good source of calcium. Top with sliced fresh fruit or berries, or syrup (see page 182). The cheesecake is best made a day before serving.

SERVES 8

HOMEMADE GRAHAM CRACKER CRUST

1½ cups crushed graham cracker crumbs

2 tablespoons light brown sugar

½ teaspoon ground cinnamon

4 tablespoons unsalted butter, melted

FILLING

1 (8-ounce) package cream cheese

1 cup part-skim ricotta cheese

½ cup confectioners' sugar

1 large egg

½ cup dairy sour cream or plain Greek yogurt

2 teaspoons pure vanilla extract

1 teaspoon freshly squeezed lemon juice (optional)

4 cups fresh raspberries and blueberries, for serving

- Preheat the oven to 350°F.
- Prepare the crust: Combine all the crust ingredients in a bowl and mix until well blended and the crumbs are moist. Transfer the mixture to a 9-inch round spring-form pan and press it evenly over the bottom. Bake for 9 minutes, or until the crust is slightly firm to the touch. Remove from the oven and let cool before filling.
- Prepare the filling: Place the cream cheese and ricotta cheese in a large bowl and beat with an electric mixer on medium speed until creamy. Add the sugar and continue to beat for 30 seconds. Add the remaining filling ingredients and beat until well blended.
- Pour the filling into the prepared graham cracker crust. Bake for 40 to 45 minutes, or until the center of the cheesecake is almost firm (it will firm up as it cools). Remove the cheesecake from the oven, and let cool to room temperature, then refrigerate for at least 4 hours before serving with the berries.

Tips for diabetes

- Reduce your portion size, or skip this recipe.

One tenth cheesecake and berries: Calories: 211 cals; Protein: 10 g; Carbohydrates: 27 g; Fat: 7 g; Fiber: 0 g; Sodium: 299 mg; 2 CARBS

MONTH 3
Fetus Forming: Construction Zone Ahead
Weeks 9 Through 13

Welcome to the last month of your first trimester. Woo-hoo! If you've been through the wringer with morning sickness (or all-day sickness), fatigue, and emotional highs and lows, you will be thrilled to move into your second trimester. Things do get better! By Week 9, your baby is the size of grape. In Week 10, he or she officially goes from an embryo to a fetus. Congrats! And, by Week 13, your gorgeous baby has grown to the size of a nectarine, about 3 inches long.

YOUR BABY'S DEVELOPMENT

- In Week 9, your baby's head continues to develop as his or her beautiful face is rounding. Muscles take form, all major limbs and joints (such as the shoulders, elbows, wrists, knees, and ankles) are working. The heart has evolved into four chambers. The valves are forming. Your baby's external sex organs are developing, but they are not visible yet. You might hear a heartbeat, but that usually happens the following week.

- In Week 10, tooth buds materialize, your baby's stomach begin to produce digestive juices, and his or her kidneys can start to produce urine. Eyelids are more developed. The ears and external features are almost formed. Your baby's heartbeat might be heard. Exciting!

- In Week 11, your baby's body is straightening. His or her skin is transparent. Hair follicles are forming. Fingers and toes have separated, and nail beds begin to appear. Tiny tooth buds form below the gums. The placenta begins to function. This amazing organ provides oxygen and nutrients to your baby.

- In Week 12, your baby's bone marrow produces white blood cells. The pituitary gland begins to produce hormones. The intestines, which have been developing outside of the baby, now have moved back into the abdomen.
- In Week 13, your baby's brain continues to develop rapidly. Vocal cords are being primed to make that first cry. Fingerprints are developed.

CHANGES IN YOUR BODY

Your body will experience changes similar to those in Month 2. Fatigue and sleepiness might continue to be your middle name. Some women may have nausea, bloating, gas, constipation, heartburn, indigestion, food aversions and cravings, sensitivity to smell, and the frequent need to pee. Headaches are common. Some bellies begin to get rounder about now. Breast fullness and heaviness is common. Tenderness, tingling, and darkening areolas might occur now, or at any time during pregnancy. Blood volume increases, giving some women that "glow."

IDEAL NUTRITION

Your nutrition focus is foods to enhance your baby's cell, brain, eye, bone, and teeth development. The following nutrients will help achieve this.

- B vitamins: cell division, brain formation, nervous system development, morning sickness
- Calcium: bones and teeth
- Magnesium: bones and muscle development
- Manganese: bone development and nerve health
- Omega-3s: brain, eye, and nervous system development
- Phosphorus: genetic material
- Potassium: nerve and muscle function
- Vitamin A: cell structure, bones, teeth, nervous system
- Vitamin C: iron absorption, healthy teeth and gums, immunity
- Vitamin D: calcium absorption
- Vitamin E: cell structure and genetic material
- Vitamin K: bone mineralization
- Zinc: cell structure and genetic material

OPTIMAL FOODS FOR MONTH 3

PROTEIN	DAIRY	GRAINS/ LEGUMES	VEGETABLES	FRUITS	FATS/OTHER
Eggs	Cheese	All-bran cereal and other fortified breakfast cereals	Artichokes	Bananas	Brewer's or nutritional yeast
Meats	Enriched plant-based milks (rice soy, and almond)	Beans: soy, black, navy, pinto, kidney, white, great northern, black-eyed, pink, cranberry, and cannellini	Asparagus	Cantaloupe	Olive oil
Nuts: almonds, cashews, pistachios, Brazil nuts, walnuts, and nut butters	Fortified dairy milk	Chickpeas	Avocados	Citrus fruits and juices: oranges, tangerines, grapefruit, lemonade	Omega-3s
Pork	Fortified orange juice and other juices	Corn and flour tortillas	Baked potato with skin on and all other potatoes	Dried apricots	Molasses
Poultry	Yogurt	Edamame	Beets	Guava	Seaweed and kelp
Seafood (fish and shellfish): salmon (wild and Atlantic), tuna, mackerel, herring, sardines in oil, halibut, cod, and catfish		Folic acid–fortified products	Broccoli and broccoli rabe	Kiwi	
Seeds: sunflower, pumpkin, chia, hemp seed, and flaxseed		Lentils	Brussels sprouts	Lychee	
Tahini		Oatmeal	Butternut squash	Mangoes	
Tofu and tempeh		Peanuts	Cabbage	Papaya	
		Wheat germ	Carrots	Pineapple	
		Whole grains: quinoa, barley, brown rice, bulgur, and whole wheat couscous	Cauliflower	Raspberries	
			Dark, leafy greens: kale, collards, mustard, Swiss chard, bok choy, and turnip greens	Strawberries	
			Mushrooms		
			Pumpkin		
			Red bell peppers		
			Romaine lettuce		
			Snow peas		
			Spinach		
			Sweet potatoes		
			Tomatoes and tomato juice		

RECIPES FOR MONTH 3

Supergreen Drink

GF DF V Q

Vitamins A, C, and K, and folate enhance your baby's cell, brain, nervous system, and bone development, plus vitamin C boosts your immunity.

BURSTING with vitamins and antioxidants, this green drink is an ideal way to start the day. Use any combination of fruits and/or vegetables. Some popular vegetables and greens include cucumbers, celery, avocado, baby spinach, and kale. Protein powders and powdered milk will give you extra nutrition. See "Freezing Bananas for Smoothies and N'ice Cream," page 176, for instructions on the best way to freeze bananas. Don't worry about making too much green drink. It's delish the next day. Give it a stir and you're good to go.

2 SERVINGS; MAKES 2 CUPS

1 medium-size banana, fresh or frozen
1 small apple, cored and quartered
2 cups packed baby spinach
1 cup orange juice or water
Ice cubes

FLAVOR AND NUTRITION BOOSTERS

Fresh mint or basil leaves
Peeled fresh ginger
Protein powder
Chia seeds
Ground flaxseeds

- Combine all the ingredients in a blender, adding your choice of flavor and nutrition boosters to taste, and mix on high speed until smooth. Adjust the consistency by adding more water. Cover and refrigerate any leftovers.

Tips for diabetes

- Reduce your portion size, or skip this recipe.
- Omit the banana to reduce the amount of carbs.

1 green drink (without any flavor and nutrition boosters): Calories: 163 cals; Protein: 3 g; Carbohydrates: 40 g; Fat: 1 g; Fiber: 5 g; Sodium: 26 mg; Vitamin A: 3,148 IU, Vitamin C: 80 mg; Vitamin K: 147 mcg; Folate: 110 mcg; Manganese: 0.5 mg; 2½ CARBS

Refreshing Fruit Salad

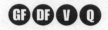

Vitamins A and C enhance your baby's cell and tooth development, plus vitamin C improves your immunity and fiber helps your digestion.

WHO can resist a fruit salad? Six cups might seem like a lot to prepare at once, but the more fruit all ready to eat, the more fruit you will eat. No time to clean and chop fruit? Pick up precut fruit or fruit from a salad bar. If you prefer to "drink your fruit," toss them into the blender (check out our smoothie and green drink recipes, pages 131, 157, 207, and 129).

SERVES 4; MAKES ABOUT 6 CUPS

1½ cups raspberries
1½ cups strawberries, halved
1 cup blueberries
2 cups cantaloupe balls
  or cubes (from about
  ½ melon)
½ cup orange juice

OPTIONAL TOPPINGS

Greek yogurt or nondairy
  yogurt (for dairy-free
  or vegan)
Chia seeds
Flaxseed
Nuts
Sunflower seeds
Ground wheat germ
Granola or muesli

- Combine all the ingredients in a large bowl and mix gently. Add your choice of toppings. If not serving immediately, cover and refrigerate without adding any toppings.

Tips for diabetes
- Reduce your portion size, or skip this recipe.

1½ cups fruit salad (no toppings): Calories: 117 cals; Protein: 2 g; Carbohydrates: 28 g; Fat: 1 g; Fiber: 6 g; Sodium: 21 mg; Vitamin A: 4,162 IU; Vitamin C: 107 mg; Manganese: 0.7 mg; 2 CARBS

Good Morning Sunshine Smoothie Bowl

GF **DF** **V**

Vitamin C optimizes the health of your teeth and gums and boosts immunity.

LOVE smoothies? Or n'ice cream? If so, this smoothie bowl will make you a happy camper at breakfast (or any time of day). Feel free to swap out the strawberries for your favorite frozen berries. See "Freezing Bananas for Smoothies and N'ice Cream," page 176, for instructions on the best way to freeze bananas. Some ideas for fabulous fixin's include granola (see page 105), coconut flakes, dried or dehydrated fruits, nuts, chia seeds, ground flaxseeds, or fresh fruit. Here is a basic recipe that you can jazz up. Yum!

MAKES 1½ CUPS

1 heaping cup frozen strawberries, raspberries, blueberries, or mixed berries

1 heaping cup frozen banana slices (from 1 banana)

2 to 3 tablespoons almond milk or fruit juice

- Place the frozen berries, frozen banana slices, and almond milk in a food processor or blender and process until smooth, scraping down the sides of the bowl as needed. Add your choice of topping and serve promptly. Freeze any leftovers.

Meal ideas

- Protein, such as natural nut butter or eggs.
- Whole grains (Perfect Homemade Granola, page 105)
- Reduced-fat milk or yogurt

Meal ideas and tips for diabetes

- Reduce your portion size, or skip this recipe.
- Protein, such as natural nut butter or eggs

¾ **cup smoothie bowl (without any toppings):** Calories: 80 cals; Protein: 1 g; Carbohydrates: 21 g; Fat: 0 g; Fiber: 3 g; Sodium: 19 mg; Vitamin C: 47 mg; 1½ CARBS

Banana Nut Muffins

The micronutrients help your baby's cell, nerve, and bone development.

NOTHING beats a great banana muffin. For a lighter muffin, substitute ¾ cup of all-purpose flour for the whole wheat flour. Gluten-free? Substitute an all-purpose gluten-free blend. Vegan? Use nondairy milk and omit the egg. Ripe bananas can be frozen whole and unpeeled (the skin will turn completely brown when frozen), or you can mash the pulp and freeze it. Before using, defrost the pulp or whole bananas at room temperature or in a microwave oven. Note: To facilitate peeling defrosted whole bananas, start at the bottom of the banana rather than at the top stem.

MAKES 12 REGULAR OR 40 MINI MUFFINS

Cooking spray (optional)
¾ cup whole wheat flour
¾ cup all-purpose flour
½ cup ground flaxseeds
2 teaspoons baking soda
¼ teaspoon salt
½ cup chopped walnuts or pecans
½ cup packed light brown sugar
⅓ cup canola oil or melted unsalted butter
1 large egg
¼ cup milk
1½ cups coarsely mashed ripe bananas (from 3 to 4 large bananas)
½ cup sunflower seeds, for sprinkling (optional)

- Preheat the oven to 350°F. Spray 12 regular or 40 mini muffin wells with cooking spray or line them with muffin liners.
- In a large bowl, whisk together the flours, flaxseeds, baking soda, salt, and walnuts until well combined.
- In a small bowl, combine the brown sugar, canola oil, egg, and milk and whisk until well blended. Add the bananas and mix well, then add to the flour mixture and mix until well blended.
- Divide the batter evenly among the prepared muffin wells. Sprinkle with sunflower seeds, if using, and bake until a tester inserted into the center comes out clean: 25 to 30 minutes for regular muffins, 10 to 12 minutes for mini muffins. Transfer the muffins to a rack and let cool slightly before eating.

Meal ideas

- Protein, such as natural nut butter or eggs
- Reduced-fat milk or yogurt (Supergreen Drink, page 129)
- Fresh fruit

Meal ideas and tips for diabetes

- Opt for the mini muffins, reduce your portion size, or skip this recipe.
- Protein, such as natural nut butters or eggs

1 regular banana muffin: Calories: 218 cals; Protein: 5 g; Carbohydrates: 29 g; Fat: 11 g; Fiber: 3 g; Sodium: 270 mg; Copper: 0.2 mg; Manganese: 1 mg; Selenium: 12 mcg; 2 CARBS

Easy Veggie Frittata

GF **LC**

Protein, vitamin A, C, and K, and B vitamins enhance your baby's cell, nerve, brain, bone, and tooth development, and boost your immune system.

THIS Italian-style omelet is basically a crustless quiche. The veggie filling is sautéed, the beaten egg is added, and the cooking is finished under the broiler. You may replace the broccoli with your favorite cooked vegetables, including zucchini, yellow squash, asparagus, mushrooms, or cooked diced potatoes. Cooked shrimp, sausage, chicken, and ham can be added for more protein. For a calcium boost, in a measuring cup, combine ⅓ cup of pasteurized instant nonfat dry milk with the whole milk. Mix until the milk powder has dissolved, then follow the directions in Step 1.

SERVES 4

5 large eggs
¼ cup whole milk
½ teaspoon salt
Freshly ground black pepper
2 tablespoons olive oil
1 tablespoon unsalted butter
1 small onion, thinly sliced
½ cup seeded and thinly
    sliced red bell pepper
1 cup small broccoli florets
2 tablespoons chopped fresh
    parsley
1 small tomato, thinly sliced
    and seeded
⅓ cup grated Parmesan or
    Cheddar cheese

- Combine the eggs, milk, salt, and pepper in a bowl and mix until well blended; set aside.
- Heat 1 tablespoon of the olive oil and the butter in a large, ovenproof 12-inch skillet over medium heat. Add the onion and bell pepper and sauté, stirring, for 4 minutes, or until light golden. Smear the oil against the sides of the skillet as you stir, to grease the pan. Add the broccoli florets and ¼ cup of water and continue to sauté for about 3 minutes, or until the broccoli is crisp-tender. Stir in the parsley during the last minute of cooking.
- While the broccoli is cooking, preheat the broiler to a high setting.

Meal ideas

- Green salad or vegetable (Creamy Asparagus-Artichoke Soup, page 136)
- Whole wheat bread or roll
- Reduced-fat milk or yogurt
- Fruit

Meal ideas and tips for diabetes

- Green salad or nonstarchy vegetable (above)
- Reduced-fat milk or unsweetened reduced-fat yogurt, 1 CARB
- Fresh fruit, 1 CARB

(continues)

One quarter of the frittata: Calories: 236 cals; Protein: 11 g; Carbohydrates: 7 g; Fat: 18 g; Fiber: 2 g; Sodium: 513 mg; Vitamin A: 1,887 IU; Vitamin C: 46 mg; Vitamin K: 44 mcg; B_{12}: 0.7 mcg; Riboflavin: 0.4 mg; Selenium: 23 mcg; ½ CARB

Easy Veggie Frittata (continued)

- Add the remaining 1 tablespoon of olive oil to the skillet, then evenly scatter the vegetables on the bottom of the pan. Add the egg mixture. Do not stir at this point. Cook on medium heat for 2 to 3 minutes, or until the bottom of the egg mixture has set. While the frittata is cooking, arrange the tomato slices on top, then sprinkle evenly with the Parmesan cheese.

- Place the frittata under the broiler for 3 to 4 minutes, or until the top has set and the cheese is light golden. Watch to prevent burning. Serve warm.

Just Plain Good Guacamole

GF DF V Q LC

Vitamin K and folate enhance your baby's cell, nerve, and bone development, and fiber aids your digestion.

WHO can turn down guacamole with vegetables or corn tortilla chips? Answer: Almost no one. This dip keeps refrigerated for one day. Some discoloration will occur, but the taste will not be affected. Enjoy!

MAKES ABOUT 2½ CUPS

3 ripe avocados, preferably Hass

3 tablespoons finely chopped red onion

1 large tomato, cut into small dice

2 tablespoons freshly squeezed lime juice, or to taste

3 tablespoons chopped fresh cilantro

1 small garlic clove, crushed, or ¼ teaspoon garlic powder

Dash of Tabasco sauce, or freshly ground black pepper

Salt

- Cut the avocados in half and remove the pits. Cut the halves into quarters, then peel them and place in a small bowl. Using the back of a fork, mash the avocados to a chunky consistency.
- Add the remaining ingredients and mix until well combined. Season to taste, cover with plastic wrap placed flush against the surface of the guacamole, and refrigerate for a couple of hours before serving.

⅓ cup guacamole: Calories: 178 cals; Protein: 2 g; Carbohydrates: 11 g; Fat: 15 g; Fiber: 7 g; Sodium: 10 mg; Folate: 97 mcg; Vitamin K: 26 mcg; Copper: 0.2 mg; 1 CARB

KITCHEN WISDOM:
HOW TO PREVENT AN AVOCADO HALF FROM BROWNING

YOU are not going to believe how easy this avocado tip is. Simply run the avocado half under water and then wrap it tightly in plastic wrap. No oil needed. Leave the pit in the half, if possible. This should prevent browning for at least 12 hours.

Creamy Asparagus-Artichoke Soup

GF DF V LC

Vitamins A, E, and K and folate foster your baby's cell, nerve, tooth, and bone development, and iron helps boost your iron stores.

A healthy green soup that is perfect for lunch or dinner, or as a snack. You can replace the asparagus with an equal amount of broccoli or zucchini. Garnish with nuts and seeds for extra nutrition. This soup keeps, refrigerated, for three days. It can be frozen for up to one month.

SERVES 4; MAKES ABOUT 5 CUPS

3 tablespoons olive oil
1 medium-size onion, chopped
½ cup canned white beans, drained and rinsed
4 cups stock or water
½ teaspoon salt, or to taste
16 ounces green asparagus, tough ends trimmed, stalks cut into 1-inch pieces (4 cups)
1 (13.75-ounce) can artichoke hearts, drained
1½ teaspoons dried tarragon (optional)
Freshly ground black pepper
Squeeze of lemon juice (optional)

- Heat the olive oil in a 6-quart saucepan over medium-high heat. Add the onion and sauté for 3 minutes. Add the beans, stock, and salt and bring to a boil. Add the asparagus, artichoke hearts, and tarragon, if using, and return to a boil, then lower the heat and simmer, uncovered, for 10 minutes. Remove from the heat.
- Allow the soup to cool slightly, then puree it. Adjust the seasoning and consistency, add the lemon juice, if desired, and serve.

Meal ideas

- Protein, such as meat, poultry, seafood, eggs, dairy, or plant-based (Chicken Salad with Dried Apricots and Almonds, page 216)
- Whole wheat bread or roll
- Reduced-fat milk or yogurt
- Fresh fruit

Meal ideas and tips for diabetes

- Protein, such as meat, poultry, seafood, eggs, dairy, or plant-based (above)
- Reduced-fat milk or unsweetened reduced-fat yogurt, 1 CARB

1 cup asparagus soup (made with water): Calories: 186 cals; Protein: 7 g; Carbohydrates: 20 g; Fat: 11 g; Fiber: 7 g; Sodium: 322 mg; Vitamin A: 1,014 IU; Vitamin E: 3 mg; Vitamin K: 69 mcg; Folate: 132 mcg; Copper: 0.3 mg; Manganese: 0.5 mg; Iron: 4 mg: 1½ CARBS

Hot and Sweet Veggie Salad

GF **DF** **V** **Q** **LC**

Vitamin C promotes healthy gums and teeth and boosts your immunity.

COLORFUL, fresh, tasty, and full of vitamin C, this salad is, well, fantastic! You can combine any veggies you like in any proportions. The cutting and slicing are the hardest part. This dish is best served soon after you prepare it, as the vegetables tend to give off liquid the longer they sit, but the flavor is still great. Refrigerate leftovers.

SERVES 4; MAKES 4 CUPS

1 small to medium-size seedless cucumber, halved lengthwise and thinly sliced (1½ cups)

½ small red onion, thinly sliced (optional)

1 small red bell pepper, cored, seeded, and sliced

1 carrot, shaved into thin strips with a vegetable peeler

2 tablespoons chopped fresh cilantro

3 tablespoons seasoned rice vinegar, or to taste

2 tablespoons sugar, or to taste

½ teaspoon toasted sesame oil, or to taste

Pinch of red pepper flakes (optional)

Salt

- Combine all the ingredients in a bowl and mix gently. Adjust the seasoning and serve.

Meal ideas

- Protein, such as meat, poultry, seafood, eggs, dairy, or plant-based (Baked or Fried Chicken Tenders, page 300)
- Whole grain or starch
- Reduced-fat milk or yogurt
- Fresh fruit

Meal ideas and tips for diabetes

- Protein, such as meat, poultry, seafood, eggs, dairy, or plant-based (above)
- Whole grain or starch, 1 CARB
- Reduced-fat milk or unsweetened reduced-fat yogurt, 1 CARB

One quarter of the veggie salad: Calories: 61 cals; Protein: 1 g; Carbohydrates: 13 g; Fat: 1 g; Fiber: 2 g; Sodium: 46 mg; Vitamin C: 27 mg; 1 CARB

Yummy Three-Bean Salad

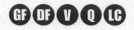

Vitamin K and folate optimize your baby's cell, brain, nerve, and bone development, and fiber helps your digestion stay on track.

SIMPLE and delicious. Chickpeas and kidney beans are called for in this recipe because they seem to be the most readily available in small ("salad topper" 7.5-ounce) can sizes. However, feel free to add your family's favorites, from black-eyed peas to cannellini beans. Need to save time? Pick up cooked beans (or your favorite veggies) from a salad bar. This salad keeps for four days refrigerated. The lime juice will cause a slight discoloration of the green beans and cilantro, but this does not affect the taste.

SERVES 4; MAKES ABOUT 4 CUPS

8 ounces green beans, sliced into thirds and cooked until crisp-tender
⅔ cup (1 [7.5-ounce can]) red kidney beans, drained and rinsed
⅔ cup (1 [7.5-ounce can]) chickpeas, drained and rinsed and
10 cherry or grape tomatoes, sliced in half
¼ cup chopped fresh cilantro
2 tablespoons olive oil
2 tablespoons freshly squeezed lime or lemon juice, or to taste
Pinch of ground cumin
Salt and freshly ground black pepper

- Combine all the ingredients in a bowl and mix well. Adjust the seasoning and serve.

Meal ideas

- Protein, such as meat, poultry, seafood, eggs, dairy, or plant-based (Steak on the Grill, page 279)
- Green salad or vegetable
- Reduced-fat milk or yogurt
- Fruit

Meal ideas and tips for diabetes

- Protein, such as meat, poultry, seafood, eggs, dairy, or plant-based (above)
- Green salad or nonstarchy vegetable
- Reduced-fat milk or unsweetened reduced-fat yogurt, 1 CARB

1 cup bean salad: Calories: 163 cals; Protein: 6 g; Carbohydrates: 19 g; Fat: 8 g; Fiber: 6 g; Sodium: 113 mg; Folate 77 mcg; Vitamin K: 35 mcg; Copper: 0.2 mg; Manganese: 0.5 mg; 1½ CARBS

Roasted New Potatoes and Bell Peppers

Vitamins A and C and B vitamins optimize your baby's cell, nerve, brain, and bone development, and vitamin C boosts your immunity.

POTATOES and bell peppers are a natural combo. Jazz things up with rosemary or garlic oil, or play around with other herbs, such as fresh thyme. The roasting time will vary according to the size of the potatoes. You can skip boiling the potatoes and increase the roasting time, if you wish. You'll keep coming back to this recipe—we promise!

SERVES 4

1½ pounds red bliss or new potatoes, scrubbed clean, dried, halved (cut any large potatoes into quarters)
1 cup seeded and diced red bell pepper
3 tablespoons olive oil
3 garlic cloves, skin on, smashed with the side of a knife
3 sprigs rosemary, or 1 tablespoon dried
Salt and freshly ground black pepper

- Preheat the oven to 450°F. Have ready a large baking sheet lined with parchment paper or foil.
- Bring a large pot of salted water to a boil. Add the potatoes and cook for 5 minutes. Drain the potatoes well and allow them to air dry for about 2 minutes. Then, spread them out on the baking sheet along with the bell pepper and drizzle with the olive oil. Add the garlic and rosemary and mix with a large spatula. Season with salt and pepper to taste and mix again.
- Roast for 15 minutes, or until the potatoes are light golden and soft in the center. If they aren't done after 15 minutes, continue to roast. Serve warm.

Meal idea

- Protein, such as meat, poultry, seafood, eggs, dairy, or plant-based (Mustard-Tarragon Pork Tenderloin, page 195)
- Green salad or vegetable
- Reduced-fat milk or yogurt
- Fruit with vitamin C

Meal ideas and tips for diabetes

- Protein, such as meat, poultry, seafood, eggs, dairy, or plant-based (above)
- Green salad or nonstarchy vegetable
- Reduced-fat milk or unsweetened reduced-fat yogurt, 1 CARB

One quarter of the potatoes: Calories: 225 cals; Protein: 3 g; Carbohydrates: 30 g; Fat: 11 g; Fiber: 5 g; Sodium: 30 mg; B_6: 0.4 mg; Copper: 0.2 mg; Vitamin C: 64 mg; 2 CARBS

Capellini with Fresh Tomatoes and Goat Cheese

Protein, vitamins C and K, B vitamins, and folate promote your baby's cell, nerve, brain, and bone development, and vitamin C boosts your immunity.

THIS no-fuss dish is especially delicious during summer's tomato season, when ripe tomatoes really taste like tomatoes. Any pasta works, even gluten-free, and ideally whole wheat. Thinner pastas cook more quickly, which is why capellini is suggested. If pasteurized goat cheese is not your thing, use Parmesan or pasteurized feta. Add cooked chicken or shrimp for extra protein.

SERVES 3 TO 4

FRESH TOMATO SAUCE

16 ounces large ripe tomatoes, cut into small dice (about 4 cups diced)
¼ cup chopped fresh dill
¼ cup thinly sliced fresh basil
2 tablespoons olive oil, or to taste
2 teaspoons freshly squeezed lemon juice, or to taste
Salt and freshly ground black pepper

8 ounces thin pasta, such as capellini or thin spaghetti
4 ounces pasteurized goat cheese (soft varieties), or to taste

- Prepare the sauce: Combine all the sauce ingredients in a bowl and mix gently. Adjust the seasoning and set aside.
- Cook the pasta according to the package directions, drain, and return to the hot pot. Add the tomato sauce and gently toss until the sauce is incorporated. Add the cheese and toss again. Serve hot.

Meal ideas

- Green salad or vegetable (Greek-Style Broccoli, page 248)
- Reduced-fat milk or yogurt
- Fresh fruit

Meal ideas and tips for diabetes

- Reduce the amount or pasta, or swap it out for zucchini noodles (see page 169).
- Ideally, use whole wheat pasta.
- Green salad or nonstarchy vegetable (above)
- Reduced-fat milk or unsweetened reduced-fat yogurt, 1 CARB

One third pasta dish (about 2 cups): Calories: 395 cals; Protein: 14 g; Carbohydrates: 46 g; Fat: 21 g; Fiber: 3 g; Sodium: 124 mg; Vitamin C: 17 mg; Vitamin K: 25 mcg; Riboflavin: 0.5 mg; Thiamine: 0.5 mg; Folate: 121 mcg; Copper: 0.2 mg; 3 CARBS

KITCHEN WISDOM: HOW TO CHOOSE OLIVE OILS

THE world of olive oils can be confusing and expensive. Different varieties of olive oils are set apart not only by the *type* of olive that's used, but the *process* used to extract the oil, the composition, and the oil's level of acidity. Confusing, right? Olive oil basically falls into two categories: *refined* and *unrefined*. Unrefined oils are pure and untreated, and therefore of higher quality. Refined oils are treated to remove flaws from the oil, but in the end, it also removes some of the health benefits. There are a few basics you need to know when choosing olive oils, and then let your taste buds and wallet guide you. Bottom line: You may want to keep two types of olive oil on hand: (1) a cheap extra-virgin olive oil, olive oil, or light olive oil for cooking and baking; and (2) a more expensive extra-virgin olive oil for drizzling on salads or flavoring special dishes.

Unrefined Olive Oils

Extra-virgin comes from the *first* pressing of green olives. It is not treated with chemicals or altered by temperature. It has a lower acidity than regular olive oil, and a peppery finish. You can cook with extra-virgin olive oil. Given the great variation in prices, some advice is to use the more flavorful and expensive extra-virgin "boutique" olive oils for dipping bread, in dressings and dips, and for drizzling on dishes that will not be cooked, and the less expensive extra-virgin oils for cooking and baking.

Virgin olive oil, also an unrefined oil, is made using a similar process as extra-virgin olive oil. Virgin olive oil has slightly more acidity and a less intense flavor than extra-virgin olive oil. Virgin is *not* commonly marketed and stocked in grocery stores.

Refined Olive Oils

Olive oil, pure olive oil, or "regular" olive oil (all the same thing) is from a *second* pressing or from chemical extraction of the olive debris after the first pressing. It is usually lighter and milder than extra-virgin and virgin olive oils. This oil is typically a blend of unrefined and refined oil.

Light olive oil does not mean it has less calories; rather, a light color and flavor, which many folks prefer. Light olive oil is a refined oil with a neutral taste and a high smoke point. It can be used for baking, sautéing, grilling, and frying.

Groovy Veggie Burgers

Protein, vitamin C, and the B vitamins foster your baby's cell, nerve, and brain development, and vitamin C boosts your immunity with fiber to aid digestion.

ALWAYS a winner, and one of our readers' favorites! Serve these burgers on a bun dressed up with tomato, lettuce, cheese, and your favorite condiments, or with a salad. Vegan? Add 2 tablespoons of ground flaxseeds in place of the egg. Coating the burgers with the bread crumbs (gluten-free, if needed) is an extra step, but it helps them keep their shape. Enjoy! To really rock these burgers, see "How to Check the Flavor of Your Meat Loaf, Burgers, or Meatballs," page 96. This includes veggie burgers!

MAKES 5 BURGERS

1½ cups cooked brown rice (from about ½ cup uncooked rice, such as Royal Blend Texmati Brown, Wild, and Red Rice)
½ cup frozen corn
¾ cup canned refried beans
2 tablespoons chopped fresh cilantro
2 tablespoons thinly sliced scallions
1 large egg
1 cup plain bread crumbs
2 tablespoons olive oil
1 cup finely sliced mushrooms (any kind)
½ cup seeded and diced red bell peppers
½ teaspoon ground cumin
¼ teaspoon salt, or to taste
Freshly ground black pepper
5 dairy-free (and gluten-free, if needed) whole wheat buns, for serving

- In a large bowl, combine the cooked brown rice, corn, refried beans, cilantro, scallions, egg, and ½ cup of the bread crumbs. Mix gently.

- Heat 1 tablespoon of the olive oil in a medium-size skillet over medium heat. Add the mushrooms and sauté, stirring occasionally, until golden brown, about 5 minutes. Add the bell pepper and cumin and cook for 1 minute longer. Remove from the heat and let cool slightly, then add the mushroom mixture to the brown rice mixture, along with the salt and black pepper to taste, and stir until well combined. Allow to cool in the refrigerator for at least 30 minutes, or overnight.

> **Meal ideas**
> - Whole grain or starch (if not using a bun)
> - Green salad or vegetable (Lemony Slaw, page 164)
> - Reduced-fat milk or yogurt
> - Fresh fruit

1 veggie burger on a whole wheat bun: Calories: 372 cals; Protein: 15 g; Carbohydrates: 55 g; Fat: 11 g; Fiber: 6 g; Sodium: 584 mg; Vitamin C: 23 mg; Niacin: 5 mg; Riboflavin: 0.3 mg; Thiamine: 0.4 mg; Copper: 0.2 mg; Manganese: 1 mg; Selenium: 17 mcg; 4 CARBS

(continued)

- Place the remaining ½ cup of the bread crumbs in a pie plate. Using a ½-cup measuring cup, scoop out the burger mixture and form it into 5 patties. Coat each patty with the bread crumbs and refrigerate until ready to cook.

- Heat the remaining 1 tablespoon of the olive oil in a large skillet over medium heat. Add the patties and cook for 5 minutes on each side, or until heated through. If they begin browning too fast, lower the heat a bit. Serve with the buns.

Meal ideas and tips for diabetes

- Skip the whole wheat bun or use only ½ bun.
- Place the burger on top of a salad, or wrap it in a large romaine lettuce leaf or two.
- Green salad or nonstarchy vegetable (Lemony Slaw, page 164)
- Reduced-fat milk or unsweetened reduced-fat yogurt, 1 CARB

Salmon with Toasted Almonds, Capers, and Herbs

Protein, vitamins D and K, B vitamins, and omega-3 DHA boost your baby's cell, nerve, brain, and bone development, and vitamin D helps your calcium absorption.

SIMPLE, tasty, and healthy. You can cut the sauce in half, but it's best to make the whole recipe and plan to have leftover sauce—it's also great on chicken. Season the fish with salt and pepper, and then pop it in the oven to bake to perfection in fifteen minutes.

SERVES 4

SAUCE

1 shallot, minced
1 tablespoon red wine vinegar
Pinch of salt
2 tablespoons capers, rinsed
½ cup finely chopped fresh flat-leaf parsley
½ cup sliced almonds, toasted
2 tablespoons olive oil
Freshly ground black pepper

4 center-cut salmon fillets, about 4 ounces each, rinsed and patted with paper towels
Salt and freshly ground black pepper

- Prepare the sauce: In a small bowl, combine the shallot, vinegar, and salt. Let sit for 30 minutes. Roughly chop the capers, parsley, and almonds and add them to the bowl along with the olive oil. Add the pepper to taste, mix, and adjust the seasoning.

- Center an oven rack and preheat the oven to 450°F. Line a baking sheet with parchment paper or foil. Season the salmon with salt and pepper. Place the salmon, skin side down, on the prepared baking sheet. Bake until the salmon is cooked through, 12 to 15 minutes, depending on the thickness. Serve with the sauce.

Meal ideas

- Salad or vegetable (Classic Creamed Spinach, page 217)
- Whole grain or starch
- Reduced-fat milk or yogurt
- Fresh fruit

Meal ideas and tips for diabetes

- Salad or nonstarchy vegetable (above)
- Whole grain or starch, 1 CARB
- Reduced-fat milk or unsweetened reduced-fat yogurt, 1 CARB
- Fresh fruit, 1 CARB

1 piece of salmon with 2 tablespoons almond sauce: Calories: 412 cals; Protein: 28 g; Carbohydrates: 5 g; Fat: 32 g; Fiber: 2 g; Sodium: 177 mg; Vitamin D: 500 IU; Vitamin K: 130 mcg; B_6: 0.7 mg; B_{12}: 3 mcg; Niacin: 10 mg; Riboflavin: 0.3 mg; Thiamine: 0.2 mg; Copper: 0.2 mg; Phosphorus: 369 mg; Magnesium: 86 mg; Selenium: 28 mcg; Omega-3 DHA: 1.2 g; 0 CARBS

Family-Friendly Chicken Curry

LC

Protein, vitamins C, E, and K, and B vitamins enhance your baby's cell, nerve, brain, and bone development, and vitamin C boosts your immunity.

OVER the years, this popular chicken curry has become a standby recipe in many homes. You can replace the red bell peppers with broccoli florets, cauliflower florets, sliced zucchini, or any other vegetable. Gluten free? Use gluten-free curry powder (check labels) and wheat-free tamari. This chicken curry keeps for three days refrigerated, and it can be frozen for up to one month.

SERVES 3

1 pound chicken tenders, cut into ½-inch slices on the diagonal

1 red bell pepper, cored, seeded, quartered, and cut into strips

1 medium-size sweet onion, halved and thinly sliced

1 tablespoon mild curry powder

1 tablespoon sugar

3 tablespoons canola oil

1 tablespoon light soy sauce or tamari

3 scallions, trimmed and sliced into large pieces

¼ cup chopped fresh cilantro, or to taste

Squeeze of lime juice

Lime wedges, for serving

- Combine the diced chicken, bell pepper, onion, curry powder, sugar, 2 tablespoons of the canola oil, and the soy sauce in a bowl. Mix well, then allow to marinate, covered and refrigerated, for at least 30 minutes, or overnight.

- Heat the remaining 1 tablespoon of canola oil in a large skillet over medium-high heat. Add half of the chicken mixture and half of the scallions and sauté for 5 to 7 minutes, or until the chicken is cooked. (Note: Use a splatter screen to reduce cleanup.) Transfer the cooked chicken to a serving bowl and cover to keep warm. Reheat the skillet, add the remaining chicken mixture and scallions, and repeat the procedure. Garnish with the cilantro and a squeeze of fresh lime juice. Serve immediately, with the lime wedges.

Meal ideas

- Salad or vegetable
- Whole grain or starch (Easy Rice and Green Lentil Side Dish, page 89)
- Reduced-fat milk or yogurt
- Fresh fruit

Meal ideas and tips for diabetes

- Salad or nonstarchy vegetable
- Whole grain or starch (above), 1 CARB
- Reduced-fat milk or unsweetened reduced-fat yogurt, 1 CARB

One third of the chicken curry: Calories: 449 cals; Protein: 34 g; Carbohydrates: 15 g; Fat: 28 g; Fiber: 4 g; Sodium: 439 mg; Vitamin C: 72 mg; Vitamin E: 4 mg; Vitamin K: 50 mcg; Niacin: 22 mg; B$_6$: 1 mg; B$_{12}$: 0.5 mcg; Phosphorus: 313 mg; Selenium: 26 mcg; 1 CARB

Favorite Fajitas on the Grill

Protein, vitamins A and C, and B vitamins enhance your baby's cell, nerve, brain, and bone development, and vitamin C boosts your immunity, plus iron adds to your iron stores.

GRILLED fajitas make life good. The beef or chicken should marinate for at least thirty minutes, or up to twelve hours. The sautéed pepper mixture can be made two days in advance, covered, and refrigerated; reheat in a microwave oven. Short on time? Cut the raw beef or chicken into strips, marinate for fifteen minutes, and broil or sauté. You can replace the beef or chicken with peeled fresh large shrimp. Marinate for about twenty minutes, then grill, broil, or sauté. For vegetarian fajitas, marinate tofu, portobello mushrooms, or your favorite vegetables for about 30 minutes, then grill or broil. Slice into strips before serving. Some topping ideas include grated cheese, guacamole (see page 135) or sliced avocado, diced tomatoes, shredded lettuce, sliced pitted black olives, jalapeño peppers, sprigs of fresh cilantro, salsa, sour cream, and lime wedges. Any leftover beef, chicken, vegetables, or tofu can be made into delicious sandwiches, quesadillas, or tacos.

SERVES 6

MARINADE

2 tablespoons olive oil

2 tablespoons seasoned rice vinegar or freshly squeezed lime juice

2 tablespoons Worcestershire sauce

1 large garlic clove, crushed, or 1 teaspoon garlic powder

½ teaspoon ground cumin

1 teaspoon chili powder

1½ pounds beef skirt steak or boneless skinless chicken breasts

- Marinate the beef: Combine all the marinade ingredients in a small bowl, mix well, and set aside. Using a fork, pierce the beef or chicken all over, then place in a large resealable plastic bag. Add the marinade, then refrigerate for at least 30 minutes, or overnight.

- Prepare the vegetables: Heat the olive oil in a large skillet over medium-high heat. Add the bell peppers and onion and sauté for 10 minutes. Remove from the heat, cover, and set aside.

Meal ideas

- Green salad or vegetable (Just Plain Good Guacamole, page 135)
- Reduced-fat milk or yogurt
- Fresh fruit that contains vitamin C

Chicken fajitas: one sixth of the fajitas (including chicken, flour tortilla, and filling): Calories: 462 cals; Protein: 34 g; Carbohydrates: 58 g; Fat: 10 g; Fiber: 2 g; Sodium: 1,007 mg; Vitamin A: 1,922 IU; Vitamin C: 82 mg; B_6: 0.7 mg; Niacin: 10 mg; Iron: 3 mg; Selenium: 18 mcg; 4 CARBS

Beef fajitas: one sixth of the fajitas (including beef, flour tortilla, and filling): Calories: 513 cals; Protein: 34 g; Carbohydrates: 58 g; Fat: 16 g; Fiber: 2 g; Sodium: 995 mg; Vitamin C: 79 mg; B_6: 0.7 mg; B_{12}: 3 mcg; Niacin: 6 mg; Riboflavin: 0.4 mg; Iron: 4 mg; Selenium: 26 mcg; Zinc: 7 mg; 4 CARBS

(continued)

VEGETABLES

1 tablespoon olive oil

2 large bell peppers, washed, cored, seeded, and cut into strips

1 sweet onion, such as Vidalia, thinly sliced

12 (7- or 8-inch) flour or corn tortillas

- To grill the beef or chicken, preheat the grill. The chicken will take longer to cook than the beef, so if you are serving both, start the chicken first. Have a clean platter ready for the cooked meat. Grill the chicken for 10 to 12 minutes on each side, or until the juices run clear when the chicken is pierced with the tip of a knife and an instant-read thermometer inserted into the center (through the side) of the chicken breast reads 165°F. Grill the beef for 6 to 8 minutes on each side, or until an instant-read thermometer inserted into the center of the meat reads 160°F. Transfer to the platter.

- To broil the beef or chicken, preheat the broiler. Arrange the beef or chicken in a broiler pan lined with parchment paper or foil. Broil the chicken for about 12 minutes on each side, the beef for about 7 minutes on each side (refer to the well-done temperatures above). Transfer to the platter.

- While the meat is cooking, heat the tortillas according to the package directions. You can also heat them on the grill just before serving, by toasting them for a minute or two on each side. Wrap the tortillas to keep them warm.

- Using a sharp knife and a chopping board with gutters to catch any juices, slice the cooked beef or chicken, against the grain, and serve. Place all of your chosen toppings, including the pepper mixture, in small bowls on the table.

Meal ideas and tips for diabetes

- Skip the tortilla and serve this as a salad on top of greens and/or vegetables.
- If you skip the tortilla, add a whole grain or starch. 1 CARB
- Salad or nonstarchy vegetable (Just Plain Good Guacamole, page 135)

Baby-Blue-Berry Buckle

Vitamin E for your baby's cell structure, plus satisfying your sweet cravings.

HAVING friends and family over and you need a special dessert? Here you go. This riff on a traditional buckle places the fruit at the bottom of the baking dish, the batter on top, and a delicious crumble on top of that. Gluten-free? Substitute with all-purpose gluten-free flour. Dairy-free? Use oil, not butter, and in place of the buttermilk, use your favorite nondairy milk mixed with 1 tablespoon of cider vinegar. Vegan? Omit the eggs, too. You can refrigerate leftovers for three days, or freeze for up to one month.

SERVES 12

FRUIT LAYER

Cooking spray
3 cups fresh or frozen
  blueberries
2 cups fresh or frozen
  blackberries
¼ cup sugar
¼ cup all-purpose flour

CRUMBLE TOPPING

⅓ cup sugar
⅓ cup all-purpose flour plus
  1 tablespoon
1 teaspoon ground cinnamon
4 tablespoons unsalted butter
1 cup sliced almonds

CAKE

2 cups all-purpose flour
¾ cup sugar
⅔ cup ground flaxseeds
1 tablespoon baking powder
⅔ cup canola oil or melted
  unsalted butter
2 large eggs
1 cup buttermilk

- Prepare the fruit layer: Preheat the oven to 350°F. Grease a 9 x 13 x 2-inch cake pan with cooking spray.
- In a bowl, mix together the berries, sugar, and flour until well combined. Transfer the mixture to the prepared cake pan and set aside.
- Prepare the crumble topping: Combine all the crumble ingredients, except the almonds, in a small bowl and quickly mix with a pastry blender or your fingers until the dough is broken into small bits. Mix in half of the almonds and refrigerate until ready to use.
- Prepare the cake batter: In a large bowl, whisk the flour, sugar, ground flaxseeds, and baking powder; set aside.
- In a separate bowl, combine the canola oil, eggs, and buttermilk and whisk until well blended. Add the egg mixture to the flour mixture and whisk until combined. Spread the batter over the fruit mixture in the cake pan.

Tips for diabetes

- Reduce your portion size, or skip this recipe.

One fifteenth of the blueberry crumble: Calories: 339 cals; Protein: 6 g; Carbohydrates: 43 g; Fat: 17 g; Fiber: 4 g; Sodium: 140 mg; Vitamin E: 3 mg; Manganese: 0.4 mg; 3 CARBS

(continued)

- Evenly distribute the crumble topping over the batter. Sprinkle the remaining ½ cup of almonds on top. Bake for 1 hour, or until the top is browned and a tester inserted into the center comes out clean (apart from a bit of blueberry juice). Remove the buckle from the oven and allow to cool before serving. Refrigerate leftovers.

Nourishing Recipes for the Second Trimester

Maturing at Full Speed

MONTH 4

Beginning to Look Like a Baby

Weeks 14 Through 17

By most accounts, the second trimester is the best. It's the golden months when you're feeling good, looking beautiful, and you might even have some of your energy back. Your appetite increases along with your need for more calories and protein. Your baby can hear noises, so talk and sing to him or her. At Week 14, your baby is the size of a lemon, progressing to a pear by Week 17.

YOUR BABY'S DEVELOPMENT

- In Week 14, your baby is getting longer and straighter. She or he has hair, eyebrows, and lanugo (body hair) to stay warm. Arms have grown to proportion with body. The sweat glands, liver, and pancreas are secreting fluids. If you have a girl, she now has 2 million eggs in her ovaries. Your baby can squint, frown, and grimace. Grasping with hands is possible.
- In Week 15, ears are more positioned. Eyes are shifting from the sides of the head to the front. Hair may be sprouting, and eyebrows show. Your baby can wiggle fingers and toes and suck his or her thumb.
- In Week 16, muscles are getting stronger. Looks more like a baby, but the skin is still translucent. Nose is fully formed. Eyelids remain sealed though they may perceive light. Toenails have started to grow.

- In Week 17, sucking and swallowing skills are evident. Cartilage is hardening to bone. Fat is forming under the skin. Ear nerve endings are developed enough to hear noises and your voice.

CHANGES IN YOUR BODY

All the work you're doing to create a beautiful baby is making you tired. Rest, mama, rest. You might have tummy issues. In addition to headaches, lightheadedness, or dizziness, some women experience nasal congestion, nosebleeds, and gum bleeding. Your belly is rounding, so you may start to show. Your ankles and feet might be rounding, too.

IDEAL NUTRITION

Your nutrition focus is to optimize your baby's cell, brain, organ, muscle, nerve, and bone development. The following nutrients will help achieve this.

- B vitamins: cell division, brain formation, nervous system development
- Calcium: bones and teeth
- Magnesium: bones and muscle development
- Manganese: bone development and nerve health
- Omega-3s: brain and eye development
- Phosphorus: bone development
- Potassium: nerve and muscle function
- Vitamin A: cell structure, bones, teeth, nervous system
- Vitamin D: calcium absorption
- Vitamin K: bone mineralization

OPTIMAL FOODS FOR MONTH 4

PROTEIN	DAIRY	GRAINS/ LEGUMES	VEGETABLES	FRUITS	FATS/OTHER
Eggs	Cheese	All-bran cereal and other fortified breakfast cereals	Artichokes	Bananas	Brewer's or nutritional yeast
Meats	Enriched plant-based milks (rice soy, and almond)	Beans: soy, black, navy, pinto, kidney, white, great northern, black-eyed, pink, cranberry, and cannellini	Asparagus	Cantaloupe	Olive oil
Nuts: almonds, cashews, pistachios, Brazil nuts, walnuts, and nut butters	Fortified dairy milk	Avocados	Citrus fruits and juices: oranges, tangerines, grapefruit, lemonade	Omega-3s
Pork	Fortified orange juice and other juices	Chickpeas	Baked potato with skin on and all other potatoes	Dried apricots	Molasses
Poultry	Yogurt	Corn and flour tortillas	Beets	Mangoes	Seaweed and kelp
Seafood (fish and shellfish): salmon (wild and Atlantic), tuna, mackerel, herring, sardines in oil, halibut, cod, and catfish		Edamame	Broccoli and broccoli rabe	Pineapple	
		Folic acid–fortified products	Brussels sprouts	Raspberries	
		Lentils	Butternut squash		
Seeds: sunflower, pumpkin, chia, hemp seed, and flaxseed		Oatmeal	Carrots		
		Peanuts	Dark, leafy greens: kale, collards, mustard, Swiss chard, bok choy, and turnip greens		
Tahini		Wheat germ	Mushrooms		
Tofu and tempeh		Whole grains: quinoa, barley, brown rice, bulgur, and whole wheat couscous	Pumpkin		
			Red bell peppers		
			Romaine lettuce		
			Spinach		
			Sweet potatoes		
			Tomatoes and tomato juice		

RECIPES FOR MONTH 4

Mango-Chia Smoothie

Vitamins A and C and B vitamins optimize your baby's cell, brain, and nervous system development, and calcium helps your bones stay strong, while vitamin C supports your immune system and oral health.

A yummy smoothie any time of day. Lactose intolerant or vegan? No worries. Lactose-free, soy or coconut yogurt can be used. For a calcium boost, add nonfat powdered milk, such as Carnation Instant Breakfast powder. One tablespoon will add 57 mg of calcium. For a protein boost, add your favorite protein powder. To sweeten, add a little bit of sugar, agave nectar, or honey (unless vegan). Use water or juice to adjust the consistency. Smoothies can last a day in the fridge and can be frozen for one month. Mix well before serving.

MAKES 1½ CUPS

1 cup sliced fresh or frozen
    mango
¾ cup plain yogurt
⅓ cup orange juice or water
2 tablespoons chia seeds
Ice cubes

- Place all the ingredients in a blender and process until smooth. Serve over ice.

Tips for diabetes

- Reduce your portion size, or skip this recipe.
- Skip the orange juice and use water instead.

¾ cup mango-chia smoothie: Calories: 218 cals; Protein: 9 g; Carbohydrates: 32 g; Fat: 7 g; Fiber: 7 g; Sodium: 69 mg; Vitamin A: 1,248 IU; Vitamin C: 60 mg; B₁₂: 0.5 mcg; Magnesium: 78 mg; Calcium: 284 mg; 2 CARBS

Dutch Baby Pancake Bliss

B vitamins enhance your baby's cell, brain, and nervous system development.

WHAT'S a Dutch baby pancake? It's one big pancake that's baked in the oven on high heat. Making the perfect puffed pancake can be hit-or-miss endeavor, so here are some cooking tips for success. The order in which you mix these ingredients is very important: the wet ingredients should be mixed before you add the dry ingredients, or the pancake may not rise sufficiently. A well-seasoned 12-inch cast-iron skillet works best and allows you to cut the pancake in the pan without damaging the finish. This pancake does not work well in a regular cake pan, so please don't attempt to use one. And finally, this pancake must be baked on the lowest oven rack to make it rise properly.

SERVES 3

½ cup milk, warmed slightly
2 large eggs
½ cup unbleached all-purpose flour
Pinch of ground cinnamon
½ teaspoon grated lemon zest (optional)
1 tablespoon unsalted butter
½ cup fresh blueberries, plus more for serving
2 tablespoons confectioners' sugar, for dusting, or to taste

- Position an oven rack on the lowest rung and preheat the oven to 425°F.
- Whisk the milk and eggs in a bowl until foamy. Add the flour, cinnamon, and lemon zest, if using, and mix until smooth.
- Melt the butter in a large, ovenproof skillet over medium-high heat. Swirl the butter around the pan to make sure it coats the bottom and sides. Pour the batter into the pan, sprinkle it with the blueberries, and increase the heat to high. Cook for 1 minute, then transfer the skillet to the oven and bake for 15 minutes, or until puffed and golden brown.
- Remove the pancake from the oven, sprinkle with the confectioners' sugar, and serve immediately with additional berries.

Meal ideas

- Protein, such as eggs, dairy, or plant-based
- Fresh fruit
- Reduced-fat milk or yogurt (Mango-Chia Smoothie, page 157)

Meal ideas and tips for diabetes

- Reduce your portion size, or skip this recipe.
- Protein, such as natural nut butter or eggs

One third of the pancake: Calories: 212 cals; Protein: 8 g; Carbohydrates: 26 g; Fat: 9 g; Fiber: 1 g; Sodium: 66 mg; B_{12}: 0.5 mcg; Niacin: 3 mg; Riboflavin: 0.3 mg; Selenium: 19 mcg; 2 CARBS

Spinach and Cheese Omelet for One ⒼⒻ Ⓠ ⓁⒸ

Protein, vitamins A, D, and K, B vitamins, and folate optimize your baby's cell, brain, nervous system, bone, and tooth development, and vitamin D helps your calcium absorption.

CAN'T go wrong with an omelet for breakfast, or any meal! Think protein and vitamins to kick-start your day! Sautéing the vegetables helps prevent a watery omelet, but if you're in a hurry, skip it. Other filling possibilities include thinly sliced mushrooms, red bell peppers, chopped broccoli florets, ham, chives, and fresh herbs.

SERVES 1

2 large eggs
Sprinkle of salt
Sprinkle of freshly ground black pepper
½ teaspoon unsalted butter
2 heaping tablespoons diced tomatoes
⅓ cup fresh baby spinach or 3 tablespoons thawed frozen spinach
2 tablespoons grated Cheddar cheese, or your favorite cheese

- Whisk together the eggs, salt, and pepper in a bowl until very light and frothy. The more you whip the eggs, the lighter the omelet will be. Set aside.
- Melt the butter in a small skillet over medium heat. Add the tomatoes and spinach and cook for 1 minute, stirring, just until hot. Transfer to a small plate or bowl and set aside. Do not rinse the skillet.
- Return the skillet to medium-low heat, add the beaten eggs, and cook for about 20 seconds. Then, while tilting the skillet, use a spatula to push the cooked egg toward the center of the pan, allowing the raw eggs to hit the hot skillet to cook. Distribute the cheese on top, followed by the cooked tomato mixture. Lower the heat and cook for 1 to 2 minutes, or until the eggs are set. Fold the omelet in half and cook for 10 to 30 seconds longer, until the omelet is cooked through.

Meal ideas

- Whole-grain bread, roll, or starch (Spiced-Up Hash Browns, page 263)
- Reduced-fat milk or yogurt
- Fresh fruit

Meal ideas and tips for diabetes

- Whole-grain bread, roll, or starch (above), 1 CARB
- Reduced-fat milk or unsweetened reduced-fat yogurt, 1 CARB

1 omelet: Calories: 226 cals; Protein: 16 g; Carbohydrates: 3 g; Fat: 16 g; Fiber: 1 g; Sodium: 244 mg; Vitamin A: 1,988 IU; Vitamin D: 85 IU; Vitamin K: 49 mcg; Folate: 74 mcg; B$_{12}$: 1 mcg; Niacin: 4 mg; Riboflavin: 0.5 mg; Choline: 299 mg; Phosphorus: 272 mg; Selenium: 35 mcg; 0 CARBS

KITCHEN WISDOM: SMART EGGS

DURING pregnancy, eggs are an excellent source of nutrition. One large egg contains 6 grams of protein, 25 mg of calcium, 0.55 mcg of vitamin B_{12} and 0.25 mg of riboflavin. That much is hard to beat. But there is a caveat with eggs—they must be fully cooked to be safe. While salmonella can be contracted a number of different ways, *Salmonella enteritidis* (SE) comes specifically from contaminated raw eggs. Proper refrigeration, cooking, and handling of raw eggs should prevent most contamination problems. People can and should enjoy eggs and egg dishes that are fully cooked (for more information on food-borne illnesses, see page 28).

Glorious Edamame Dip

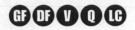

Vitamins A and K and folate foster your baby's cell, brain, nervous system, and bone and tooth development.

EASY to make and supertasty, this green dip is glorious! Keep a stash in the fridge to snack on any time of day. Serve with fresh cut vegetables, vegan whole-grain crackers, or romaine leaves as scoopers. Corn chips are also yummy! This dip keeps refrigerated for three days.

MAKES ABOUT 1 CUP

3 tablespoons olive oil
1½ cups shelled edamame
2 cups lightly packed baby spinach
2 tablespoons freshly squeezed lemon juice, or to taste
1 tablespoon tahini
Pinch of garlic powder
Pinch of red pepper flakes
Salt and freshly ground black pepper

- Place all the ingredients in a blender or the bowl of a food processor and process until smooth, scraping down the sides as needed. Process to your desired consistency. Add water, 1 tablespoon at a time, to thin the dip, if needed. Adjust the seasoning and serve.

½ cup edamame dip: Calories: 189 cals; Protein: 8 g; Carbohydrates: 7 g; Fat: 15 g; Fiber: 4 g; Sodium: 21 mg; Vitamin A: 2,176 IU; Vitamin K: 124 mcg; Folate: 226 mcg; Copper: 0.2 mg; Manganese: 0.6 mg; ½ CARB

Turkish-Style Red Lentil Soup

Protein, B vitamins, and folate promote your baby's cell, brain, and nervous system development, and iron boosts your iron stores, while fiber moves things along.

PACKED with nutrition and fiber, this red lentil soup is ideal for lunch or dinner, or as a snack. The orange lentils will lose some of their color during cooking; the finished soup will be a golden yellow color. Add diced tomatoes and cucumbers as a garnish, or swirl in some plain Greek yogurt. This soup keeps refrigerated for about one week, and it can be frozen for up to one month.

SERVES 6; MAKES ABOUT 7 CUPS

2 tablespoons olive oil

1 medium-size onion, chopped

2 garlic cloves, crushed

3 carrots, peeled and sliced

1½ cups dried red lentils, picked over and rinsed

2 teaspoons dried mint

1 teaspoon ground cumin (optional)

Pinch of paprika or red pepper flakes

7 cups stock (any kind) or water

Salt and freshly ground black pepper

- Heat the olive oil in a 6-quart saucepan over medium-high heat. Add the onion and sauté for 3 minutes. Add the garlic, carrots, red lentils, mint, cumin, if using, paprika, and stock and bring to a boil. Lower the heat and simmer, uncovered, for 30 minutes, or until the carrots are soft and the lentils are mushy.
- Remove the soup from the heat and cool slightly. Then, with an immersion blender or regular blender, puree it to a slightly chunky consistency. Thin with water, if needed. Adjust the seasoning and serve.

Meal ideas

- Green salad or vegetable (Asian-Inspired Spinach Salad, page 186)
- Whole wheat bread or roll
- Reduced-fat milk or yogurt
- Fresh fruit

Meal ideas and tips for diabetes

- Reduce your portion size, if necessary.
- Green salad or nonstarchy vegetable (above)
- Whole wheat bread or roll, 1 CARB
- Reduced-fat milk or unsweetened reduced-fat yogurt, 1 CARB

1 generous cup lentil soup (made with stock): Calories: 341 cals; Protein: 19 g; Carbohydrates: 47 g; Fat: 9 g; Fiber: 7 g; Sodium: 433 mg; B_6: 0.5 mg; Niacin: 9 mg; Riboflavin: 0.3 mg; Thiamine: 0.4 mg; Folate: 125 mcg; Copper: 1 mg; Iron: 4 mg; Manganese: 1 mg; Zinc: 3 mg; 3 CARBS

My Big Fat Greek Salad

Vitamins A, C, E, and K, B vitamins, and folate boost your baby's cell, brain, nervous system, bone, and tooth development, while vitamin C keeps you healthy.

IF you like olives, tomatoes, feta, artichokes, and images of the gorgeous beaches of Greece, this salad is for you. Mix in some cooked whole grains or serve a hearty whole-grain bread on the side. Vegan or lactose intolerant? Leave out the cheese. Refrigerate leftovers.

SERVES 2

½ cup artichoke hearts, drained, and cut into wedges (about 5 hearts)

1 large tomato, diced, or 12 cherry or grape tomatoes, halved

⅓ cup crumbled pasteurized feta cheese

12 pitted black or green olives

3 tablespoons olive oil

1 tablespoon cider vinegar, or to taste

1 tablespoon freshly squeezed lemon juice, or to taste

Generous pinch of dried oregano

Salt and freshly ground black pepper

4 cups mixed baby greens, for serving

- Combine all the ingredients, except the mixed greens, in a bowl and toss gently. Adjust the seasoning. Divide the mixed greens between two plates. Divide the Greek salad in half and arrange it on top of the greens. Serve promptly.

Meal ideas

- Protein, such as meat, poultry, seafood, eggs, dairy, or plant-based (Grilled or Broiled Lamb Chops, page 228)
- Whole grain, bread, or starch
- Reduced-fat milk or yogurt
- Fresh fruit

Meal ideas and tips for diabetes

- Protein, such as meat, poultry, seafood, eggs, dairy, or plant-based (above)
- Whole grain, bread, or starch, 1 CARB
- Reduced-fat milk or unsweetened reduced-fat yogurt, 1 CARB

One half of the Greek salad: Calories: 326 cals; Protein: 7 g; Carbohydrates: 13 g; Fat: 29 g; Fiber: 5 g; Sodium: 464 mg; Vitamin A: 1,751 IU; Vitamin C: 22 mg; Vitamin K: 115 mcg; Vitamin E: 4 mg; Riboflavin: 0.3 mg; Folate: 133 mcg; Copper: 0.3 mg; 1 CARB

Lemony Slaw

GF DF V Q LC

Vitamins A, C, and K enhance your baby's cell, brain, nervous system, bone, and tooth development, and boost your immunity.

PACKED with vitamins A, C, and K, this coleslaw is a popular sidekick for anything from hamburgers to roasted chicken. Use white or red cabbage, or a mixture of both. To save time, buy a packaged coleslaw mix, or pick up shredded cabbage and carrots from a grocery store salad bar. Grated or sliced carrots, jicama, fennel bulb, and radishes are all great additions. Need more protein in your day? Toss in some nuts and/or seeds. Vegan? Use vegan mayonnaise. Dress the slaw at the last minute. Refrigerate leftovers, but they will tend to get a bit soggy.

SERVES 4

1 tablespoon olive oil
2 tablespoons freshly squeezed lemon juice, or to taste
1 tablespoon light mayonnaise
Salt and freshly ground black pepper
8 ounces thinly sliced cabbage, or 1 (8-ounce) package coleslaw mix (about 4 cups)
¼ cup grated carrot
¼ chopped celery
2 tablespoons chopped fresh dill (optional)

- Combine the olive oil, lemon juice, mayonnaise, and salt and pepper to taste in a small bowl and whisk until emulsified. Refrigerate until ready to use.
- Combine the cabbage, carrot, celery, and dill, if using, in a large bowl and toss gently. Dress the slaw with the mayonnaise mixture and adjust the seasoning before serving.

Meal ideas

- Protein, such as meat, poultry, seafood, eggs, dairy, or plant-based (Crab Cakes with Homemade Tartar Sauce, page 193)
- Whole grain or starch
- Reduced-fat milk or yogurt
- Fresh fruit

Meal ideas and tips for diabetes

- Protein, such as meat, poultry, seafood, eggs, dairy, or plant-based (above)
- Whole grain or starch, 1 CARB
- Reduced-fat milk or unsweetened reduced-fat yogurt, 1 CARB

1 cup slaw: Calories: 68 cals; Protein: 1 g; Carbohydrates: 6 g; Fat: 5 g; Fiber: 2 g; Sodium: 58 mg; Vitamin A: 1,461 IU; Vitamin C: 30 mg; Vitamin K: 68 mcg; ½ CARB

Orzo Salad with Ginger-Sesame Dressing   **DF** **V**

Vitamins A, C, and E, B vitamins, and folate optimize your baby's cell, brain, nervous system, bone, and tooth development, and vitamin C keeps your immune system strong.

A winner with our testers! Adults and kids love this dressing, which can be used on anything from greens to grains. The ginger is what makes it special. Feel free to replace the orzo with any other small pasta, or any whole grain, such as quinoa or farro. Need veggie subs? Add lightly cooked asparagus, green beans, edamame, or broccoli florets. Gluten-free? Use your favorite gluten-free pasta or grain. No time? Pick up veggies, cooked pasta, and proteins (such as cooked shrimp, chicken—or tofu—to keep it vegan) from a salad bar. More fiber? You can toss in greens, such as spinach, arugula, or mizuna. Add 2 tablespoons of chia and/or flaxseeds for some real power.

SERVES 6

GINGER-SESAME DRESSING (MAKES ABOUT ½ CUP)

2 teaspoons minced fresh ginger
1 garlic clove, halved
2 tablespoons cider vinegar
1½ tablespoons light soy sauce or wheat-free tamari
½ teaspoon light brown sugar
1 teaspoon toasted sesame oil
¼ cup canola oil

- Prepare the dressing: Combine all the dressing ingredients plus 2 tablespoons of water in the bowl of a mini food processor, or use an immersion blender, and puree until smooth, scraping down the sides of the bowl as needed. Adjust the seasoning, transfer to a bowl or jar, cover, and refrigerate. Whisk or shake before serving.

Meal ideas

- Protein, such as meat, poultry, seafood, eggs, dairy, or plant-based (Steak on the Grill, page 279)
- Reduced-fat milk or yogurt
- Fresh fruit

Meal ideas and tips for diabetes

- Protein, such as meat, poultry, seafood, eggs, dairy, or plant-based (above)
- Reduced-fat milk or unsweetened reduced-fat yogurt, 1 CARB

(continues)

⅔ cup orzo salad: Calories: 262 cals; Protein: 6 g; Carbohydrates: 27 g; Fat: 14 g; Fiber: 3 g; Sodium: 270 mg; Vitamin A: 4,228 IU; Vitamin C: 34 mg; Vitamin E: 5 mg; Niacin: 5 mg; Thiamine: 0.4 mg; Folate: 104 mcg; Copper: 0.3 mg; Manganese: 0.5 mg; Selenium: 22 mcg; 2 CARBS

Orzo Salad with Ginger-Sesame Dressing (continued)

SALAD

1 cup uncooked orzo

2 cups snow peas

1 cup shredded carrot

1 cup seeded and diced red
    bell pepper

¼ cup sliced scallion

Salt

⅓ cup sunflower or pumpkin
    seeds, for garnish

- Prepare the salad: Add the orzo to the boiling water and cook until done, following the package directions.
- Cook the snow peas in boiling water for 5 minutes, or until crisp-tender, and drain. Place them in a bowl and add the carrot, bell pepper, scallions, cooked orzo, and ⅓ cup of the dressing. Toss, adjust the seasoning, and add more dressing, if desired, 1 tablespoon at a time. Top with the seeds.

Easy Lemon Garlic Spinach

GF DF V Q LC

Vitamins A, C, and K and folate promote your baby's cell, brain, nervous system, bone, and tooth development, and vitamin C keeps you healthy, too.

BURSTING with folate, spinach is awesome during pregnancy. This easy dish is a partner to just about any main course.

SERVES 4

12 ounces baby spinach leaves
    (2 [6-ounce bags])
2 tablespoons olive oil
2 garlic cloves, minced,
    or to taste
Salt and freshly ground black
    pepper
Squeeze of lemon juice,
    or to taste

- Rinse the spinach and spin it dry in a salad spinner, leaving just a little water clinging to the leaves.
- In a large skillet or pot, heat the olive oil over medium-high heat and sauté the garlic for about 30 seconds. Add the spinach (you may need to add it in batches, depending on the size of your skillet), season with salt and pepper, and stir. Cook for 2 minutes. Adjust the seasoning. Transfer the spinach to a serving bowl and top with a squeeze of lemon.

Meal ideas

- Protein, such as meat, poultry, seafood, eggs, dairy, or plant-based
- Whole grain or starch (Lentil, Brown Rice, and Mushroom Pilaf, page 249)
- Reduced-fat milk or yogurt
- Fresh fruit

Meal ideas and tips for diabetes

- Protein, such as meat, poultry, seafood, eggs, dairy, or plant-based
- Whole grain or starch (above)
- Reduced-fat milk or unsweetened reduced-fat yogurt, 1 CARB

½ cup spinach: Calories: 82 cals; Protein: 3 g; Carbohydrates: 4 g; Fat: 7 g; Fiber: 2 g; Sodium: 68 mg; Vitamin A: 7,975 IU; Vitamin C: 26 mg; Vitamin K: 415 mcg; Folate: 166 mcg; Manganese: 0.7 mg; 0 CARBS

Maple Glazed Carrots

Vitamin A fosters your baby's bone and tooth development.

TAKE carrots to a new level with a simple drizzle of maple syrup and a pinch of spices. Dairy-free or vegan? Replace the butter with coconut oil or olive oil. Use your favorite spices in place of the ones called for. Garnish with fresh herbs, if you have them on hand.

SERVES 4

2 tablespoons unsalted butter

5 large carrots, peeled and sliced into ¼-inch rounds (almost 4 cups)

Salt and freshly ground black pepper

1 teaspoon ground star anise, cardamom, or cinnamon, or a mixture of spices, or to taste

½ cup water or stock

2 tablespoons pure maple syrup, or to taste

- In a medium-size skillet, melt the butter over medium heat. Add the carrots, salt, pepper to taste, and the star anise and sauté for 2 minutes, or just until the carrots begin to give off their juices. Add the water and bring to a boil, then lower the heat to a strong simmer and cook, covered, for 7 to 10 minutes, or until the carrots are tender and almost all the water has evaporated.

- Add the maple syrup and stir to coat, adjust the seasoning, and serve.

Meal ideas

- Protein, such as meat, poultry, seafood, eggs, dairy, or plant-based (Chili-Rubbed Pork Chops, page 174)
- Whole grain
- Reduced-fat milk or yogurt
- Fresh fruit

Meal ideas and tips for diabetes

- Protein, such as meat, poultry, seafood, eggs, dairy, or plant-based (above)
- Whole grain or starch, 1 CARB
- Reduced-fat milk or unsweetened reduced-fat yogurt, 1 CARB

¾ **cup carrots:** Calories: 133 cals; Protein: 1 g; Carbohydrates: 20 g; Fat: 6 g; Fiber: 4 g; Sodium: 97 mg; Vitamin A: 23,106 IU; Manganese: 0.5 mg; 1 CARB

Zucchini Noodles with Spicy Shrimp

Protein, vitamins C and E, folate, and B vitamins boost your baby's cell, brain, nervous system, and bone development, and vitamin C keeps your immune system strong.

LOW-CARB and gluten-free, these zucchini noodles (sometimes called "zoodles") are topped with tender, spicy shrimp for a tasty and light meal. You may be able to find spiralized zucchini in your grocery store, or if you've got a spiralizer, you can make them. You can replace the shrimp with cubed chicken breast, tofu, or anything else. For more heat, add a pinch of cayenne or pepper flakes. Garnish with your favorite herbs. To all our moms with diabetes during pregnancy, this low-carb recipe was created for you, with love!

SERVES 4

1½ pounds peeled and deveined medium or large shrimp, rinsed

2 teaspoons seafood seasoning mix, or to taste

3 tablespoons olive oil

2 large garlic cloves, minced

8 ounces mushrooms, stems trimmed and sliced (1½ cups)

Salt and freshly ground black pepper

1½ cups cherry tomatoes, sliced in half

5 medium-size zucchini, spiralized (about 5 cups)

- In a bowl, mix the shrimp with the seafood seasoning; set aside.
- In a large skillet, heat 1 tablespoon of the olive oil over medium-high heat. Add the garlic and sauté for 30 seconds. Add the mushrooms, stir, season with salt and pepper, and cook for 1 minute, then add the cherry tomatoes and cook for 2 minutes longer. Transfer to a large bowl and cover to keep warm. Do not rinse the skillet.
- Add 1 tablespoon of the olive oil to the skillet and heat over high heat. When the oil is hot, add the seasoning-coated shrimp in a single layer and cook until pink and slightly golden on the first side, about 2 minutes, then flip the shrimp and cook for 2 to 3 minutes, or until cooked through. Transfer the shrimp and any juices to the cooked vegetables. Cover to keep warm. Do not rinse the skillet.

Meal ideas

- Reduced-fat milk or yogurt
- Green salad (Everyone's Favorite Caesar Salad, page 84)
- Fresh fruit

(continues)

One quarter of the zucchini noodles: Calories: 253 cals; Protein: 26 g; Carbohydrates: 9 g; Fat: 13 g; Fiber: 2 g; Sodium: 979 mg; Vitamin C: 33 mg; Vitamin E: 4 mg; Folate: 79 mcg; B_6: 0.6 mcg; B_{12}: 2 mcg; Niacin: 10 mg; Riboflavin: 0.3 mg; Choline: 160 mg; Copper: 0.5 mg; Phosphorus: 513 mg; Selenium: 54 mcg, Zinc: 2 mg; 1 CARB

Zucchini Noodles with Spicy Shrimp (continued)

- Add the remaining tablespoon of olive oil to the skillet and heat over high heat. Add the spiralized zucchini and cook for 3 minutes, until crisp-tender. If sticking occurs, add up to 2 tablespoons of water.
- Add the veggies and shrimp and all of the juices back to the skillet. Gently mix with the zucchini. Adjust the seasoning and serve.

Meal ideas and tips for diabetes
- Reduced-fat milk or unsweetened reduced-fat yogurt, 1 CARB
- Green salad (Everyone's Favorite Caesar Salad, page 84)
- Fruit, 1 CARB

Sheet Pan Roasted Chicken Dinner

Protein, vitamins A, C, and K, and B vitamins enhance your baby's cell, brain, nervous system, and bone development, and vitamin C keeps your immune system healthy.

THIS healthy sheet pan dish makes dinner a cinch. To keep the vegetables from overcooking, they are added after the chicken has been in the oven for 20 minutes. Feel free to make as many substitutions as you wish. Scoring the chicken with a knife, which means making a surface slice about ¼ inch deep in the meaty parts (about 4 slices per piece), will allow the meat to absorb the flavor and cook more quickly. Trick: The smaller you cut the potatoes, the faster they will cook. Leftovers can be stored in the refrigerator for up to four days.

SERVES 6

2 pounds bone-in chicken thighs and drumsticks, scored with a knife about ¼ inch deep (see headnote)

3 tablespoons olive oil

2 teaspoons poultry or steak seasoning

1½ cups peeled and sliced carrot (sliced 1-inch thick)

2 cups Brussels sprouts, halved if large

2 cups baby potatoes, cut in half or quartered

3 garlic cloves, minced, or ½ teaspoon garlic powder

1 tablespoon dried oregano or Italian seasoning

Salt and freshly ground black pepper

- Position a rack in the middle of the oven and heat to 425°F. Line a large, rimmed baking sheet with parchment paper or foil.
- Place the chicken in a large bowl. Add 1 tablespoon of the olive oil and the poultry seasoning, toss and then transfer to the middle of the baking sheet. Place the carrot, Brussels sprouts, and baby potatoes in the same bowl. Add the remaining 2 tablespoons of olive oil, garlic, and oregano, and toss.
- Roast the chicken for 20 minutes. Remove the baking sheet from the oven and add the vegetables, spreading them out in a single layer around the chicken. Season everything with salt and pepper. Return to the oven and continue to roast for 30 minutes, or until the chicken is cooked through and the potatoes are soft.

Meal ideas

- Salad (Tomato-Mozzarella Salad, page 188)
- Reduced-fat milk or yogurt
- Fresh fruit

Meal ideas and tips for diabetes

- Salad (above)
- Reduced-fat milk or unsweetened reduced-fat yogurt, 1 CARB
- Fresh fruit, 1 CARB

One sixth of the chicken dish: Calories: 308 cals; Protein: 20 g; Carbohydrates: 16 g; Fat: 18 g; Fiber: 3 g; Sodium: 108 mg; Vitamin A: 5,360 IU; Vitamin C: 34 mg; Vitamin K: 64 mcg; Niacin: 9 mg; B_6: 0.6 mg; Copper: 0.2 mg; Selenium: 20 mcg; 1 CARB

Indian-Spiced Salmon with Cucumber-Tomato Salsa

GF **LC**

Protein, vitamins D and E, B vitamins, and omega-3 DHA enhance your baby's cell, brain, nervous system, and bone development, and vitamin D helps your calcium absorption.

A supremely healthy and tasty main course. This delicious Indian-spiced marinade can be used for almost anything. Don't let the number of different spices scare you—use whatever ones you have on hand or are willing to purchase. They are used in other recipes throughout this book. Short on time? Skip the cucumber-tomato salsa and top the salmon with a squeeze of lemon juice and fresh cilantro or your favorite herb.

SERVES 4

INDIAN-SPICED MARINADE

1 teaspoon roasted ground cumin

¼ teaspoon ground cinnamon

1 teaspoon garam masala

2 teaspoons paprika

½ teaspoon ground turmeric

¼ teaspoon cayenne pepper, or to taste

1 teaspoon sugar

½ teaspoon salt

1 teaspoon garlic powder

3 tablespoons plain Greek-style yogurt

1 tablespoon freshly squeezed lemon juice

4 skinless center-cut salmon fillets, about 4 ounces each, rinsed and patted with paper towels

- Marinate the salmon: Combine all the marinade ingredients in a small bowl and mix until smooth.
- Place the salmon fillets in a Pyrex baking dish. Cover each with some of marinade, then gently turn them until all sides are well coated. Cover with plastic wrap and refrigerate for at least 2 hours, or up to 8.
- When ready to cook the salmon, prepare the salsa: Combine all the ingredients in a small bowl and mix gently. Adjust the seasoning and set aside.

Meal ideas

- Green salad or vegetable (Roasted Asparagus, page 189)
- Whole grain or starch
- Reduced-fat milk or yogurt
- Fresh fruit

Meal ideas and tips for diabetes

- Green salad or nonstarchy vegetable (above)
- Whole grain or starch, 1 CARB
- Reduced-fat milk or unsweetened reduced-fat yogurt, 1 CARB

1 piece of salmon and 5 tablespoons salsa: Calories: 276 cals; Protein: 24 g; Carbohydrates: 2 g; Fat: 19 g; Fiber: 1 g; Sodium: 70 mg; Vitamin D: 500 IU; Vitamin E: 5 mg; B$_6$: 0.7 mg; B$_{12}$: 4 mcg; Niacin: 14 mg; Phosphorus: 287 mg; Selenium: 27 mcg; Omega-3 DHA: 1.2 g; 0 CARBS

(continued)

CUCUMBER-TOMATO SALSA (MAKES 1½ CUPS)

1 cup diced tomatoes

⅔ cup diced seedless cucumber

1 tablespoon minced green chiles (optional)

3 tablespoons chopped fresh cilantro, sliced fresh mint leaves, or a mixture of both

1 tablespoon olive oil

Squeeze of lemon juice, or to taste

Salt and freshly ground black pepper

SALMON

Cooking spray

- To broil the salmon, adjust an oven rack two rungs down from the heating element and preheat the broiler to HIGH. Line a rimmed baking sheet with parchment paper or foil, spray it with cooking spray, and arrange the fillets on it, skinned side down. Place the salmon under the broiler and cook for 10 to 12 minutes, depending on the thickness. (There is no need to turn the fish.)

- Transfer the salmon to a serving platter or individual plates and serve promptly with the salsa.

Chili-Rubbed Pork Chops

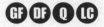

Protein and B vitamins optimize your baby's cell, brain, and nervous system development.

HAVING a supply of rubs can make flavoring meat, poultry, and seafood a snap. Don't be put off by the number of steps in this recipe—they include instructions for either grilling or broiling the pork chops.

MAKES 4 CHOPS

SPICE RUB

1 teaspoon Italian seasoning
½ teaspoon chili powder
½ teaspoon garlic powder, or 1 small garlic clove, crushed
½ teaspoon ground ginger
½ teaspoon ground cumin
2 teaspoons canola oil

1 pound pork chops (about 4 chops)
Cooking spray (optional)

- Prepare the spice rub: Combine the rub ingredients in a small bowl or measuring cup and mix well.
- Smear one side of the pork chops with half of the spice rub. Using a fork, pierce the meat all over to allow the spices to seep in, and repeat on the other side. Place the pork chops in a 1-gallon resealable plastic bag, seal, and refrigerate for at least 1 hour, or up to 48.
- To grill the pork chops, preheat the grill. Have a clean plate ready for the cooked meat. Spray the grill rack with cooking spray. Grill the pork chops for about 7 minutes on each side (depending on their thickness), or until an instant-read thermometer inserted into the center of the meat close to the bone reads 160°F.
- To broil the pork chops, preheat the broiler and line a shallow baking pan or a rimmed baking sheet with parchment paper or foil. Arrange the pork chops in the pan and broil for 5 to 7 minutes on each side, watching carefully to prevent burning.

Meal ideas

- Green salad or vegetable
- Whole grain or starch (Orzo Salad with Ginger-Sesame Dressing, page 165)
- Reduced-fat milk or yogurt
- Fresh fruit

Meal ideas and tips for diabetes

- Green salad or nonstarchy vegetable
- Whole grain or starch (above), 1 CARB
- Reduced-fat milk or unsweetened reduced-fat yogurt, 1 CARB

One 4-ounce pork chop: Calories: 237 cals; Protein: 29 g; Carbohydrates: 0 g; Fat: 13 g; Fiber: 0 g; Sodium: 62 mg; B_6: 1 mg; B_{12}: 0.7 mcg; Niacin: 14 mg; Riboflavin: 0.3 mg; Thiamine: 0.7 mg; Phosphorus: 249 mg; Selenium: 49 mcg; Zinc: 2 mg; 0 CARBS

Best-Ever Flank Steak with Salsa Verde

Protein and B vitamins promote your baby's cell, brain, and nervous system development.

THIS steak and salsa verde recipe has been a favorite among readers since day one. In addition to protein and vitamins, the steak is also a good source of iron. The flank steak should marinate for at least one hour, or up to twenty-four. The cooked flank steak and salsa verde keep for three days refrigerated.

SERVES 6

1 (1½-pound) flank steak

MARINADE

¼ cup light soy sauce or wheat-free tamari (for gluten-free)

1 teaspoon canola oil

2 teaspoons seasoned rice vinegar or freshly squeezed lime juice

1 tablespoon Worcestershire sauce

1 garlic clove, minced

1 tablespoon minced fresh ginger, or 1 teaspoon ground ginger

1 tablespoon chopped fresh rosemary

SALSA VERDE (MAKES ⅓ CUP)

1½ cups packed fresh cilantro leaves

1½ tablespoons capers

1 garlic clove

2 tablespoons freshly squeezed lemon juice, or to taste

¼ cup olive oil

Freshly ground black pepper

- Remove any visible fat from the flank steak. Using a fork, pierce the steak all over, then place it in a 1-gallon resealable plastic bag or in a pie dish and set aside.
- Prepare the marinade: Combine all of the marinade ingredients in a small bowl or measuring cup and mix well. Add the marinade to the flank steak, turning to make sure that it is completely covered with the marinade, and refrigerate for at least 1 hour, or up to 24.
- Prepare the salsa verde: Combine all the salsa ingredients in the bowl of a food processor and process until pureed and the sauce is slightly emulsified, scraping down the sides of the bowl as needed. Transfer to a serving bowl, cover with plastic wrap, placing it directly against the surface of the sauce (this is to prevent discoloration), and refrigerate.
- Preheat the grill. Have a serving platter ready for the cooked flank steak. Grill the flank steak for 12 to 15 minutes, or until well done (an instant-read thermometer should read 160°F). Transfer the cooked meat to the platter. Slice the steak against the grain and serve with the salsa.

Meal ideas

- Green salad or vegetable (Tomato, Hearts of Palm, and Asparagus Salad, page 244)
- Whole grain or starch
- Reduced-fat milk or yogurt
- Fresh fruit

Meal ideas and tips for diabetes

- Green salad or nonstarchy vegetable (above)
- Whole grain or starch, 1 CARB
- Reduced-fat milk or unsweetened reduced-fat yogurt, 1 CARB
- Fresh fruit, 1 CARB

4 ounces steak with 1 tablespoon sauce: Calories: 289 cals; Protein: 22 g; Carbohydrates: 1 g; Fat: 22 g; Fiber: 0; Sodium: 139 mg; B_6: 0.5 mg; B_{12}: 3 mcg; Niacin: 8 mg; Selenium: 24 mcg; Zinc: 8 mg; 0 CARBS

Strawberry-Banana N'ice Cream

Vitamin C and fiber keep you fit and healthy.

THINK: gelato. Think: healthy. Think: refreshing. And yes, think: vegan! All you need is a food processor or blender and some frozen fruit, and you're good to go. See "Freezing Bananas for Smoothies and N'ice Cream," below, for instructions on the best way to freeze bananas. Top your n'ice cream with fresh or dried fruit, nuts, seeds, coconut flakes, or goji berries. Or add a spoon of nut butter for more protein.

MAKES ABOUT 2 CUPS

2 medium-size bananas, sliced and frozen (see headnote)
1½ cups frozen strawberries
3 tablespoons almond milk or fruit juice
¼ cup chia seeds (optional)

- Combine all the ingredients, except the chia seeds, in a food processor or blender and pulse until completely smooth, scraping down the sides as necessary. If the mixture is too thick, thin it with more almond milk, 1 tablespoon at a time. It should be the consistency of gelato. Serve topped with a sprinkle of the chia seeds.

> **Tips for diabetes**
> - Reduce your portion size, or skip this recipe.

½ cup n'ice cream (with chia seeds): Calories: 141 cals; Protein: 3 g; Carbohydrates: 24; Fat: 5 g; Fiber: 7; Sodium: 12 mg; Vitamin C: 37 mg; Copper: 0.2 mg; Manganese: 0.8 mg; 2 CARBS

KITCHEN WISDOM: FREEZING BANANAS FOR SMOOTHIES AND N'ICE CREAM

FROZEN bananas make preparing smoothies, green drinks, and n'ice cream a cinch. The best way to store frozen bananas is to slice them into ½-inch rounds, place them in a single layer on a plate, and freeze them for 4 hours or overnight. You can make a bunch of banana slices and keep them in a resealable bag. This way they are ready when you are.

MONTH 5
Boy, Girl, or Secret?
Weeks 18 Through 22

Month 5 is a time for steady growth and development. In Week 18, your baby is the length of a red bell pepper and weighs about 7 ounces. By Week 22, your little angel has grown to about 11 inches long, and almost 1 pound. Your baby is beginning to look like a real baby, even though she or he is only the size of a large mango.

YOUR BABY'S DEVELOPMENT

- In Week 18, kicks usually start. You may also feel hiccups. They are related to normal development and not the foods you eat. Vocal cords are developing. By now, the sex organs of your child can be determined by ultrasound. Fingerprints have developed.
- In Week 19, as your baby grows, a greasy white protective substance called vernix caseosa covers him or her.
- In Week 20, your baby's sensory nerve cells are developing in the brain.
- In Week 21, arms and legs are more in proportion to the body. Cartilage is turning to bone. Your baby's moves are more coordinated and less jerky.
- In Week 22, all primary teeth have formed. The liver is fully functioning, and the pancreas produces insulin. Senses continue to develop. Your baby can perceive light and dark, and he or she hears the real world beyond the womb.

CHANGES IN YOUR BODY

You might have more energy and you probably have a bigger appetite. As your belly grows, so does the likelihood that you will feel bloating, gas, constipation, heartburn, and indigestion. Achiness in lower abdomen, sides, back, or legs is common. Annoyances below the belt remain much the same: white vaginal discharge, hemorrhoids, swelling of feet and ankles, varicose veins, leg cramps. Skin color can change. You might get stretch marks and itchy skin. Occasional headaches, lightheadedness, and dizziness are all common. You might feel Braxton Hicks contractions.

IDEAL NUTRITION

Your nutrition highlights your baby's cell, nerve, bone, and brain development. The following nutrients will help achieve this.

- B vitamins: cell division, brain formation, nervous system development
- Calcium: bones and teeth
- Magnesium: bones and muscle development
- Manganese: bone development and nerve health
- Omega-3s: brain, eye, nervous system development
- Phosphorus: bone development
- Selenium: cell structure
- Vitamin A: cell structure, bones, teeth, nervous system
- Vitamin D: calcium absorption
- Vitamin K: bone mineralization
- Vitamin E: cell structure
- Zinc: cell structure

OPTIMAL FOODS FOR MONTH 5

PROTEIN	DAIRY	GRAINS/ LEGUMES	VEGETABLES	FRUITS	FATS/OTHER
Eggs	Cheese	All-bran cereal and other fortified breakfast cereals	Artichokes	Bananas	Brewer's or nutritional yeast
Meats	Enriched plant-based milks (rice soy, and almond)	Beans: soy, black, navy, pinto, kidney, white, great northern, black-eyed, pink, cranberry, and cannellini	Asparagus	Cantaloupe	Olive oil
Nuts: almonds, cashews, pistachios, Brazil nuts, walnuts, and nut butters	Fortified dairy milk		Avocados	Citrus fruits and juices: oranges, tangerines, grapefruit, lemonade	Omega-3s
Pork	Fortified orange juice and other juices	Chickpeas	Baked potato with skin on and all other potatoes	Dried apricots	Molasses
Poultry	Yogurt	Corn and flour tortillas	Beets	Mangoes	Seaweed and kelp
Seafood (fish and shellfish): salmon (wild and Atlantic), tuna, mackerel, herring, sardines in oil, halibut, cod, and catfish		Edamame	Broccoli and broccoli rabe	Pineapple	
		Folic acid–fortified products	Brussels sprouts	Raspberries	
Seeds: sunflower, pumpkin, chia, hemp seed, and flaxseed		Lentils	Butternut squash		
		Oatmeal	Carrots		
Tahini		Peanuts	Dark, leafy greens: kale, collards, mustard, Swiss chard, bok choy, and turnip greens		
Tofu and tempeh		Wheat germ	Mushrooms		
		Whole grains: quinoa, barley, brown rice, bulgur, and whole wheat couscous	Pumpkin		
			Red bell peppers		
			Romaine lettuce		
			Spinach		
			Sweet potatoes		
			Tomatoes and tomato juice		

RECIPES FOR MONTH 5

Easy Whole Wheat Pancakes

Q

Protein, B vitamins, and folate optimize your baby's cell, brain, and nervous system development.

LIGHT and delicious, these pancakes will brighten up any morning. Don't have buttermilk? No sweat. Add 1 tablespoon of cider vinegar to 1 cup of milk and let sit for 10 minutes. Need more fiber? Add 3 tablespoons of ground flaxseeds to the batter. Gluten-free? Use gluten-free flour or oat flour. Need a calcium boost? Add up to ⅓ cup of powdered milk. Any leftover pancakes should be covered and refrigerated, or frozen, with layers of parchment paper in between each pancake. Reheat them in an ungreased skillet over medium-low heat until hot, one to two minutes per pancake. Don't use the microwave, which will make the pancakes unpleasantly rubbery.

MAKES ABOUT NINE 5-INCH PANCAKES

1 large egg
1¼ cups buttermilk
½ teaspoon pure vanilla extract
½ cup unbleached all-purpose flour
½ cup whole wheat flour
1 tablespoon baking powder
2 tablespoons sugar
Pinch of salt
2 tablespoons melted unsalted butter
Cooking spray or canola oil

- In a large bowl, whisk together the egg, buttermilk, and vanilla. Add the flours, baking powder, sugar, and salt and whisk until smooth. Add the melted butter and whisk until well incorporated.

- Heat a medium-size skillet over medium to medium-high heat until hot. Using a heatproof brush, lightly oil the skillet with cooking spray or canola oil. Add a scant ⅓-cup of batter and immediately swirl the batter to form a pancake. Cook until the surface bubbles and sets and the underside is golden brown, usually a little longer than 1 minute. Flip the pancake with a wide spatula and cook for 1 minute more, or until cooked through. Transfer to a plate or platter.

- Repeat this procedure with the remaining batter, lightly oiling the skillet as needed. You can keep the pancakes warm in a low oven.

Meal ideas

- Reduced-fat milk or yogurt (Pineapple-Banana-Calcium Smoothie, page 207)
- Fresh fruit

Meal ideas and tips for diabetes

- Reduce your portion size, or skip this recipe.
- Use a low-sugar jam (such as Polaner All Fruit; 2 teaspoons are FREE)
- Protein, such as natural nut butter or eggs, 1 CARB

3 pancakes: Calories: 241 cals; Protein: 10 g; Carbohydrates: 44 g; Fat: 3 g; Fiber: 3 g; Sodium: 699 mg; Riboflavin: 0.4 mg; Niacin: 4 mg; Thiamine: 0.3 mg; Folate: 82 mcg; Manganese: 1 mg; Selenium: 27 mcg; 2½ CARBS

Quick Strawberry-Raspberry Syrup

GF DF V Q

Vitamin C for your overall health.

THIS syrup is delicious served with any type of store-bought or homemade pancakes (page 237), waffles (page 208), French toast (page 104), or oatmeal. It is also a wonderful accompaniment to yogurt, frozen yogurt, or ice cream (including dairy-free and vegan brands), and it is great on top of the cheesecake (page 124). You can use 4 cups of one kind of berry instead of mixing strawberries and raspberries. Frozen berries work well, too. Leftovers will keep refrigerated for three days.

MAKES ABOUT 2¼ CUPS

1 cup sugar
2 cups fresh strawberries, hulled and quartered
2 cups fresh raspberries
½ teaspoon pure vanilla extract, or to taste

- Combine the sugar and berries in a large pot. Use a potato masher or a large fork to break up the berries a bit to help thicken the syrup.
- Bring to a boil. Lower the heat and simmer, uncovered, for 10 minutes, or until the syrup reaches your desired consistency. Remove from the heat and stir in the vanilla.

Tips for diabetes
- Reduce your portion size, or skip this recipe.

2 tablespoons berry syrup: Calories: 100 cals; Protein: 0.5 g; Carbohydrates: 25 g; Fat: 0.2 g; Fiber: 2 g; Sodium: 1 mg; Vitamin C: 23 mg; 1½ CARBS

KITCHEN WISDOM: HOW TO COOK DIFFERENT TYPES OF OATS

THE world of oats can be confusing. There are three basic types: quick-cooking, old-fashioned, and steel-cut, which are the least processed, and therefore most nutritious.

Quick-cooking oats: These thin, small flakes, which cook in a matter of minutes, are commonly eaten for breakfast. They are not suitable for granola. They are suitable for "overnight oats" usually made with equal amounts of oats and water (or dairy or plant-based milk) combined in a jar or bowl, covered, and left in the refrigerator overnight. You can also mix in raisins or dried fruit. Nuts and seeds ideally should be added at the last minute, to keep their crunch.

Rolled oats (also called old-fashioned rolled oats): These thicker, rounder flakes are also eaten as porridge. They have a longer cooking time, usually about 10 minutes over low heat. They are used in granola, crisp toppings, and other baked goods. Follow the package directions to prepare. Add your favorite fixin's and spices to jazz things up.

Steel-cut oats: Shaped like tiny pellets, these oats take the longest to cook, about 25 minutes on a low simmer. Follow the package directions to cook. The good news is that a big batch can be cooked in advance and then reheated for breakfast throughout the week (in a microwave oven, thinned with a little water or milk, if needed).

Great Green Broccoli-Spinach Soup

GF LC

Protein, vitamins A, C, and K, B vitamins, and folate promote your baby's cell, brain, nervous system, and bone development, plus the vitamin C helps boost your immunity.

VITAMINS, minerals, and hydration are all part of this great soup! Lactose intolerant or vegan? Use vegetable stock and skip the cheese. Garnish with nuts, seeds, or croutons (gluten-free, if necessary). This soup keeps refrigerated for about three days. It can be frozen for up to one month.

SERVES 6; MAKES ABOUT 7 CUPS

3 tablespoons olive oil
1 medium-size onion, chopped
4 cups broccoli florets (8 ounces)
1 medium-size potato, peeled and diced
5 cups stock (any kind)
½ teaspoon salt, or to taste
4 cups baby spinach (1 [6-ounce package])
Freshly ground black pepper
1 cup shredded sharp Cheddar cheese, or your favorite cheese, for garnish

- Heat the olive oil in a 6-quart saucepan over medium-high heat. Add the onion and sauté for 3 minutes. Add the broccoli, potato, stock, and salt and bring to a boil, then lower the heat and simmer, covered, for about 15 minutes, or until the potato is tender.

- Remove from the heat and allow the soup to cool slightly. Then, add the spinach and puree the soup in batches in a blender or food processor. Return the pureed soup to the rinsed-out saucepan. Adjust the seasoning, garnish with the cheese, and serve immediately.

Meal ideas

- Protein, such as meat, poultry, seafood, eggs, dairy, or plant-based (Tasty Tuna Salad Sandwich, page 187)
- Whole wheat bread or roll
- Reduced-fat milk or yogurt
- Fresh fruit

Meal ideas and tips for diabetes

- Protein, such as meat, poultry, seafood, eggs, dairy, or plant-based (above)
- Whole wheat bread or roll, 1 CARB
- Reduced-fat milk or unsweetened reduced-fat yogurt, 1 CARB

1 cup broccoli-spinach soup (made with chicken stock): Calories: 260 cals; Protein: 12 g; Carbohydrates: 18 g; Fat: 16 g; Fiber: 3 g; Sodium: 444 mg; Niacin: 3 mg; B_6: 0.4 mg; Riboflavin: 0.4 mg; Folate: 105 mcg; Vitamin K: 223 mcg; Copper: 0.2 mg; Selenium: 12 mcg; Vitamin A: 4,005 IU; Vitamin C: 55 mg; 1 CARB

Cucumber-Tomato Yogurt Salad

Protein and B vitamins enhance your baby's cell, brain, and nervous system development.

THIS Indian-inspired salad, also known as *raita*, is commonly eaten as an accompaniment to hot curries and dal (page 192). It is delicious as a side dish for grilled foods and stews. And it makes a wonderful dip for pita (if no need to be gluten-free), corn chips, and veggies. For an extra boost, throw in some sunflower seeds. This salad keeps for two days refrigerated.

MAKES ABOUT 2 CUPS

1½ cups plain Greek yogurt
1 garlic clove, minced, or
    ½ teaspoon garlic powder
½ teaspoon roasted ground
    cumin
2 tablespoons thinly sliced
    fresh mint leaves, or
    2 teaspoons dried
1 cup grated cucumber
    (gently squeeze out
    the juice)
½ cup tomatoes, seeded and
    cut into a small dice
Salt and freshly ground black
    pepper

- Combine all the ingredients in a bowl and stir. Refrigerate for 1 hour before serving to allow the flavors to develop.

Heaping ½ cup tomato-cucumber salad: Calories: 147 cals; Protein: 13 g; Carbohydrates: 8 g; Fat: 7 g; Fiber: 1 g; Sodium: 52 mg; B_{12}: 1 mcg; Riboflavin: 0.4 mg; Selenium: 14 mcg; ½ CARB

Asian-Inspired Spinach Salad

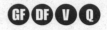

Protein, vitamins A and C, and folate promote your baby's cell, brain, and nervous system development, and fiber helps your digestion.

THE crunch of nuts and seeds combined with sweet juicy oranges plays perfectly against the baby spinach leaves. Need more protein? Add cooked chicken, shrimp, or tofu (to keep it vegan), plus some cooked quinoa or your favorite whole grain to turn this salad into a full meal. Use fresh mandarins when in season; otherwise, drained canned mandarins in natural juices are just fine.

SERVES 2

DRESSING

1 teaspoon light soy sauce or wheat-free tamari (for gluten-free)
1 tablespoon seasoned rice vinegar
3 tablespoons canola oil
A few drops of toasted sesame oil
1 very small garlic clove, crushed
Freshly ground black pepper

SPINACH SALAD

4 cups baby spinach (1 [6-ounce bag])
⅓ cup sliced or slivered almonds, toasted
⅓ cup raw pumpkin or sunflower seeds
1 tablespoon chia seeds
1 cup fresh mandarin oranges or canned in juice (no added sugar)

- Prepare the dressing: Combine all the dressing ingredients in a small bowl and mix well.
- Prepare the salad: Combine all the salad ingredients in a salad bowl. Add the dressing, toss gently, adjust the seasoning, and serve.

Meal ideas

- Protein, such as meat, poultry, seafood, eggs, dairy, or plant-based (Grilled Chicken Kebabs, page 196)
- Whole grain or starch
- Reduced-fat milk or yogurt
- Fresh fruit

Meal ideas and tips for diabetes

- Protein, such as meat, poultry, seafood, eggs, dairy, or plant-based (above)
- Whole grain or starch, 1 CARB
- Reduced-fat milk or unsweetened reduced-fat yogurt, 1 CARB

One half spinach salad (about 3 cups): Calories: 558 cals; Protein: 16 g; Carbohydrates: 25 g; Fat: 47 g; Fiber: 9 g; Sodium: 151 mg; Vitamin A: 9,071 IU; Vitamin C: 20 mg; Niacin: 6 mg; Folate: 191 mcg; Copper: 0.6 mg; Magnesium: 297 mg; Manganese: 2 mg; Phosphorus: 411 mg; Zinc: 3 mg; 2 CARBS

Tasty Tuna Salad Sandwich

Protein, vitamin K, B vitamins, and folate enhance your baby's cell, brain, nervous system, and bone development, and the iron builds up your iron stores.

LIGHT, fresh, and high in protein, this deli-style tuna salad is perfect between two slices of whole wheat or sprouted bread, stuffed in a pita pocket, or atop crackers. It's also amazing on a bed of your favorite greens. Rinsing and draining the canned tuna removes some of the fishy taste. Pickles and celery add a nice crunch, but feel free to add your favorite ingredients, such as capers, red bell peppers, cucumbers, and tomatoes.

MAKES 2 SANDWICHES

1 (6- to 6½-ounce) can light tuna in spring water, drained and rinsed
1 scallion, thinly sliced
2 tablespoons finely diced celery
1 dill pickle, finely diced
3 tablespoons light mayonnaise, or to taste
1 tablespoon freshly squeezed lemon juice, or to taste
Salt and freshly ground black pepper
4 slices hearty calcium-enriched or whole-grain bread

- In a bowl, combine all the ingredients, except the bread, and mix until well blended. Adjust the seasoning and assemble the sandwiches.

Meal ideas

- Green salad or raw veggies
- Reduced-fat milk or yogurt
- Fresh fruit

Meal ideas and tips for diabetes

- Reduce the amount of bread to one slice, if necessary.
- Skip the bread and place the tuna salad on top of lettuce or in half of an avocado
- Green salad or raw veggies
- Reduced-fat milk or unsweetened reduced-fat yogurt, 1 CARB

1 tuna sandwich with calcium-enriched bread: Calories: 378 cals; Protein: 24 g; Carbohydrates: 46 g; Fat: 11 g; Fiber: 3 g; Sodium: 837 mg; Vitamin K: 53 mcg; B_{12}: 2 mcg; B_6: 0.3 mg; Niacin: 16 mg; Thiamine: 0.4 mg; Riboflavin: 0.4 mg; Folate: 100 mcg; Iron: 4 mg; Selenium: 79 mcg; 3 CARBS

Tomato-Mozzarella Salad

Protein, vitamin K, and B vitamins boost your baby's cell, brain, nervous system, and bone development, while the calcium strengthens your bones.

A classic salad that can easily be transformed into a full meal by adding greens and a whole grain or bread. On the move? Make a tasty baguette or pita pocket for an awesome lunch. Vegan? Use your favorite vegan cheese or skip the cheese. This salad is best eaten the same day it is made. Refrigerate leftovers.

MAKES ABOUT 4 CUPS

3 large tomatoes, cubed, or 2 cups halved cherry tomatoes
8 ounces pasteurized mozzarella cheese, cut into cubes or rounds
⅓ cup thinly sliced fresh basil leaves, or 1 tablespoon dried
1 tablespoon cider vinegar, or to taste
A couple of drops of balsamic vinegar
3 tablespoons olive oil
Salt and freshly ground black pepper

- Combine all the ingredients in a bowl, mix gently, allow to sit for 15 minutes for the flavors to develop, then serve.

Meal ideas

- Protein, such as meat, poultry, seafood, eggs, dairy, or plant-based (Lemon-Herb Grilled Chicken, page 253)
- Whole grain or starch
- Reduced-fat milk or yogurt
- Fresh fruit

Meal ideas and tips for diabetes

- Protein, such as meat, poultry, seafood, eggs, dairy, or plant-based (above)
- Whole grain or starch, 1 CARB
- Reduced-fat milk or unsweetened reduced-fat yogurt, 1 CARB

1 cup tomato-mozzarella salad: Calories: 275 cals; Protein: 14 g; Carbohydrates: 7 g; Fat: 22 g; Fiber: 1 g; Sodium: 383 mg; Vitamin K: 28 mcg; B$_{12}$: 1 mcg; Niacin: 6 mg; Calcium: 411 mg; Phosphorus: 335 mg; Selenium, 16 mcg; Zinc: 2 mg; ½ CARB

Roasted Asparagus

GF **DF** **V** **Q** **LC**

Vitamin K enhances your baby's bone development.

ROASTING asparagus is quick and easy. Leftovers can be sliced and tossed into a salad. A sprinkle of Parmesan is a welcome garnish, if you are not avoiding dairy or vegan.

SERVES 3

12 ounces green asparagus, tough bottom ends trimmed

2 tablespoons olive oil

Salt and freshly ground black pepper

1 teaspoon grated lemon zest, or to taste

2 tablespoons chopped fresh dill

- Center an oven rack and preheat the oven to 425°F. Line a baking sheet with parchment paper or foil.
- Place the asparagus spears on the baking sheet and gently toss them, keeping their tops and bottoms facing the same direction, with the olive oil and salt and pepper to taste, until well coated. Spread out in a single layer.
- Roast for 6 to 8 minutes, or until crisp-tender (the time will depend on the thickness of the spears). Remove from the oven. Add the lemon zest and dill and transfer to a serving dish. Serve warm or at room temperature.

Meal ideas

- Protein, such as meat, poultry, seafood, eggs, dairy, or plant-based (Baked Salmon with Mustard-Dill Sauce, page 224)
- Whole grain or starch
- Reduced-fat milk or yogurt
- Fresh fruit

Meal ideas and tips for diabetes

- Protein, such as meat, poultry, seafood, eggs, dairy, or plant-based (above)
- Whole grain or starch, 1 CARB
- Reduced-fat milk or unsweetened reduced-fat yogurt, 1 CARB

¾ cup (or one third) of the asparagus: Calories: 102 cals; Protein: 2 g; Carbohydrates: 4 g; Fat: 9 g; Fiber: 2 g; Sodium: 2 mg; Vitamin K: 53 mcg; Copper: 0.2 mg; 0 CARBS

Lima Beans with Artichoke Hearts and Dill

Folate enhances your baby's brain and nervous system development, while vitamin C boosts your immunity and fiber supports digestion.

IF you like lima beans and artichokes, you'll love this nutrient-filled side dish. If you've never had this combo, it's worth a try. This dish keeps for three days refrigerated. It does not freeze well.

MAKES ABOUT 2½ CUPS

1 cup vegetable stock
8 ounces frozen lima beans (about 1¾ cups)
1 (14-ounce) can artichoke hearts, drained and cut into quarters, or 1 (8-ounce) package frozen sliced artichoke hearts
½ cup half-and-half
1½ tablespoons quick-dissolving flour, such as Wondra, or to desired consistency
¼ cup chopped fresh dill
Salt and freshly ground black pepper
Squeeze of lemon juice

- In a large saucepan, bring the stock to a boil. Add the lima beans and artichoke hearts and return to a boil. Lower the heat and simmer, covered, for 5 minutes.
- Add the half-and-half and return to a simmer, then sprinkle in the flour, stir, and continue to simmer for 2 minutes. Add the dill and season to taste with salt and pepper and lemon juice. Serve warm.

Meal ideas

- Protein, such as meat, poultry, seafood, eggs, dairy, or plant-based (Mustard-Tarragon Pork Tenderloin, page 195)
- Whole grain or starch
- Reduced-fat milk or yogurt
- Fresh fruit

Meal ideas and tips for diabetes

- Protein, such as meat, poultry, seafood, eggs, dairy, or plant-based (above)
- Green salad
- Reduced-fat milk or unsweetened reduced-fat yogurt, 1 CARB

Heaping ½ cup lima beans with artichoke hearts: Calories: 172 cals; Protein: 8 g; Carbohydrates: 29 g; Fat: 4 g; Fiber: 8 g; Sodium: 98 mg; Vitamin C: 17 mg; Folate: 90 mcg; Copper: 0.3 mg; Magnesium: 88 mg; Manganese: 1 mg; 2 CARBS

Mac and Cheese with Broccoli

Protein, vitamins C and K, B vitamins, folate, and calcium boost your baby's cell, brain, nervous system, and bone development, while the calcium strengthens your bones, too.

A legendary classic made healthier with the addition of chopped broccoli. It's still creamy, gooey, and easy to make, and will likely become a go-to dish when you're looking for a soothing comfort food. Chop the broccoli florets in a food processor using the Pulse button. This dish keeps refrigerated for three days.

SERVES 6

3 tablespoons unsalted butter
2 tablespoons all-purpose flour
2 cups whole milk
8 ounces uncooked macaroni noodles (2 cups)
3 cups finely chopped broccoli florets
1½ cups grated sharp Cheddar cheese (about 5 ounces)
¼ teaspoon garlic powder
½ teaspoon onion powder
Salt and freshly ground black pepper

- In a large skillet, melt the butter over medium heat. Add the flour and whisk until it begins to bubble. Cook for 2 minutes. Add the milk, bring to a simmer, and cook, stirring constantly, until it reaches the consistency of a thin pudding. Remove from the heat and set aside.
- Cook the pasta according to the package directions until al dente. During the last minute of cooking, add the broccoli. Drain the mixture in a fine-mesh colander and add it to the milk mixture. Mix well, then add the cheese and spices. Stir until the cheese has fully melted. Adjust the seasoning and serve promptly.

Meal ideas

- Protein, such as meat, poultry, seafood, eggs, dairy, or plant-based (BBQ Chicken, page 120)
- Green salad or nonstarchy vegetable
- Reduced-fat milk or yogurt
- Fruit

Meal ideas and tips for diabetes

- Reduce your portion size, if necessary.
- Protein, such as meat, poultry, seafood, eggs, dairy, or plant based (above)
- Green salad or nonstarchy vegetable

1¼ cups mac and cheese: Calories: 329 cals; Protein: 16 g; Carbohydrates: 38 g; Fat: 13 g; Fiber: 2 g; Sodium: 237mg; Vitamin C: 41 mg; Vitamin K: 47 mcg; B₂: 0.6 mg; Riboflavin: 0.4 mg; Thiamine: 0.4 mg; Folate: 135 mcg; Calcium: 322 mg; Phosphorus: 301 mg; 3 CARBS

Delicious Dal

 GF DF V

Protein, B vitamins, and folate optimize your baby's cell, brain, and nervous system development, while iron adds to your stores and fiber keeps your digestion on track.

YES, this Indian dish requires numerous spices, but if you've got them on hand—go for it. Many of them are used in recipes throughout this book, so it's worth picking them up on your next grocery run or grocery order. You can serve this dal with rice, quinoa, any whole grain, or with whole wheat naan (if you do not need it to be gluten-free). A classic side dish to accompany dal is the Cucumber-Tomato Yogurt Salad (page 172). This dal will keep refrigerated for three days, and it can be frozen for up to one month.

MAKES ABOUT 4 CUPS

1½ cups dried red lentils, picked over and rinsed
2 tablespoons canola oil
½ cup chopped onion
2 tablespoons minced fresh ginger
2 garlic cloves, minced
1 teaspoon garam masala or curry powder
1 teaspoon roasted ground cumin
1 teaspoon ground turmeric
1½ cups diced tomatoes (from about 2 large tomatoes)
Salt and freshly ground black pepper
¼ cup chopped fresh cilantro leaves, for garnish

- Combine the lentils and 4 cups of water in a medium-size saucepan. Bring to a boil, then lower the heat and simmer strongly for 15 to 20 minutes, or until the lentils are tender. (The mixture should be the consistency of a very thick pea soup.) Cover and set aside.
- Heat the canola oil in a medium-size skillet over medium heat until hot. Add the onion and cook until golden brown, about 7 minutes. Add the ginger, garlic, garam masala, cumin, and turmeric and sauté, stirring constantly, for 1 minute. Stir in the tomatoes and cook for 2 minutes. Remove from the heat and stir this onion mixture into the lentils. Adjust the seasonings, garnish with the cilantro, and serve.

Meal ideas

- Protein, such as meat, poultry, seafood, eggs, dairy, or plant-based
- Green salad or nonstarchy vegetable (Kale with Cranberries and Walnuts, page 115)
- Reduced-fat milk or yogurt
- Fruit

Meal ideas and tips for diabetes

- Protein, such as meat, poultry, seafood, eggs, dairy, or plant-based
- Green salad or nonstarchy vegetable (above)

⅔ **cup dal:** Calories: 229 cals; Protein: 12 g; Carbohydrates: 34 g; Fat: 6 g; Fiber: 6 g; Sodium: 7 mg; Thiamine: 0.3 mg; Folate: 108 mcg; Copper: 1 mg; Manganese: 1 mg; Iron: 4 mg; 2 CARBS

Crab Cakes with Homemade Tartar Sauce 🅓🅕 🅛🅒

Protein and B vitamins promote your baby's cell, brain, and nervous system development.

OUR readers have raved about this crab cake recipe for years. We love it, too! When your budget allows for a serious splurge, there is nothing better than these jumbo lump cakes laced with fresh herbs, served with a zippy homemade tartar sauce. Any leftover crab cakes can be eaten cold with a salad or made into delectable sandwiches. Gluten-free? Be sure to use gluten-free bread crumbs. The recipes for both the sauce and the crab cakes can be cut in half for a smaller yield. One pound of jumbo lump or back fin crabmeat (which equals about 2 cups of crabmeat) can be used in place of 8 ounces of each. Generally, back fin crabmeat needs to be picked over more carefully, as it contains bits of shell. The crab cakes can be formed up to twelve hours in advance, covered, and refrigerated. The tartar sauce can be made two days in advance, covered, and refrigerated.

MAKES 7 CRAB CAKES

HOMEMADE TARTAR SAUCE (MAKES ABOUT ½ CUP)

¼ cup light mayonnaise
1½ tablespoons dill pickle relish (not sweet pickle relish)
1 teaspoon freshly squeezed lemon or lime juice, or to taste
Freshly ground black pepper

- Prepare the tartar sauce: Combine all the ingredients in a small bowl and mix well. Adjust the seasoning and transfer to a serving bowl. Cover and refrigerate until ready to use.

Meal ideas

- Whole grain or starch
- Green salad or green vegetable (Favorite Broccoli Slaw, page 291)
- Reduced-fat milk or yogurt
- Fresh fruit

Meal ideas and tips for diabetes

- Whole grain or starch, 1 CARB
- Green salad or nonstarchy vegetable (above)
- Reduced-fat milk or unsweetened reduced-fat yogurt

(continues)

One crab cake (about 3 ounces): Calories: 154 cals; Protein: 15 g; Carbohydrates: 6 g; Fat: 8 g; Fiber: 0 g; Sodium: 393 mg; B_{12}: 2 mcg; Niacin: 5 mg; Copper: 1 mg; Selenium: 34 mcg; Zinc: 3 mg; ½ CARB
2 tablespoons tartar sauce: Calories: 51 cals; Protein: 0 g; Carbohydrates: 2 g; Fat: 5 g; Fiber: 0 g; Sodium: 200 mg; 0 CARBS

CRAB CAKES

8 ounces jumbo lump crabmeat, picked over to remove any shells

8 ounces back fin crabmeat, picked over to remove any shells

½ cup plain bread crumbs

2 tablespoons sliced scallion or fresh chives

¼ cup chopped fresh dill, cilantro, or basil, or a mixture, or to taste

2 teaspoons grated lemon zest

2 teaspoons Dijon mustard

2 large eggs, lightly beaten

2 tablespoons light mayonnaise

2 tablespoons olive oil

Lemon or lime wedges, for serving

- Prepare the crab cakes: Combine all the crab cake ingredients, except the olive oil and lemon wedges, in a bowl. Mix gently until well incorporated. To form the crab cakes, use a ⅓-cup measuring cup to portion out each crab cake, then form it into a patty and place it on a large plate. Cover and refrigerate until ready to cook.

- Heat the olive oil in a large skillet over medium-high heat. Add three crab cakes (avoid overcrowding) and cook on one side for about 3 minutes, or until golden brown. Carefully flip and cook the other side for about 3 minutes, or until golden brown and thoroughly heated. (Note: You may need to adjust the heat if the crab cakes begin browning too quickly.) Transfer the cooked crab cakes to a serving plate. Cook the remaining crab cakes and serve promptly, with the lemon wedges.

Mustard-Tarragon Pork Tenderloin

Protein and B vitamins boost your baby's cell, brain, nervous system, and muscle development.

LOVE pork? Here you go. And, if chicken is more to your taste, this tasty marinade also works well with chicken. Because there is almost no fat in pork tenderloin, please watch the cooking time, as the meat can dry out quickly. If you don't have fresh tarragon, add 1 extra teaspoon of dried. Leftovers are fabulous in a sandwich, salad, or reheated.

SERVES 6

MUSTARD-TARRAGON MARINADE

1 tablespoon olive oil
2 tablespoons light soy sauce or wheat-free tamari (for gluten-free)
2½ tablespoons honey
3 tablespoons Dijon mustard
2 tablespoons chopped fresh tarragon
1 tablespoon dried tarragon
1 teaspoon garlic powder
Freshly ground black pepper

2 pounds pork tenderloin (1 or 2 tenderloins, depending on the size)

- Marinate the pork: In a medium-size bowl, combine all the marinade ingredients plus 2 tablespoons of water and mix well. Add the pork tenderloin, turning to coat until it is well covered, then poke the meat all over with a fork. Cover, or transfer to a resealable plastic bag, and refrigerate for at least 6 hours, or up to 24.

- When ready to cook, center an oven rack and preheat the oven to 400°F. Transfer the pork to a baking dish (reserve the marinade in the bowl) and roast for 25 to 30 minutes, depending on the thickness. As the pork cooks, baste it once or twice with the reserved marinade. This will help keep it moist.

- Once cooked, remove the pork from the oven and preheat the broiler to HIGH. Broil for 5 minutes to give the outside a nice color. Discard all leftover marinade.

Meal ideas

- Whole grain or starch (Couscous Salad with Chickpeas and Artichokes, page 272)
- Green salad or vegetable
- Reduced-fat milk or yogurt
- Fresh fruit

Meal ideas and tips for diabetes

- Whole grain or starch (above), 1 CARB
- Green salad or nonstarchy vegetable
- Reduced-fat milk or unsweetened reduced-fat yogurt, 1 CARB

One sixth of the tenderloin: Calories: 183 cals; Protein: 33 g; Carbohydrates: 0 g; Fat: 6 g; Fiber: 0 g; Sodium: 348 mg; B$_6$: 1 mg; B$_{12}$: 0.7 mcg; Niacin: 17 mg; Riboflavin: 0.5 mg; Thiamine: 1 mg; Phosphorus: 476 mg; Selenium: 68 mcg; Zinc: 3 mg; 0 CARBS

Grilled Chicken Kebabs

Protein, vitamin C, and B vitamins foster your baby's cell, brain, and nervous system development and promote your overall good health.

THE combination of Dijon mustard, fresh basil, garlic, and Italian seasoning can make any chicken dish taste great. Add mushrooms, onions, red bell peppers, and sweet pineapple and you have a spectacular kebab. No time to prep? Pick up precut pineapple from a salad bar or in the produce section of the grocery store. Try to keep all the ingredients on the skewer about the same size to avoid bits burning.

MAKES ABOUT 12 KEBABS

DIJON-BASIL MARINADE

1 tablespoon olive oil
1 tablespoon Dijon mustard
3 tablespoons chopped fresh
   basil
1 teaspoon garlic powder
1 tablespoon Italian seasoning
½ teaspoon salt
1 teaspoon sugar
Freshly ground black pepper

1½ pounds skinless, boneless
   chicken breasts, cut into
   1½-inch pieces
2 to 3 medium-size onions,
   cut into large cubes
About 10 ounces fresh
   pineapple, cut into pieces
   (2 cups)
1 large red bell pepper, cored,
   seeded, and cut into pieces
About 8 ounces cremini or
   button mushrooms
Cooking spray

- Marinate the chicken: In a medium-size bowl, whisk together all the marinade ingredients. Add the chicken, stir until well coated, and then, using a fork, prick the chicken to allow the marinade to seep in. Cover with plastic wrap and refrigerate for at least 3 hours, and up to 12 hours.

- Have ready twelve 12-inch metal or bamboo skewers. If using bamboo skewers, soak them in water for 30 minutes before grilling.

- To make the kebabs, thread the chicken, onions, pineapple, bell peppers, and mushrooms, alternating them, onto the skewers. Leave enough room at the ends of the skewers so you can hold them comfortably during grilling. Keep the extra marinade for basting the skewers as they cook.

Meal ideas

- Whole grain or starch
- Green salad or green vegetable (Grilled or Roasted Vegetables, page 246)
- Reduced-fat milk or yogurt
- Fresh fruit

Meal ideas and tips for diabetes

- Whole grain or starch, 1 CARB
- Green salad or nonstarchy vegetable (above)
- Reduced-fat milk or unsweetened reduced-fat yogurt, 1 CARB

2 chicken skewers: Calories: 257 cals; Protein: 25 g; Carbohydrates: 14 g; Fat: 11 g; Fiber: 2 g; Sodium: 76 mg; Vitamin C: 40 mg; B_6: 1 mg; Niacin: 17 mg; Riboflavin: 0.3 mg; Copper: 0.2 mg; Phosphorus: 243 mg; Selenium: 22 mcg; 1 CARB

(continued)

- To cook, have a serving platter ready for the cooked kebabs. Preheat the grill to high. When hot, lower the heat to medium. Spray the grill grate with the cooking spray. Grill the kebabs, uncovered, basting them occasionally with the reserved marinade. Turn and move the pieces and adjust the heat as needed, until the vegetables and chicken are nicely browned and the chicken is cooked through, 5 to 7 minutes. Cut a piece of chicken in half to check for doneness. Transfer the kebabs to the platter and serve promptly. Discard all leftover marinade.

Favorite Spaghetti and Meat Sauce

Protein, vitamin C, B vitamins, and folate boost your baby's cell, brain, and nervous system development, and fiber maintains your healthy digestive tract.

SPAGHETTI with meat sauce is always a crowd-pleaser. Feel free to add your favorite sauce ingredients and omit any of the items that your children or others might not like, such as the mushrooms, red bell peppers, or fresh herbs. Top your spaghetti with lots of Parmesan cheese, for calcium. And if you're pressed for time, you can use jarred pasta sauce. The meat sauce keeps for three days refrigerated, and it can be frozen for up to one month.

SERVES 8

SAUCE (MAKES ABOUT 8 CUPS)

2 tablespoons olive oil
1 onion, finely diced
2 garlic cloves, minced, or
    1 teaspoon garlic powder
2 teaspoons dried oregano
2 teaspoons Italian seasoning
1 pound lean ground beef
1 cup whole milk
8 ounces mushrooms (any
    kind), stems trimmed and
    thinly sliced
1 small red bell pepper, cored,
    seeded, and cut into
    small dice
1 (15-ounce) can tomato
    sauce
1 (14.5-ounce) can diced
    tomatoes (do not drain)
Salt and freshly ground black
    pepper

- Prepare the sauce: In a large, heavy-bottomed nonreactive saucepan, heat the olive oil over medium-high heat. Add the onion and sauté for 3 minutes. Add the garlic, oregano, and Italian seasoning and sauté for 1 minute longer.
- Crumble the ground beef into the saucepan and sauté for 5 minutes, stirring and breaking up any large lumps of meat with the back of a wooden spoon. Add the milk, mushrooms, and bell pepper and simmer gently for 30 minutes, or until most of the liquid has evaporated.

Meal ideas

- Green salad or green vegetable (Greek-Style Broccoli, page 248)
- Reduced-fat milk or yogurt
- Fresh fruit

Meal ideas and tips for diabetes

- Reduce your portion size of the pasta.
- Instead of pasta, serve the sauce on zucchini noodles (see page 169) or cauliflower rice (see page 271).
- Green salad or nonstarchy vegetable (above)

One eighth of the sauce and whole wheat pasta (without garnishes): Calories: 350 cals; Protein: 23 g; Carbohydrates: 50 g; Fat: 8 g; Fiber: 7 g; Sodium: 275 mg; Vitamin C: 22 mg; B_6: 0.6 mg; B_{12}: 1 mcg; Niacin: 13 mg; Riboflavin: 0.4 mg; Thiamine: 0.3 mg; Copper: 0.5 mg; Magnesium: 104 mg; Manganese: 2 mg; Phosphorus: 380 mg; Zinc: 5 mg; 4 CARBS

(continued)

16 ounces whole wheat
  spaghetti or your favorite
  pasta, cooked according to
  the package directions
3 to 4 tablespoons chopped
  fresh basil, parsley, or dill,
  for garnish
Grated Parmesan cheese,
  for serving

- Add the tomato sauce and diced tomatoes and simmer for 30 minutes longer, or until the sauce has thickened to your desired consistency. (Cook the pasta while the sauce is simmering.) Adjust the seasoning, add the basil, and serve over the spaghetti. Pass the cheese at the table.

Carrot Cake with Cream Cheese Frosting

Vitamin A enhances your baby's cell and nerve development.

WHEN your sweet tooth calls, head to the kitchen to bake this delicious cake. Frost it for a celebration or keep it simple for a family dessert or snack. Some grocery stores have salad bars that carry grated carrots, which makes the cake a cinch to make. An equal amount of all-purpose flour can be substituted for the whole wheat flour. Gluten-free? Use an equal amount of gluten-free all-purpose flour.

MAKES ONE 9 X 13-INCH CAKE; SERVES 12

CARROT CAKE

Cooking spray
¾ cup all-purpose flour, plus more for pan
¾ cup whole wheat flour
2 teaspoons baking soda
1½ teaspoons baking powder
2 teaspoons ground cinnamon
½ teaspoon salt
¾ cup canola oil
4 large eggs
1 cup granulated sugar
2 cups grated carrot (about 4 large carrots)
1 (8-ounce) can crushed pineapple, drained
½ cup chopped walnuts or pecans

- Preheat the oven to 350°F. Lightly spray with cooking spray and flour a 9 x 13 x 2-inch baking pan.
- In a large bowl, combine the flours, baking soda, baking powder, cinnamon, and salt, stir, and set aside.
- In a separate large bowl, combine the canola oil and eggs and beat with an electric mixer on medium speed for 3 minutes. Add the granulated sugar and beat for another 3 minutes. Add the flour mixture in three batches, beating on low speed and scraping the sides of the bowl after each addition. Mix just until the flour is absorbed. With a rubber spatula, fold in the carrot, pineapple, and walnuts until evenly distributed.
- Fill the baking pan with the batter and tap gently to release any air bubbles. Bake for about 45 minutes, or until a tester inserted into the center comes out clean. Remove from the oven and let stand for 5 minutes, then invert onto a wire rack. Let cool completely.

Tips for diabetes
- Skip the frosting.
- Reduce your portion size, or skip this recipe.

One twelfth of the cake: Calories: 309 cals; Protein: 5 g; Carbohydrates: 32 g; Fat: 19 g; Fiber: 2 g; Sodium: 315 mg; Vitamin A: 3,490 IU; Manganese: 0.6 mg; Selenium: 13 mcg; 2 CARBS

3 tablespoons (one twelfth) of the frosting: Calories: 197 cals; Protein: 1 g; Carbohydrates: 26 g; Fat: 10 g; Fiber: 0 g; Sodium: 60 mg; 2 CARBS

(continued)

CREAM CHEESE FROSTING (MAKES ABOUT 2½ CUPS)

1 (8-ounce) package
   cream cheese, at room
   temperature
4 tablespoons unsalted
   butter, at room
   temperature
1 tablespoon pure vanilla
   extract
3 cups confectioners' sugar

- Prepare the frosting: Combine the cream cheese and butter in a large bowl and beat with an electric mixer on medium speed for 2 minutes, or until creamy. Add the vanilla and 1½ cups of the confectioners' sugar and beat for 1 minute longer, scraping down the sides of the bowl as necessary. Add the remaining 1½ cups of the confectioners' sugar and beat until the frosting is smooth and creamy. If the frosting is too thin to spread, add a bit more confectioners' sugar. If it is too thick, thin it with 1 teaspoon of water at a time.

MONTH 6

Face, Hair, Lungs, Eyes, and Taste

Weeks 23 Through 27

This month is a time for exciting growth and development on the inside and out. By Week 23, your tiny tot is about 11 inches long from crown to rump, the size of a papaya. By Week 27, he or she has reached about 14 inches and weighs almost 2 pounds. Think about a head of cauliflower.

YOUR BABY'S DEVELOPMENT

- In Week 23, your baby's hearing is more acute. His or her body starts to gain fat, but the skin is still translucent.
- In Week 24, your baby's organs continue to develop. His or her gorgeous face is fully formed, and your little one might have hair.
- In Week 25, the bones are hardening, and hair continues to grow. The lungs are developing air sacs. Nostrils are opening. The vocal cords are forming.
- In Week 26, lungs have developed to the point where your baby begins to practice breathing. All oxygen goes through the placenta and umbilical cord until birth. Your baby's eyes open and blink.
- In Week 27, lungs are continuing to develop as breathing matures.

CHANGES IN YOUR BODY

The changes from Month 5 continue into Month 6. You will be navigating a growing belly and the joys and pitfalls that go along with it. Your baby will be very active.

IDEAL NUTRITION

Your nutrition focus is foods to enhance your baby's cell, brain, eye, organ, and bone development. The following nutrients will help achieve this.

- B vitamins: cell division, brain formation, nervous system development
- Calcium: bones and teeth
- Iron: maternal blood volume
- Magnesium: heart functioning, blood glucose regulation, blood pressure control
- Manganese: bone development, thyroid, blood glucose regulation, nervous system
- Omega-3s: brain, eye, nervous system development
- Potassium: nerve and muscle function
- Vitamin A: cell formation, bones, teeth, central nervous system, vision
- Vitamin C: iron absorption, healthy teeth and gums, immunity
- Vitamin D: calcium absorption

OPTIMAL FOODS FOR MONTH 6

PROTEIN	DAIRY	GRAINS/ LEGUMES	VEGETABLES	FRUITS	FATS/OTHER
Eggs	Cheese	All-bran cereal and other fortified breakfast cereals	Artichokes	Bananas	Brewer's or nutritional yeast
Meats	Enriched plant-based milks (rice soy, and almond)	Beans: soy, black, navy, pinto, kidney, white, great northern, black-eyed, pink, cranberry, Lima, and cannellini	Asparagus	Cantaloupe	Olive oil
Nuts: almonds, cashews, pistachios, Brazil nuts, walnuts, and nut butters	Fortified dairy milk	Chickpeas	Avocados	Citrus fruits and juices: oranges, tangerines, grapefruit, lemonade	Omega-3s
Pork	Fortified orange juice and other juices	Corn and flour tortillas	Baked potato with skin on and all other potatoes	Dried apricots and figs	Molasses, blackstrap
Poultry	Yogurt	Cream of Wheat	Beets	Guava	Seaweed, kelp, spirulina
Seafood (fish and shellfish): salmon (wild and Atlantic), tuna, mackerel, herring, sardines in oil, halibut, cod, catfish, canned oysters		Edamame	Broccoli and broccoli rabe	Kiwi	
		Folic acid–fortified products	Brussels sprouts	Lychee	
Seeds: sunflower, pumpkin, chia, hemp seed, and flaxseed		Lentils	Butternut squash	Mangoes	
		Oatmeal	Cabbage	Papaya	
Tahini		Peanuts	Carrots	Prune juice	
Tofu and tempeh		Wheat germ	Cauliflower	Pineapple	
		Whole grains: quinoa, barley, brown rice, bulgur, and whole wheat couscous	Dark, leafy greens: kale, collards, mustard, Swiss chard, bok choy, and turnip greens	Raspberries	
			Hearts of palm	Strawberries	
			Mushrooms		
			Pumpkin		
			Red bell peppers		
			Romaine lettuce		
			Snow peas		
			Spinach		
			Sweet potatoes		
			Tomatoes and tomato juice		

RECIPES FOR MONTH 6

Pineapple-Banana-Calcium Smoothie

Vitamin C and B vitamins enhance your baby's cell, brain, and nervous system development, and the calcium builds strong bones.

A delicious boost of energy to start your day—or get you through the day! Lactose intolerant or vegan? No worries. Lactose-free, soy, or coconut yogurt can be used. To sweeten, add a little bit of sugar, agave nectar, or honey. Need more protein? Add your favorite protein powder. Use water or juice to adjust the consistency. This will keep a day in the fridge and can be frozen. Mix well before serving. See "Freezing Bananas for Smoothies and N'ice Cream," page 176, for instructions on the best way to freeze bananas.

MAKES 3 CUPS

¾ cup plain yogurt
1 medium-size fresh or
    frozen banana
½ cup fresh pineapple,
    chopped, or canned
    pineapple in natural juices,
    drained
3 tablespoons powdered milk
½ cup orange juice or water
Ice cubes

- Place all the ingredients, except the ice, in a blender and process until smooth. Serve over ice.

Tips for diabetes

- Reduce your portion size, or skip this recipe.
- Use water instead of orange juice, and reduce or skip the bananas.

1½ **cups pineapple-banana-calcium smoothie:** Calories: 196 cals; Protein: 9 g; Carbohydrates: 38 g; Fat: 2 g; Fiber: 2 g; Sodium: 101 mg; Vitamin C: 43 mg; B$_{12}$: 0.5 mcg; Riboflavin: 0.3 mg; Calcium: 263 mg; 2½ CARBS

Weekend Pecan Waffles

Protein, B vitamins, and folate promote your baby's cell, brain, and nervous system development and muscle building.

THESE waffles are a weekend treat that can be refrigerated or frozen for weekday breakfast bliss. If you do not have whole wheat flour, you can use 1¾ cups of all-purpose flour or oat flour (page 265); gluten-free flour works, too. Dairy-free or vegan? Use your favorite nondairy milk and coconut oil instead of butter and omit the eggs. Need more calcium? In a measuring cup, mix ⅓ cup of pasteurized instant nonfat dry milk with the milk until dissolved, then follow the directions in Step 2. (Waffles made with instant nonfat dry milk tend to be heavier.) Need more fiber? Add 2 tablespoons of ground flaxseeds to the batter in Step 1. To prevent cooked waffles from getting soggy, lean them up against each other in a tentlike position to allow the steam to escape. If they do get soggy or cold, toast them briefly in a toaster or place them directly on the rack of a 350°F oven for a few minutes.

MAKES ABOUT EIGHTEEN 5½ X 2¼-INCH WAFFLES

¾ cup whole wheat flour
1 cup all-purpose flour
1 tablespoon baking powder
1 tablespoon sugar
½ teaspoon salt
2 large eggs
1 large egg white
6 tablespoons unsalted butter, melted, plus more for waffle iron (optional)
2 cups reduced-fat milk
½ cup chopped pecans, toasted
2 tablespoons ground flaxseeds (optional)
Cooking spray (optional)

- Place the flours, baking powder, sugar, and salt in a large bowl and whisk together.
- In a second bowl or large measuring cup, whisk together the eggs, egg white, melted butter, and milk.
- Add the wet ingredients to the dry and whisk together until well blended. Stir in the pecans and ground flaxseeds, if using.
- Preheat the waffle iron on its HIGH setting. Spray the waffle grids with cooking spray or brush with melted butter. Spoon some batter onto the hot iron and spread to within ¼ inch of the edges. Close the lid and cook until the waffles are golden brown. Repeat with the remaining batter. Serve immediately.

Meal ideas

- Protein, such as eggs, dairy, or plant-based
- Reduced-fat milk or yogurt
- Fresh fruit (Refreshing Fruit Salad, page 130)

Meal ideas and tips for diabetes

- Reduce your portion size, or skip this recipe.
- Use a low-sugar jam (such as Polaner All Fruit; 2 teaspoons are FREE), or low-sugar syrup.
- Protein, such as natural nut butter or eggs, 1 CARB

3 waffles: Calories: 371 cals; Protein: 10g; Carbohydrates: 35 g; Fat: 22 g; Fiber: 4 g; Sodium: 247 mg; Niacin: 4 mg; B$_{12}$: 0.5 mg; Thiamine: 0.3 mg; Riboflavin: 0.3 mg; Folate: 82 mcg; Copper: 0.2 mg; Manganese: 1 mg; Selenium: 23 mcg: 2 CARBS

Pasta, Bean, and Vegetable Soup

Protein, vitamins A, C, and K, B vitamins, and folate optimize your baby's cell, brain, nervous system, bone, and muscle development.

THIS nourishing soup is sure to become a family favorite. For a real treat, garnish it with pesto and grated Parmesan cheese. On the veggie scene, add your favorites that require a long cooking time, such as potatoes, winter squash, or leeks, in Step 1. Add any quick-cooking vegetables, such as broccoli or cauliflower florets, summer squash, corn, peas, and green beans, in Step 2. Need more protein? Add sautéed tofu or diced cooked meat. Gluten-free? Use rice or your favorite grain instead of pasta. Refrigerate leftovers for three days or freeze for up to one month. Slow cooker instructions follow.

SERVES 8; MAKES ABOUT 8 CUPS

3 tablespoons olive oil
1 medium-size onion, diced
2 garlic cloves, crushed
5 carrots, cut lengthwise in half, and sliced, or 2 cups sliced peeled baby carrots
2 teaspoons dried thyme, oregano, basil, or a mixture, or herbes de Provence
1 teaspoon salt, or to taste
5 cups stock (6 cups if not using the V8 juice, or more if needed)
1½ cups V8 or tomato juice
1 (14.5-ounce) can diced tomatoes (do not drain), or 2 cups diced fresh tomatoes

- Heat the olive oil in a 6-quart saucepan over medium-high heat. Add the onion and sauté for 2 minutes. Add the garlic, carrots, and thyme and sauté for 3 minutes. Add the salt, stock, and V8 juice, and bring to a boil. Lower the heat and simmer, uncovered, for 10 minutes.
- Add the tomatoes, beans, zucchini, and pasta, lower the heat, and simmer for 15 to 20 minutes, or until the pasta is cooked. Add the baby spinach during the last 10 minutes of cooking.
- Adjust the seasoning, and thin the soup with stock or water, if desired. Serve immediately and pass the pesto and cheese at the table, if desired.

Meal ideas

- Protein, such as meat, poultry, seafood, eggs, dairy, or plant-based (Chicken Salad with Dried Apricots and Almonds, page 216)
- Reduced-fat milk or yogurt
- Fresh fruit

Meal ideas and tips for diabetes

- Skip the ditalini pasta in the soup or use less, if necessary.
- Protein, such as meat, poultry, seafood, eggs, dairy, or plant-based (above)
- Fresh fruit, 1 CARB

(continues)

1 cup pasta bean soup (made with chicken stock): Calories: 235 cals; Protein: 11 g; Carbohydrates: 32 g; Fat: 8 g; Fiber: 5 g; Sodium: 549 mg; Vitamin A: 7,041 IU; Vitamin C: 48 mg; Vitamin K: 82 mcg; Thiamine: 0.3 mg; Riboflavin: 0.3 mg; Folate: 120 mcg; Copper: 0.3 mg; Manganese: 0.5 mg; Selenium: 10 mcg: 2 CARBS

1 (15.5-ounce) can great
    northern beans, drained
    and rinsed
1 medium-size zucchini,
    quartered lengthwise, and
    sliced
¾ cup ditalini pasta, or other
    small dried pasta
4 cups baby spinach
    (1 [6-ounce] bag)
Freshly ground black pepper
Pesto or fresh herbs, for
    serving (optional)
Grated Parmesan cheese or
    your favorite cheese, for
    serving (optional)

SLOW COOKER INSTRUCTIONS:

- Reduce the stock by ½ cup. Use only ½ cup of dried pasta.

- Using a skillet instead of a saucepan, or your Instant Pot, sauté the onion as directed in Step 1, then add the garlic, carrots, and thyme and sauté for 3 more minutes.

- Transfer the contents of the skillet to the slow cooker, and add the salt, stock, V8 juice, and diced tomatoes. Cover and cook on HIGH for 6 hours. During the last 30 minutes of cooking, add the beans, pasta, and Swiss chard. (Note: Do not leave the slow cooker unattended while cooking the pasta.) Finish the soup as directed in Step 3.

Creamy Cauliflower Soup

Protein, vitamins A and K, and B vitamins promote your baby's cell, brain, nervous system, bone, and muscle development.

CHEESE and cauliflower are a perfect match, and a healthy one, too. For a chunkier soup, puree all but 2 cups of the soup. Garnish with chopped fresh cilantro or parsley. This soup keeps refrigerated for three days. It does not freeze well.

SERVES 6; MAKES ABOUT 7 CUPS

3 tablespoons olive oil
1 medium-size onion, chopped
4 cups cauliflower florets (about 1 pound)
1 medium-size potato, peeled and diced
½ teaspoon salt, or to taste
4 cups chicken or vegetable stock
4 cups baby spinach
1½ cups whole milk
1 cup grated sharp Cheddar cheese, Fontina, or Monterey Jack
Freshly ground black pepper
¼ cup chopped fresh parsley or cilantro, for garnish

- Heat the olive oil in a 6-quart saucepan over medium-high heat. Add the onion and sauté for 3 minutes. Add the cauliflower florets, potato, salt, and chicken stock and bring to a boil, then lower the heat and simmer for 15 to 20 minutes, or until the potato and cauliflower are tender. During the last 5 minutes of cooking, add the spinach. Remove from the heat.

- Allow the soup to cool slightly, then puree it, using an immersion or regular blender. Return the pureed soup to the rinsed-out saucepan. Add the milk and bring just to a boil over medium-high heat. Add the cheese, lower the heat to low, and stir until the cheese is melted—do not let the soup boil after adding the cheese.

- Adjust the seasoning, garnish with the parsley, and serve.

Meal ideas

- Protein, such as meat, poultry, seafood, eggs, dairy, or plant-based (Asian-Inspired Spinach Salad, page 186)
- Whole wheat bread or roll
- Reduced-fat milk or yogurt
- Fresh fruit

Meal ideas and tips for diabetes

- Protein, such as meat, poultry, seafood, eggs, dairy, or plant-based (above)
- Reduced-fat milk or unsweetened reduced-fat yogurt, 1 CARB

1 cup cauliflower soup (made with chicken stock): Calories: 269 cals; Protein: 12 g; Carbohydrates: 18 g; Fat: 17 g; Fiber: 1 g; Sodium: 591 mg; Vitamin A: 2,428 IU, Vitamin K: 144 mcg; B_{12}: 0.5 mcg; Copper: 0.2 mg; Selenium: 12 mcg; 1 CARB

Salad in a Jar with Classic Vinaigrette

GF

Protein, vitamins A, C, E, and K, B vitamins, folate, calcium, and iron promote your baby's overall growth and development, as well as provide nutrients for you, plus fiber.

THIS salad wins the award for one of the most nutrient-dense recipes in this book! Jarred salads are a healthy craze—you'll love them when you're on the go. Having a supply of homemade salad dressings (see page 214) on hand is ideal, but in a pinch, store-bought dressings are great. Feel totally free to add what you like and take out what you don't. Vegans and those who are lactose intolerant can skip the cheese or add a nondairy cheese. See "Shelf Life for Common Salad Ingredients," page 213, to help you determine how to combine ingredients according to their shelf life for ultimate freshness. You will need a 1-quart (32-ounce) mason jar, or any jar of similar size.

MAKES 1 SALAD

3 tablespoons Classic Vinaigrette (page 214), or your favorite dressing
⅓ cup cooked or canned kidney beans, chickpeas, or your favorite beans or lentils
½ cup diced tomatoes or cherry tomatoes
⅓ cup diced cucumber
¼ cup crumbled pasteurized feta or your favorite cheese
½ cup cooked quinoa, or your favorite grain
2 tablespoons seeds, such as pumpkin or sunflower
2 tablespoons nuts, such as walnuts or pecans
About 2 to 3 cups baby spinach, to fill the jar
Fresh herbs (optional)

- Place the dressing at the bottom of the mason jar. Layer with the beans, tomatoes, cucumber, feta, quinoa, seeds, and nuts. Finish with the spinach on top and fresh herbs, if using. Place a lid on the mason jar and refrigerate until ready to dump into a large bowl and enjoy.

Meal ideas
- Whole wheat bread or roll
- Reduced-fat milk or yogurt

Meal ideas and tips for diabetes
- Skip or swap out the beans for a protein, such as cooked chicken or eggs.
- Reduced-fat milk or unsweetened reduced-fat yogurt, 1 CARB

1 jarred salad with 3 tablespoons classic vinaigrette: Calories: 747 cals; Protein: 24 g; Carbohydrates: 43 g; Fat: 55 g; Fiber: 11 g; Sodium: 657 mg; Vitamin A: 7,375 IU; Vitamin C: 31 mg; Vitamin E: 6 mg; Vitamin K: 371 mcg; B_6: 0.5 mg; B_{12}: 0.6 mcg; Riboflavin: 0.5 mg; Thiamine: 0.3 mg; Folate: 243 mcg; Copper: 0.8 mg; Calcium: 327 mg; Iron: 7 mg; Magnesium: 229 mg; Manganese: 2 mg; Phosphorus: 644 mg; Selenium: 12 mcg; Zinc: 5 mg; 2½ CARBS

KITCHEN WISDOM: SHELF LIFE FOR COMMON SALAD INGREDIENTS

HAVING a salad every day as part of your meal plan is an excellent idea. Prepping the ingredients for the week makes assembling a delicious salad a cinch. Here are some tips for the shelf-life of salad ingredients. Please check out our recipes for Awesome Homemade Salad Dressings on pages 214 to 215, and our Salad in a Jar with Classic Vinaigrette on page 212.

Add on the same day
  Peeled hard-boiled eggs (unpeeled last longer)
  Avocado
  Nuts and seeds

Prep 2 days in advance
  Cooked vegetables: asparagus, broccoli, cauliflower, green beans, zucchini, peas, corn, edamame
  Fresh vegetables: mushrooms, carrots, broccoli, cauliflower, tomatoes
  Fresh greens (unless prewashed)
  Onions, scallions, fresh herbs
  Fresh fruit (unless they brown, such as freshly cut apples and pears)

Prep 5 days in advance
  Cheese: feta, mozzarella, Cheddar, goat, Swiss, Parmesan
  Cooked beans
  Unpeeled hard-boiled eggs
  Whole grains, pasta, and rice
  Salad dressings

Awesome Homemade Salad Dressings GF DF V LC

Zero-carb homemade goodness for mom and baby.

OUR Classic Vinaigrette and Balsamic Dressing are perfect for all salads and vegetables. The hearty sun-dried tomato and basil dressing is great on vegetables (especially cooked potatoes), on pasta, or drizzled on a sandwich. Once you've tried these homemade dressings, and you see just how easy they are to make, you'll find it hard to go back to the store-bought stuff.

CLASSIC VINAIGRETTE

MAKES ABOUT ⅔ CUP

1 tablespoon Dijon mustard
¼ cup cider vinegar
½ teaspoon dried tarragon, basil, or oregano (optional)
Pinch of salt
Pinch of sugar
Pinch of garlic powder (optional)
Freshly ground black pepper
¼ cup canola oil
¼ cup olive oil, or your favorite oil

- Combine all the ingredients, except the oil, in a jar with a lid or in a small bowl and shake or whisk until well blended. Cover and refrigerate for up to 1 week. Whisk or shake before serving.

1 tablespoon vinaigrette: Calories: 81 cals; Protein: 0 g; Carbohydrates: 0 g; Fat: 9 g; Fiber: 0 g; Sodium: 10 mg; 0 CARBS

BALSAMIC DRESSING

MAKES ABOUT ⅔ CUP

1 teaspoon Dijon mustard
Salt and freshly ground black pepper
2 tablespoons balsamic vinegar
2 teaspoons freshly squeezed lemon juice, or to taste
Pinch of garlic powder
¼ cup canola oil

- Combine the mustard, salt, pepper, vinegar, lemon juice, and garlic powder and 2 tablespoons of water in a small bowl and mix well. In a slow stream, whisk in the canola oil until emulsified. Adjust the seasoning. Cover and refrigerate for up to 1 week. Whisk or shake before serving.

1 tablespoon balsamic dressing: Calories: 51 cals; Protein: 0 g; Carbohydrates: 1 g; Fat: 5 g; Fiber: 0 g; Sodium: 12 mg; 0 CARBS

(continued)

SUN-DRIED TOMATO AND BASIL DRESSING

MAKES ABOUT ¾ CUP

⅓ cup sun-dried tomatoes packed in oil
2 teaspoons red wine vinegar
2 teaspoons balsamic vinegar
¼ cup canola oil
¼ cup boiling water, plus 3 to 4 tablespoons as needed
½ teaspoon dried oregano or Italian seasoning
Salt and freshly ground black pepper

- Combine all the ingredients in a blender or food processor and process until smooth. The dressing can be thinned to your desired consistency with up to 4 tablespoons of additional hot water, added 1 tablespoon at a time. Cover and refrigerate for up to 5 days. Whisk or shake before serving.

1 tablespoon sun-dried tomato dressing: Calories: 110 cals; Protein: 0 g; Carbohydrates: 2 g; Fat: 4 g; Fiber: 0 g; Sodium: 7 mg; 0 CARBS

Chicken Salad with Dried Apricots and Almonds

GF DF LC

Protein, vitamins A, C, and E, and B vitamins boost your baby's cell, brain, nervous system, bone, and muscle development.

A favorite chicken salad that is terrific on toasted whole-grain bread (gluten-free if necessary) or on a bed of mixed greens. Buy a rotisserie chicken or packaged cooked chicken in the deli section. Feel free to add your favorite spices, herbs, and other ingredients. Some nice additions are cooked edamame, diced celery, toasted pine nuts, and a dash of curry powder. You'll keep coming back to this recipe—many of our readers do.

MAKES ABOUT 3 CUPS SALAD

2½ cups diced cooked
　　chicken
⅓ cup chopped dried apricots
2 tablespoons chopped fresh
　　herbs, such as dill
½ red bell pepper, seeded
　　and finely diced, or ¼ cup
　　chopped jarred roasted red
　　peppers
⅓ cup sliced almonds, toasted
2 tablespoons pumpkin or
　　sunflower seeds
½ cup light mayonnaise,
　　or to taste
Squeeze of lemon juice,
　　or to taste
Salt and freshly ground black
　　pepper

- Combine all the ingredients in a bowl and mix well. Adjust the seasoning. Refrigerate if not serving immediately.

Meal ideas

- Green salad or vegetable (Gazpacho [Without the Gas], page 289)
- Whole wheat bread or roll
- Reduced-fat milk or yogurt
- Fresh fruit

Meal ideas and tips for diabetes

- Green salad or nonstarchy vegetable (above)
- Whole wheat bread or roll, 1 CARB

1 cup chicken salad: Calories: 371 cals; Protein: 42 g; Carbohydrates: 11 g; Fat: 16 g; Fiber: 4 g; Sodium: 108 mg; Vitamin A: 1,358 IU; Vitamin C: 34 mg; Vitamin E: 5 mg; B$_6$: 1 mg; Niacin: 26 mg; Riboflavin: 0.3 mg; Choline: 115 mg; Copper: 0.4 mg; Magnesium: 119 mg; Manganese: 0.6 mg; Phosphorus: 432 mg; Zinc: 2 mg; 1 CARB

Classic Creamed Spinach

LC

Vitamins A, C, and K, B vitamins, folate, and calcium enhance your baby's cell, brain, nervous system, and bone development, plus it offers you calcium.

FEELING like you need some healthy comfort food? This creamed spinach is going to make you happy. Filled with vitamins and minerals, it's delicious and nutritious. Leftovers keep refrigerated for three days.

SERVES 3; MAKES ABOUT 1½ CUPS

1 (10-ounce) package frozen chopped spinach, cooked and drained, or 1 (10- or 12-ounce) package fresh baby spinach

2 tablespoons unsalted butter

¼ cup chopped onion (preferably a sweet onion, such as Vidalia)

2 tablespoons all-purpose flour

½ cup whole milk

½ cup shredded Monterey Jack cheese or an easy melting cheese

Salt and freshly ground black pepper

- If using fresh spinach, place about 2 cups of water in a large saucepan, add a pinch of salt, and bring to a boil. Add the spinach and cook for about 3 minutes, or just until wilted. Drain and cool, then squeeze dry, coarsely chop, and set aside.

- Melt the butter in a large saucepan (you can use the same saucepan used to cook the fresh spinach) over medium-high heat. Add the onion and sauté for 3 minutes, or until lightly browned. Add the flour and continue to sauté for 30 seconds, then add the milk, stirring constantly, and cook, stirring, until smooth and slightly thickened, 1 to 3 minutes. Add the spinach and cheese and stir to heat through. Season, then serve immediately.

Meal ideas

- Protein, such as meat, poultry, seafood, eggs, dairy, or plant-based (Make It Again Meat Loaf, page 95)
- Whole grain or starch
- Reduced-fat milk or yogurt
- Fresh fruit

Meal ideas and tips for diabetes

- Protein, such as meat, poultry, seafood, eggs, dairy, or plant-based (above)
- Whole grain or starch, 1 CARB
- Reduced-fat milk or unsweetened reduced fat yogurt, 1 CARB

½ cup creamed spinach: Calories: 209 cals; Protein: 9 g; Carbohydrates: 11 g; Fat: 15 g; Fiber: 2 g; Sodium: 207 mg; Vitamin A: 9,309 IU; Vitamin C: 28 mg; Vitamin K: 458 mcg; Riboflavin: 0.4 mg; Folate: 201 mcg; Calcium: 286 mg; Magnesium: 86 mg; Manganese: 1 mg; 1 CARB

Light and Healthy Vegetable Ragout

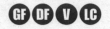

Vitamins A, C, and K enhance your baby's cell, brain, nervous system, and bone development, plus vitamin C for your immunity.

THIS versatile ragout works with anything—from eggs in the morning to a grilled steak at night. Thinned with some tomato sauce or crushed tomatoes, it turns into a fabulous sauce for vegetarian or vegan lasagne. Use your favorite veggies in whatever amounts you want. Adjust the liquid to your desired consistency. Short on time? Pick up veggies at a salad bar. Refrigerate for three days or freeze for up to one month. Slow cooker or Instant Pot instructions follow.

SERVES 8; MAKES ABOUT 8 CUPS

⅓ cup olive oil
1 medium-size onion, chopped
2 garlic cloves, minced
1 tablespoon dried oregano
1 large carrot, peeled and coarsely grated
1 red bell pepper, cored, seeded, and diced
2 small purple eggplant (about 1 pound total), diced
2 (14.5-ounce) cans diced tomatoes, drained
1¼ cups tomato or V8 juice
1½ teaspoons sugar
1 medium-size zucchini, diced
1 (14-ounce) can quartered-artichoke hearts
¼ cup chopped fresh basil or cilantro
Salt and freshly ground black pepper

- Heat the olive oil in a 6-quart nonreactive saucepan over medium-high heat. Add the onion and sauté for 3 minutes. Add the garlic, oregano, carrot, and bell pepper and continue to sauté for 3 minutes, stirring frequently.

- Add the eggplant and cook, stirring constantly, for 3 minutes. Add the tomatoes, tomato juice, and sugar, stir, then lower the heat and gently simmer, uncovered, for 15 minutes, stirring occasionally. Add the zucchini and artichoke hearts, stir, and cook for about 25 minutes, or until the vegetables are tender and the sauce has reached the desired consistency.

- Add the basil and season with salt and pepper to taste.

Meal ideas

- Protein, such as meat, poultry, seafood, eggs, dairy, or plant-based (Grilled or Broiled Lamb Chops, page 228)
- Whole grain or starch
- Reduced-fat milk or yogurt
- Fresh fruit

Meal ideas and tips for diabetes

- Protein, such as meat, poultry, seafood, eggs, dairy, or plant-based (above)
- Whole grain or starch, 1 CARB
- Reduced-fat milk or unsweetened reduced-fat yogurt, 1 CARB

1 cup vegetable ragout: Calories: 160 cals; Protein: 3 g; Carbohydrates: 18 g; Fat: 9 g; Fiber: 5 g; Sodium: 365 mg; Vitamin A: 4,463 IU; Vitamin C: 83 mg; Vitamin K: 24 mcg; 1 CARB

(continued)

SLOW COOKER OR INSTANT POT INSTRUCTIONS:

- Follow Step 1, use your Instant Pot if you have one, then add the eggplant and cook, stirring constantly, for 3 minutes.

- Transfer the contents of the skillet to the slow cooker and add the tomatoes, tomato juice, sugar, and zucchini. Cover and cook on HIGH for 5 hours. Note: If you prefer a slightly thicker sauce, add 2 tablespoons of quick-dissolving flour during the last 15 minutes of cooking. Finish the ragout as directed in Step 3.

Mexican-Style Rice and Beans

B vitamins and folate optimize your baby's cell, brain, and nervous system development.

THIS new recipe for Mexican-style rice is a winner among family and friends. The squeeze of fresh lime and cilantro brighten the dish. Lots of ingredients are listed here, but many of them are spices. So, give it a try; you'll be really happy you did. Leftovers keep for three days refrigerated and can be frozen for one month.

SERVES 6

2 tablespoons olive oil
1 onion, chopped
2 garlic cloves, minced
1 tablespoon minced fresh or jarred serrano or jalapeño chiles (optional)
1 teaspoon roasted ground cumin
1 teaspoon dried oregano
1 teaspoon paprika
Pinch of red pepper flakes (optional)
1½ cups long-grain white rice
1 (14.5-ounce) can diced tomatoes, or 1½ cups diced ripe tomatoes
½ teaspoon salt, or to taste
¾ cup canned black beans, or any kind of canned bean, drained and rinsed
Grated zest and juice of 1 lime, or to taste
3 tablespoons chopped fresh cilantro

- In a large saucepan, heat the olive oil over medium heat until hot. Add the onion, garlic, and chiles and sauté, stirring occasionally, for 3 minutes. Add the cumin, oregano, paprika, and red pepper flakes, if using, and sauté for 30 seconds longer, then add the rice and sauté, stirring, for 2 minutes.

- Mix in the tomatoes, add 1½ cups of water and the salt, then stir and bring to a boil. Lower the heat and gently simmer, covered, for 15 to 20 minutes, or until the rice is tender and all the water has been absorbed. Remove from the heat, stir in the black beans, and let stand, covered, for 10 minutes. Adjust the seasoning, then add the lime zest and juice. Sprinkle with the cilantro and serve.

Meal ideas

- Protein, such as meat, poultry, seafood, eggs, dairy, or plant-based (Chili-Rubbed Pork Chops, page 174)
- Green salad or vegetable
- Reduced-fat milk or yogurt
- Fresh fruit

Meal ideas and tips for diabetes

- Reduce your portion size, if necessary.
- Protein, such as meat, poultry, seafood, eggs, dairy, or plant-based (above)
- Green salad
- Reduced-fat milk or unsweetened reduced-fat yogurt, 1 CARB

⅔ **cup rice and beans:** Calories: 258 cals; Protein: 6 g; Carbohydrates: 47 g; Fat: 5 g; Fiber: 4 g; Sodium: 200 mg; Niacin: 4 mg; Thiamine: 0.4 mg; Folate: 152 mcg; Copper: 0.2 mg; Manganese: 0.7 mg; 3 CARBS

Twenty-Minute Tomato Sauce

GF **DF** **V** **Q** **LC**

Vitamins A and C promote cell health and immunity.

THIS quick tomato sauce is a great stand-in when you're out of jarred sauce or you have gorgeous ripe tomatoes that are begging to be made into a light sauce. Make a big batch and freeze it.

MAKES ABOUT 2½ CUPS

¼ cup olive oil
2 garlic cloves, minced
2 pounds tomatoes
    (about 7 large), cut into
    ½-inch dice
1 tablespoon Italian seasoning
1 tablespoon light brown sugar
1 teaspoon salt
Freshly ground black pepper
2 tablespoons tomato puree
⅓ cup chopped basil or your
    favorite fresh herbs

- In a large saucepan, combine the olive oil and garlic and sauté over medium-high heat, stirring occasionally, for 2 minutes, or until light golden. Add the tomatoes, Italian seasoning, brown sugar, and salt and pepper to taste and simmer for 10 minutes, stirring occasionally.
- Stir in the tomato puree and continue to simmer for 10 minutes. Add the basil, adjust the seasoning, and serve.

Meal ideas

- Protein, such as meat, poultry, seafood, eggs, dairy, or plant-based (Easy-Bake Meatballs, page 222)
- Whole wheat pasta or grains
- Reduced-fat milk or yogurt
- Green salad or vegetable

Meal ideas and tips for diabetes

- Protein, such as meat, poultry, seafood, eggs, dairy, or plant-based (above)
- Whole wheat pasta or grains, 1 or 2 CARBS
- Green salad or nonstarchy vegetable, 1 CARB

½ cup tomato sauce: Calories: 117 cals; Protein: 2 g; Carbohydrates: 8 g; Fat: 9 g; Fiber: 2 g; Sodium: 398 mg; Vitamin A: 1,409 IU; Vitamin C: 20 mg; ½ CARB

Easy-Bake Meatballs

Protein, vitamins A and K, and B vitamins foster your baby's cell, brain, nervous system, and bone development.

IF you're a meatball fan, you just gotta try these amazing baked balls! Freeze some for busy nights when you're exhausted and can't face the kitchen. Pinched for time? Frozen spinach, thawed and drained, can be substituted for the fresh; skip sautéing it in Step 2. If you don't have small muffin pans, roll the meatballs by hand and cook them in a skillet, or in tomato sauce. The meatballs can be refrigerated for three days or frozen for one month. To really rock these meatballs, see "How to Check the Flavor of Your Meat Loaf, Burgers, or Meatballs" on page 96.

**MAKES 24 MEATBALLS;
ABOUT 8 SERVINGS**

1 tablespoon olive oil
4 cups fresh baby spinach
    (1 [6-ounce] bag)
8 ounces ground lean pork
8 ounces ground lean beef
½ cup finely grated Parmesan
    cheese
2 large eggs
2 teaspoons dried oregano or
    Italian seasoning
1 teaspoon garlic powder
1 teaspoon salt
½ teaspoon red pepper flakes
½ cup bread crumbs or panko
¼ cup ground flaxseeds
    (optional)
Cooking spray

- Heat the olive oil in a large skillet and sauté the spinach until just wilted. Remove from the heat.
- In a large mixing bowl, combine the pork, beef, Parmesan, eggs, oregano, garlic powder, salt, red pepper flakes, bread crumbs, and flaxseeds, if using, and the spinach. Using your hands, mix all the ingredients until well incorporated and refrigerate if not using immediately.
- When ready to cook, place a baking pan or piece of aluminum on the middle oven rack to catch any juices that run off. Preheat the oven to 400°F. Spray a twenty-four-well mini muffin pan with cooking spray, or if you have a smaller mini muffin pan, bake in batches.

Meal ideas

- Green salad or vegetable (Twenty-Minute Tomato Sauce, page 221)
- Whole wheat pasta or whole grains
- Reduced-fat milk or yogurt
- Fresh fruit

Meal ideas and tips for diabetes

- Green salad or nonstarchy vegetable (above)
- Whole wheat pasta or whole grains, 1 CARB
- Reduced-fat milk or unsweetened reduced-fat yogurt, 1 CARB

3 meatballs: Calories: 170 cals; Protein: 17 g; Carbohydrates: 7 g; Fat: 8 g; Fiber: 2 g; Sodium: 495 mg; Vitamin A: 1,120 IU; Vitamin K: 53 mcg; B$_6$: 0.4 mg; B$_{12}$: 1 mcg; Niacin: 7 mg; Riboflavin: 0.3 mg; Thiamine: 0.3 mg; Selenium: 23 mcg; Zinc: 3 mg; ½ CARB

(continued)

- Using a heaping tablespoon or a mini ice-cream scooper, portion out the meatball mixture on a large plate (it's okay to stack the portions). Using your hands, shape the meatballs into rounds, and place one ball in each prepared muffin well. The meat should rise above the rim of the cup like a fully baked crowned muffin.

- Bake for 20 minutes, or until golden and cooked through. Remove from the oven and serve on top of pasta with your favorite sauce.

Baked Salmon with Mustard-Dill Sauce

Protein, vitamin D, B vitamins, and omega-3 DHA enhance your baby's muscle, bone, brain, and nerve development.

AN easy and satisfying dish when salmon is on your shopping list. The sauce can be made two days in advance. If you don't have whole-grain Dijon mustard, use regular Dijon. The salmon can be baked, broiled, panfried, or grilled (check our other salmon recipes for ideas and instructions). Serve on top of a bed of greens for a lovely presentation and healthy meal.

SERVES 4

DILL MARINADE

3 tablespoons freshly
  squeezed lemon juice
1½ tablespoons olive oil
3 tablespoons chopped
  fresh dill
Sprinkle of salt
Sprinkle of freshly ground
  black pepper

4 skinless center-cut salmon
  fillets, about 4 ounces
  each, rinsed and patted
  with paper towels

- Marinate the salmon: Combine all the marinade ingredients in a Pyrex baking dish and mix well, then add the salmon and turn to coat evenly with the marinade. Cover and refrigerate for at least 1 hour, or up to 6.

- Prepare the sauce: Combine all the sauce ingredients in a small bowl and mix well. Cover and refrigerate.

- Center an oven rack and preheat the oven to 400°F. Line a rimmed baking sheet with parchment paper or foil.

Meal ideas

- Whole grain or starch
- Green salad or vegetable (Beets with Goat Cheese and Greens, page 269)
- Reduced-fat milk or yogurt
- Fresh fruit

Meal ideas and tips for diabetes

- Whole grain or starch, 1 CARB
- Green salad or nonstarchy vegetable (above)
- Reduced-fat milk or unsweetened reduced-fat yogurt, 1 CARB

1 salmon fillet with 2 tablespoons sauce: Calories: 268 cals; Protein: 23 g; Carbohydrates: 0 g; Fat: 18 g; Fiber: 0 g; Sodium: 268 mg; Vitamin D: 500 IU; B_6: 0.7 mg; B_{12}: 4 mcg; Niacin: 10 mg; Thiamine: 0.2 mg; Phosphorus: 282 mg; Selenium: 28 mcg; Omega-3 DHA: 1.2 g; 0 CARBS

(continued)

MUSTARD-DILL SAUCE (MAKES A LITTLE LESS THAN ½ CUP)

2 tablespoons Dijon mustard, or to taste

¼ cup sour cream or Greek yogurt

3 tablespoons finely chopped fresh dill or your favorite fresh herb

2 teaspoons capers (optional)

Freshly squeezed lemon or lime juice

Freshly ground black pepper

- Place the salmon, skin side down, on the prepared baking sheet. Bake for 10 to 15 minutes (depending on the thickness), or until cooked through when flaked with the tip of a knife in the thickest part of the flesh. (There is no need to turn the fish, but you can if you want to.) Transfer the salmon to individual plates or a serving platter and evenly divide the sauce over the top, or serve it on the side.

Terrific Turkey Chili

DF

Protein, vitamins A and C, B vitamins, and folate optimize your baby's muscle, bone, and overall development, plus fiber helps your digestion stay on track.

A great fix-it-and-forget-it recipe. This light and flavorful turkey chili pairs well with rice or any whole grain, or serve it on a bun. Possible garnishes include diced avocado, grated reduced-fat Cheddar cheese or fat-free sour cream (use dairy-free, if necessary), diced ripe tomatoes, sliced scallions, and chopped cilantro. It can be frozen in single-serving portions for easy weeknight dinners that make you a happy camper.

SERVES 8

2 (15.25-ounce) cans kidney beans, drained and rinsed (about 3 cups)
1 (14.5-ounce) can diced tomatoes, with juice
2 tablespoons olive oil
1½ pounds ground turkey
1 large onion, chopped
1 red bell pepper, cored, seeded, and diced
1½ tablespoons chili powder
1 teaspoon roasted ground cumin
1 teaspoon dried oregano or Italian seasoning
1 teaspoon paprika
2 teaspoons garlic powder
1 teaspoon salt
2 teaspoons light brown sugar
1 (8-ounce) can tomato sauce
1½ cups tomato juice
1 to 2 tablespoons cornstarch, if needed

- Place the kidney beans in a bowl, then transfer one third of them to the bowl of a food processor. Add the diced tomatoes and their juices and process until fairly smooth; set aside.
- Heat 1 tablespoon of the olive oil in a large, heavy-bottomed saucepan over medium-high heat. Add the turkey and sauté, breaking it up with a wooden spoon, until it loses its raw color, about 5 minutes. Transfer to a heatproof bowl and set aside. (Do not rinse the pot.)

Meal ideas

- Whole-grain or whole wheat bun
- Green salad or vegetables (Favorite Broccoli Slaw, page 291)
- Reduced-fat milk or yogurt
- Fresh fruit

Meal ideas and tips for diabetes

- Reduce the amount of kidney beans or skip them.
- Whole grain, 1 CARB
- Green salad or nonstarchy vegetable (above)

1 cup turkey chili: Calories: 255 cals; Protein: 27 g; Carbohydrates: 25 g; Fat: 6 g; Fiber: 6 g; Sodium: 579 mg; Vitamin A: 1,236 IU; Vitamin C: 60 mg; B_6: 0.9 mg; B_{12}: 0.4 mcg; Niacin: 10 mg; Thiamine: 0.2 mg; Folate: 122 mcg; Copper: 0.2 mg; Phosphorus: 320 mg; Selenium: 20 mcg; Zinc: 2 mg; 2 CARBS

(continued)

- Add the remaining 1 tablespoon of olive oil to the pot and heat over medium heat. Add the onion and bell pepper and sauté, stirring, for 3 minutes. Add the chili powder, cumin, oregano, paprika, garlic powder, salt, and brown sugar and cook for 2 minutes. Add the whole kidney beans, the pureed kidney bean mixture, and the cooked turkey and stir until well combined. Add the tomato sauce and tomato juice, bring to a boil, then lower the heat and gently simmer for 30 to 40 minutes, or until the meat is very tender. If the chili becomes too thick, add some water, about ¼ cup at a time. If the chili is too thin, mix 3 tablespoons of water with 1 to 2 tablespoons of cornstarch, then stir it into the chili and cook to thicken. Adjust the seasoning and serve.

Grilled or Broiled Lamb Chops

Protein and B vitamins promote your baby's muscle, cell, brain, and nerve development.

IF you like lamb, this marinade has pleased many readers over the years (and it also works beautifully with chicken or seafood). The combination of garlic, lemon, olive oil, and rosemary is magical. Add a squeeze of lemon and a sprinkle of chopped fresh parsley for the perfect finishing touch to the grilled lamb. Discard all excess marinade.

SERVES 4

1¼ pounds lamb chops (about 4), each 2 inches thick

MARINADE

2 garlic cloves, minced
2 tablespoons freshly squeezed lemon juice
1 to 2 tablespoons chopped fresh rosemary, mint, or thyme
1 tablespoon olive oil
Freshly ground black pepper

Cooking spray
2 tablespoons freshly squeezed lemon juice
Salt
¼ cup chopped fresh parsley, for garnish

- Marinate the lamb: Trim any visible fat from the lamb chops, then, using a fork, pierce the meat all over to allow the marinade to seep in. Place the lamb chops in a 1-gallon resealable plastic bag. Add the garlic, lemon juice, rosemary, olive oil, and pepper to the bag and squish it around to make sure that the chops are completely covered with the marinade. Seal the bag and refrigerate for at least 1 hour, or up to 24.
- To grill the lamb chops, preheat the grill. Have a clean plate ready for the cooked meat. Spray the grill with cooking spray. Grill the lamb chops for about 7 minutes per side (depending on their thickness), or until an instant-read thermometer inserted into the center of the meat close to the bone reads 160°F.
- To broil the lamb chops, preheat the broiler and line a shallow baking pan or a rimmed baking sheet with parchment paper or foil. Arrange the lamb chops in the prepared pan and broil for 5 to 7 minutes per side, or until an instant-read thermometer inserted into the center of the meat close to the bone reads 160°F. Watch carefully to prevent burning.
- Arrange the cooked lamb chops on the plate and sprinkle with the lemon juice, a pinch of salt, and chopped parsley.

Meal ideas

- Whole grain or starch (Yummy Three-Bean Salad, page 138)
- Green salad or vegetable
- Reduced-fat milk or yogurt
- Fresh fruit

Meal ideas and tips for diabetes

- Whole grain or starch (above)
- Green salad or nonstarchy vegetable
- Reduced-fat milk or unsweetened reduced-fat yogurt, 1 CARB

1 lamb chop: Calories: 136 cals; Protein: 23 g; Carbohydrates: 0 g; Fat: 5 g; Fiber: 0 g; Sodium: 56 mg; B_{12}: 2 mcg; Niacin: 8 mg; Phosphorus: 251 mg; Zinc: 2 mg; 0 CARBS

Peach and Blackberry Cobbler

A sweet and healthy treat, plus the fiber is good for your digestion.

THIS simple dessert is bursting with beautiful summery flavors. When fresh peaches are in season, by all means use them. Off-season, or if you are short on time, use frozen or canned peaches. The blackberries (or you can use blueberries) can be fresh or frozen. An equal amount of all-purpose flour can be substituted for the whole wheat flour. One pound of sliced frozen peaches, or one 29-ounce can of yellow sliced cling peaches in light syrup may be substituted for the fresh peaches. Drain the canned peaches.

MAKES ONE 9-INCH COBBLER; SERVES 8

COBBLER DOUGH

¾ cup all-purpose flour
¾ cup whole wheat flour
2 teaspoons baking powder
¼ cup sugar
Pinch of salt
6 tablespoons cold unsalted butter, cut into pieces
¾ cup whole milk
1½ teaspoons pure vanilla extract

PEACH AND BLACKBERRY FILLING

1½ pounds peaches (about 5), pitted, peeled, and sliced
8 ounces fresh blackberries or blueberries (about 2 cups), or 2 cups frozen berries
½ cup sugar
2 tablespoons all-purpose flour, or 1½ tablespoons cornstarch
½ teaspoon ground cinnamon

- Preheat the oven to 425°F. Have ready a 9-inch baking dish.
- Prepare the dough: Combine the flours, baking powder, sugar, and salt in a large bowl and stir to mix. Add the butter, then, using your fingers, rub the mixture until it resembles coarse meal. Stir in the milk and vanilla just until the dough comes together; set aside.
- Prepare the filling: Combine all of the ingredients in a large bowl and mix well. (Note: You do not need to thaw the frozen fruit before baking; however, if using frozen fruit, your baking time will increase by 10 to 15 minutes.) Transfer the filling to the baking dish, then drop heaping spoonfuls of the cobbler dough over the fruit, leaving some empty spaces for the fruit to show through.
- Bake for 12 minutes, then lower the heat to 400°F and continue to bake for 30 to 35 minutes, or until the peaches are tender when pierced with the tip of a knife and the juices are bubbling. Remove the cobbler from the oven and allow to cool slightly before serving.

> **Tips for diabetes**
> - Reduce your portion size, or skip this recipe.

One eighth of the cobbler: Calories: 300 cals; Protein: 5 g; Carbohydrates: 51 g; Fat: 10 g; Fiber: 6 g; Sodium: 103 mg; Copper: 0.2 mg; Manganese: 1 mg; Selenium: 15 mcg; 3 CARBS

Body-Building Recipes
For the Third Trimester

Grow, Baby, Grow

MONTH 7
Intense Brain Development
Weeks 28 Through 31

During the seventh month, your baby's brain is rapidly developing, and the best thing you can do is fuel it with omega-3s and B vitamins. You will find your appetite spike as your baby's body fills out with muscle and fat. By Week 28, your bundle of joy is the size of a large eggplant. At Week 31, she or he has reached the length of a pineapple, about 16 inches, and weighs about 3.3 pounds.

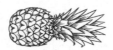

YOUR BABY'S DEVELOPMENT

- In Week 28, your baby's brain is developing at lightning speed. She or he may cough, suck, or hiccup more often.
- In Week 29, your baby is continuing to store fat.
- In Week 30, your baby's central nervous system continues to develop.
- In Week 31, your baby's brain receives signals from all five senses. He or she has defined patterns of sleep and wakeful hours.

CHANGES IN YOUR BODY

You will experience more of the same as you navigate your growing belly. Your baby will be active. You may feel breathless. If you have concerns about whether your baby is active, you can perform kick counts after meals. Typically, you start counting baby kicks during the third trimester, or at 28 weeks. Your doctor may recommend that you begin as early as the 24th week if you have a high-risk pregnancy. According to the American Congress of Obstetricians and Gynecologists, most healthy babies should take less than two hours for ten kicks.

IDEAL NUTRITION

Your nutrition focus is foods to enhance your baby's brain and nerve development and blood volume. The following nutrients will help achieve this.

- B vitamins: cell division, brain formation, nervous system development
- Copper: iron utilization
- Iron: supporting blood volume
- Magnesium: heart functioning, blood glucose regulation, blood pressure control
- Manganese: bone development, thyroid, blood glucose regulation, nervous system
- Omega-3s: brain and eye development
- Phosphorus: bone development
- Potassium: nerve and muscle function
- Protein: support fetal muscle growth
- Vitamin A: cell formation, bones, teeth, central nervous system, vision
- Vitamin C: iron absorption, healthy teeth and gums, immunity
- Vitamin K: bone mineralization

OPTIMAL FOODS FOR MONTH 7

PROTEIN	DAIRY	GRAINS/ LEGUMES	VEGETABLES	FRUITS	FATS/OTHER
Eggs	Cheese	All-bran cereal and other fortified breakfast cereals	Artichokes	Bananas	Brewer's or nutritional yeast
Meats	Enriched plant-based milks (rice soy, and almond)	Beans: soy, black, navy, pinto, kidney, white, great northern, black-eyed, pink, cranberry, and cannellini	Asparagus	Cantaloupe	Olive oil
Nuts: almonds, cashews, pistachios, Brazil nuts, walnuts, and nut butters	Fortified dairy milk	Chickpeas	Avocados	Citrus fruits and juices: oranges, tangerines, grapefruit, lemonade	Omega-3s
Pork	Fortified orange juice and other juices	Corn and flour tortillas	Baked potato with skin on and all other potatoes	Dried apricots and figs	Molasses, blackstrap
Poultry	Yogurt	Cream of Wheat	Beets	Guava	Seaweed, kelp, spirulina
Seafood (fish and shellfish): salmon (wild and Atlantic), tuna, mackerel, herring, sardines in oil, halibut, cod, catfish, canned oysters		Edamame	Broccoli and broccoli rabe	Kiwi	
		Folic acid–fortified products	Brussels sprouts	Lychee	
Seeds: sunflower, pumpkin, chia, hemp seed, and flaxseed		Lentils	Butternut squash	Mangoes	
		Oatmeal	Cabbage	Papaya	
Tahini		Peanuts	Carrots	Prune juice	
Tofu and tempeh		Wheat germ	Cauliflower	Pineapple	
		Whole grains: quinoa, barley, brown rice, bulgur, and whole wheat couscous	Dark, leafy greens: kale, collards, mustard, Swiss chard, bok choy, and turnip greens	Raspberries	
			Hearts of palm	Strawberries	
			Mushrooms		
			Pumpkin		
			Red bell peppers		
			Romaine lettuce		
			Snow peas		
			Spinach		
			Sweet potatoes		
			Tomatoes and tomato juice		

RECIPES FOR MONTH 7

Ricotta Pancakes with Blueberry Sauce

Protein and B vitamins enhance your baby's cell, brain, nervous system, and muscle development.

IT'S hard to turn down a bite of these protein-packed ricotta pancakes topped with blueberry sauce and throw on some chia seeds, if you have them. The key to making these delicate pancakes is to use as little flour as possible. They might be harder to flip, but the slightly creamy consistency of the finished pancakes is worth the effort. The blueberry sauce is also an excellent topping for ice cream or yogurt. An equal amount of pasteurized farmer cheese can be substituted for the ricotta cheese, although the calcium value will decrease. They do not freeze well.

**BLUEBERRY SAUCE
(MAKES ABOUT 1 CUP)**

1 pint fresh blueberries (about 2 cups), or 8 ounces frozen unsweetened blueberries

⅓ cup sugar, or to taste

- Prepare the sauce: Combine the blueberries and sugar in a saucepan and bring to a boil, stirring occasionally, over high heat. Continue to cook until the syrup has thickened slightly, about 5 minutes. Set aside.

Meal ideas

- Reduced-fat milk or yogurt
- Fresh fruit (Refreshing Fruit Salad, page 130)

Meal ideas and tips for diabetes

- Reduce your portion size, or skip this recipe.
- Instead of the blueberry sauce, use a low-sugar jam (such as Polaner All Fruit; 2 teaspoons are FREE).

(continues)

3 ricotta pancakes: Calories: 243 cals; Protein: 13 g; Carbohydrates: 29 g; Fat: 8 g; Fiber: 0 g; Sodium: 108 mg; Niacin: 4 mg; Riboflavin: 0.3 mg; Selenium: 24 mcg; 2 CARBS

⅓ cup blueberry sauce: Calories: 141 cals; Protein: 1 g; Carbohydrates: 36 g; Fat: 0 g; Fiber: 0 g; Sodium: 1 mg; 2 CARBS

PANCAKES (MAKES NINE 3-INCH PANCAKES)

1 cup part-skim ricotta cheese
1 large egg
2 tablespoons sugar
1 teaspoon pure vanilla extract
6 tablespoons all-purpose
 flour
1 tablespoon orange
 marmalade or apricot jam
2 tablespoons canola oil or
 unsalted butter

- Prepare the pancakes: Mix the ricotta cheese, egg, sugar, and vanilla in a bowl until smooth. Add the flour and orange marmalade and mix until well blended.

- Heat 1 tablespoon of the canola oil in a large skillet over medium-high heat. Add 1 heaping tablespoon of the pancake batter for each pancake and flatten slightly with the back of the spoon; do not crowd the pancakes in the pan. Cook for 2 minutes, or until the bottoms are golden brown. With a wide spatula, very carefully flip each pancake (use a blunt knife to push the pancake onto the spatula) and continue to cook until golden brown on the second side, about 2 minutes longer. Repeat with the rest of the batter, greasing the skillet with the remaining canola oil, as needed. Top the finished pancakes with the blueberry sauce, or your favorite topping, and serve promptly.

Yummy Granola Parfait

Q

Protein, vitamin E, B vitamins, and folate optimize your baby's cell, brain, nervous system, and muscle development, while calcium builds bone and fiber helps your digestion.

LOVELY for breakfast, or as a snack. On the run? Make this parfait in a mason jar with a lid. If you have some time and energy to spend in the kitchen, try our awesome Perfect Homemade Granola (page 105).

SERVES 1

¾ cup plain Greek yogurt
½ cup fresh fruit or berries or your favorite fruit sauce
½ cup store-bought or homemade granola

- In a glass, small bowl, or jar with a lid, make layers of the yogurt, sauce, and granola. Keep refrigerated if not eating promptly.

Tips for diabetes
- Reduce your portion size, or skip this recipe.

1 granola parfait: Calories: 455 cals; Protein: 19 g; Carbohydrates: 56 g; Fat: 18 g; Fiber: 7 g; Sodium: 145 mg; Vitamin E: 7 mg; B$_6$: 0.4 mg; B$_{12}$: 1 mcg; Niacin: 5 mg; Riboflavin: 0.6 mg; Thiamine: 0.4 mg; Folate: 76 mcg; Calcium: 387 mg; Copper: 0.5 mg; Magnesium: 138 mg; Manganese: 3 mg; Phosphorus: 536 mg; Selenium: 22 mcg; Zinc: 4 mg; 4 CARBS

KITCHEN WISDOM: HEALTHY SNACKS FOR AROUND 100 TO 200 CALORIES

1 mozzarella cheese stick = 80

1 medium-size apple = 90

2 tablespoons raisins = 90

5 pieces dried apricot = 90

1 cup grapes = 100

1 medium-size banana = 105

1 cup fresh strawberries with 2 tablespoons By Nature Sweetened Light Whipped
   Cream = 105

8 ounces Naked Protein Juice Smoothie = 110

18 dry-roasted whole almonds = 120

¼ cup trail mix (1 ounce) = 130

¼ cup hummus with 8 baby carrots = 136

2 tablespoons guacamole with 3 whole wheat crackers = 144

1 slice of whole wheat bread with 1 teaspoon jam = 165

1 brown rice cake with 1 tablespoon almond butter = 171

½ cup fruit salad in light syrup (drained) with ½ cup reduced-fat vanilla yogurt = 177

½ cup cottage cheese with 5 whole wheat crackers = 189

1 celery stalk with 2 tablespoons peanut butter = 199

1 ounce Cheddar cheese with 5 whole wheat crackers = 201

1 hard-boiled egg with 1 whole wheat pita = 207

¼ cup dry-roasted peanuts = 213

Green Split Pea Soup

Protein, vitamin A, B vitamins, and folate promote your baby's cell, brain, nervous system, and muscle development, plus fiber for your digestion.

IF you insist that green split pea soup needs a ham bone for flavor, this lighter recipe might convince you otherwise. But, if you love the flavor of the ham bone, go for it. Here are some easy soaking options: Pick over and rinse the peas, then soak them for eight to twelve hours in 5 cups of water. Or, for faster results, place the peas in a 3-quart saucepan, add water to cover by at least 2 inches, and bring to a boil. Cook for two minutes, then remove from the heat and let stand, covered, at room temperature, for at least one hour, or up to three. Drain and rinse the peas, then proceed with the recipe. This soup keeps refrigerated for about five days, and it can be frozen for up to one month. Slow cooker/Instant Pot instructions follow.

SERVES 6; MAKES ABOUT 7 CUPS

3 tablespoons olive oil
1 medium-size onion, finely chopped
2 garlic cloves, crushed
3 carrots, peeled and sliced (2 cups)
2 celery stalks, sliced
1 teaspoon dried thyme
1 teaspoon dried marjoram (optional)
2 bay leaves
8 cups stock or water, plus more as needed
1⅓ cups dried green split peas (10 ounces)
Salt and freshly ground black pepper

- Heat the olive oil in a 6-quart saucepan over medium heat. Add the onion and sauté for 3 minutes. Add the garlic, carrots, celery, thyme, marjoram, if using, and bay leaves and sauté for 3 minutes longer.
- Add the stock and split peas, stir, and bring to a boil. Skim off the foam with a spoon, then lower the heat and simmer for about 2 hours, or until the peas are tender.
- If the soup is too thick, add more stock or water, 2 tablespoons at a time. Adjust the seasoning, remove the bay leaves, and serve immediately.

Meal ideas

- Whole wheat bread (Best-Ever Bruschetta, page 266)
- Reduced-fat milk or yogurt
- Fresh fruit

Meal ideas and tips for diabetes

- Reduce your portion size, if necessary.
- Green salad or nonstarchy vegetable (Tomato-Mozzarella Salad, page 188)

(continues)

1 cup split pea soup: Calories: 373 cals; Protein: 20 g; Carbohydrates: 49 g; Fat: 11 g; Fiber: 14 g; Sodium: 505 mg; Vitamin A: 6,934 IU; B_6: 0.4 mg; Niacin: 4 mg; Folate: 163 mcg; Thiamine: 0.5 mg; Riboflavin: 0.4 mg; Zinc: 2 mg; Copper: 0.6 mg; Manganese: 0.7 mg; 3 CARBS

Green Split Pea Soup (continued)

SLOW COOKER OR INSTANT POT INSTRUCTIONS:

- It is essential to soak the peas before adding them to the slow cooker or Instant Pot. The amount of time it takes for the peas to cook will vary; it may take up to 10 hours. Use 6 cups of stock instead of eight.

- Using a large skillet instead of a saucepan, or your Instant Pot, follow the instructions in Step 1.

- Transfer the contents of the skillet to the slow cooker. Add the drained soaked peas and the stock, cover, and cook on HIGH for 8 hours, or possibly up to 10 hours, until the peas are soft. Finish the soup as directed in Step 3.

Easy Cheese-y Toast

Ⓠ ⓁⒸ

Protein, B vitamins, and calcium foster your baby's cell, brain, nervous system, muscle and skeletal development, plus it keeps your bones strong.

CHEESE toasts are open-faced grilled cheese sandwiches, nothing fancy, just plain good. You can use any type of bread or cheese. If you like your bread crisp, toast both sides. For more punch, sprinkle the toasts with chopped fresh basil, dried Italian seasoning, or a pinch of paprika or chili flakes. Enjoy any time of day.

SERVES 1

1 slice country-style
    whole-grain bread
Dijon mustard (optional)
2 slices hard cheese, such as
    Swiss or provolone
2 tomato slices
4 cucumber slices
¼ cup baby greens

- Preheat the broiler or toaster oven to HIGH. Lightly toast the bread on both sides. Spread a bit of Dijon, if using, on one side of the bread, then top with the cheese and broil just until the cheese melts and bubbles. Top with the tomato and cucumber slices and the baby greens.

Meal ideas

- Protein, such as meat, poultry, seafood, eggs, dairy, or plant-based
- Green salad or vegetable (Quick Romaine and Avocado Salad, page 109)
- Reduced-fat milk or yogurt
- Fresh fruit

Meal ideas and tips for diabetes

- Protein, such as meat, poultry, seafood, eggs, dairy, or plant-based
- Green salad or nonstarchy vegetable (above)
- Reduced-fat milk or unsweetened reduced-fat yogurt, 1 CARB

1 cheese-y toast: Calories: 190 cals; Protein: 12 g; Carbohydrates: 14 g; Fat: 10 g; Fiber: 2 g; Sodium: 155 mg; B$_{12}$: 0.9 mcg; Niacin: 4 mg; Manganese: 0.6 mg; Selenium: 17 mcg; Calcium: 290 mg; 1 CARB

Tomato, Hearts of Palm, and Asparagus Salad

GF **DF** **V** **Q** **LC**

Vitamins A, C, E, and K, and folate boost your baby's cell, brain, nervous system, muscle and skeletal development, plus iron helps maintain your iron supply.

A favorite salad among our pregnant moms, both for flavor and nutrition! Canned or jarred hearts of palm can be found in the international food section of many grocery stores. If you've never had them, give them a try. No time? You can replace the asparagus with your favorite vegetables that don't need to be cooked, such as cucumber or avocado, or with more baby greens.

SERVES 4; MAKES ABOUT 4 CUPS

1 pound asparagus, tough ends trimmed, cut into 2-inch pieces
1 (14-ounce) can hearts of palm, drained and cut into 1-inch slices (1 cup)
2 ripe tomatoes, diced
4 cups baby greens
2 tablespoons cider vinegar
½ teaspoon Dijon mustard
¼ cup olive or canola oil
Salt and freshly ground black pepper

- Boil, steam, or microwave the asparagus until crisp-tender. The cooking time will depend on the cooking method, but the average cooking time is about 5 minutes. Drain, place in a bowl, and let cool.

- Add the hearts of palm and tomatoes to the asparagus; set aside. Arrange the baby greens on a serving platter; set aside.

- In a small bowl, stir together the vinegar and mustard. Add the olive oil and mix until well blended. Add most of the dressing to the salad and toss gently. Adjust the seasoning. Drizzle the remaining dressing evenly over the baby greens, place the asparagus salad in the center, and serve immediately.

Meal ideas

- Protein, such as meat, poultry, seafood, eggs, dairy, or plant-based (Lemon-Herb Grilled Chicken, page 253)
- Whole wheat roll, bread, or starch
- Reduced-fat milk or yogurt
- Fresh fruit

Meal ideas and tips for diabetes

- Protein, such as meat, poultry, seafood, eggs, dairy, or plant-based (above)
- Whole wheat roll, bread, or starch, 1 CARB
- Reduced-fat milk or unsweetened reduced-fat yogurt, 1 CARB

1 cup asparagus and hearts of palm salad: Calories: 172 cals; Protein: 5 g; Carbohydrates: 10 g; Fat: 14 g; Fiber: 5 g; Sodium: 168 mg; Vitamin A: 1,881 IU; Vitamin C: 21 mg; Vitamin E: 4 mg; Vitamin K: 106 mcg; Folate: 121 mcg; Iron: 4 mg; Manganese: 0.9 mg; Copper: 0.4 mg; 1 CARB

Snappy Mediterranean-Style Chicken Salad

Protein, vitamins E and K, B vitamins, and folate boost your baby's cell, brain, nervous system, muscle, and skeletal development.

A divine chicken salad for a divine pregnant diva! If you don't have sun-dried tomatoes, fresh will do. You can replace the pasta with whole grains, such as quinoa, farro, bulgur, couscous, or rice. No dairy? Skip the feta. But keep throwing nuts and seeds into everything.

SERVES 4

2 cups uncooked bow-tie or other pasta, preferably whole wheat

5 tablespoons olive oil

8 ounces chicken breasts or tenders, diced (2 cups)

⅓ cup sun-dried tomatoes in oil, drained and cut into a small dice

½ cup coarsely chopped pitted black olives

¼ cup pasteurized feta cheese, crumbled

4 cups baby arugula or baby greens

2 tablespoons pumpkin seeds

2 tablespoons sunflower seeds

3 tablespoons cider or balsamic vinegar, or to taste

- Cook the pasta according to the package directions. Drain, then transfer the pasta to a large serving bowl. Add 1 tablespoon of the olive oil (this will prevent the pasta from sticking together), mix, and set aside.

- Heat 2 tablespoons of the olive oil in a large skillet over medium-high heat. Add the chicken and sauté, stirring occasionally, for 5 minutes, or until completely cooked and nicely browned.

- Transfer the cooked chicken to the pasta, then add the remaining ingredients, including the remaining 2 tablespoons of olive oil, and gently mix until well combined. Adjust the seasoning and serve at room temperature.

Meal ideas

- Reduced-fat milk or yogurt
- Fresh fruit

Meal ideas and tips for diabetes

- Reduced-fat milk or unsweetened reduced-fat yogurt, 1 CARB
- Fresh fruit, 1 CARB

One quarter of the chicken salad: Calories: 389 cals; Protein: 26 g; Carbohydrates: 20 g, Fat: 23 g, Fiber: 3 g, Sodium: 301 mg; Vitamin E: 4 mg; Vitamin K: 29 mcg; B₆: 0.5 mg; Niacin: 10 mg; Riboflavin: 0.3 mg; Folate: 85 mcg; Copper: 0.4 mg; Magnesium: 100 mg; Manganese: 0.7 mg; Phosphorus: 333 mg; Selenium: 32 mcg; 1½ CARBS

Grilled or Roasted Vegetables

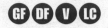

Vitamins A, C, and E enhance your baby's cell, brain, nervous system, and skeletal development.

IF you've got your grill fired up for poultry, meat, or fish, throw on these marinated veggies, too. Sautéing the onion and garlic separately brings out their sweetness. Add or delete any veggies. This is a blueprint to get you started. There are optional roasting instructions.

SERVES 6; MAKES ABOUT 4 CUPS

1 medium-size red bell pepper, cored, seeded, and quartered (1 cup)
1 medium-size purple eggplant (about 8 ounces), cut into ½-inch-thick slices
1 medium-size zucchini (about 8 ounces), cut into ½-inch-thick slices
8 ounces large mushrooms, stems trimmed
1 tablespoon dried oregano
1 tablespoon dried basil or Italian seasoning
1 teaspoon salt
Freshly ground black pepper
1 tablespoon freshly squeezed lemon juice
⅓ cup plus 2 tablespoons olive oil
1 medium-size sweet onion, preferably Vidalia, diced
2 garlic cloves, minced
1 (14.5-ounce) can diced tomatoes, drained
¼ cup chopped fresh basil or cilantro leaves

- Place the bell pepper, eggplant, zucchini, and mushrooms in a very large bowl (or in a large roasting pan if roasting). Add the oregano, dried basil, salt, black pepper to taste, lemon juice, and ⅓ cup of the olive oil, then gently toss until all the vegetables are well coated. Allow the vegetables to marinate at room temperature for 10 to 20 minutes.

- Heat the remaining 2 tablespoons of olive oil in a small skillet over medium-high heat. Add the onion and sauté, stirring occasionally, for 5 to 7 minutes, or until light golden. Add the garlic and sauté for 1 minute more. Add the canned tomatoes and cook just until heated; set aside, covered to keep warm.

- Preheat the grill (or see the roasting instructions). Grill the vegetables over medium-high heat for about 15 minutes, or until nicely browned and cooked through. Turn and move the vegetables around on the grill as necessary to promote even cooking and to avoid scorching.

Meal ideas

- Protein, such as meat, poultry, seafood, eggs, dairy, or plant-based (BBQ Chicken, page 120)
- Green salad
- Reduced-fat milk or yogurt
- Fresh fruit

Meal ideas and tips for diabetes

- Protein, such as meat, poultry, seafood, eggs, dairy, or plant-based (above)
- Green salad
- Reduced-fat milk or unsweetened reduced-fat yogurt, 1 CARB

⅔ cup grilled vegetables: Calories: 195 cals; Protein: 3 g; Carbohydrates: 10 g; Fat: 17 g; Fiber: 3 g; Sodium: 10 mg; Vitamin A: 1,372 IU; Vitamin C: 50 mg; Vitamin E: 3 mg; Copper: 0.2 mg; 1 CARB

(continued)

- Discard the marinade, then return the grilled vegetables to the bowl in which they were marinated. While they are still warm, chop the cooked vegetables into small dice. Place the diced vegetables in a serving bowl, add the tomato mixture and the fresh basil, and mix gently. Serve immediately.

- To roast the vegetables, preheat the oven to 475°F. Meanwhile, combine the prepared vegetables in a large roasting pan and marinate them as in Step 1. Roast the vegetables for 20 to 30 minutes, stirring them after 15 minutes of cooking. The vegetables are done when the eggplant and bell peppers are soft. Meanwhile, prepare the tomato mixture, following the instructions in Step 2. Finish the vegetables as in Step 4.

Greek-Style Broccoli

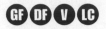

Vitamins C and K optimize your baby's bone development.

A drizzle of olive oil and lemon can lift broccoli and other vegetables (think: cauliflower, green beans, and spinach) to new heights. It is important to add the olive oil first, and then the lemon juice to prevent discoloration. Finish with a sprinkle of fresh herbs, if desired. A finishing salt, such as Maldon, is a wonderful touch.

SERVES 4

12 ounces broccoli florets
2 tablespoons olive oil, or to taste
1 tablespoon freshly squeezed lemon juice, or to taste
Salt and freshly ground black pepper
2 tablespoons chopped fresh parsley, dill, or your favorite fresh herb

- Boil or steam the broccoli florets until crisp-tender. Drain well and blot well with paper towels. (This is important, as extra water will dilute the dressing.)
- Place the broccoli in a bowl, add the olive oil, and gently mix. Add the remaining ingredients and mix again. Adjust the seasoning and serve warm or at room temperature.

Meal ideas

- Protein, such as meat, poultry, seafood, eggs, dairy, or plant-based (Tilapia Mediterranean Style, page 252)
- Whole grain or starch
- Reduced-fat milk or yogurt
- Fresh fruit

Meal ideas and tips for diabetes

- Protein, such as meat, poultry, seafood, eggs, dairy, or plant-based (above)
- Whole grain or starch, 1 CARB
- Reduced-fat milk or unsweetened reduced-fat yogurt, 1 CARB

¾ cup broccoli: Calories: 90 cals; Protein: 2 g; Carbohydrates: 6 g; Fat: 7 g; Fiber: 2 g; Sodium: 29 mg; Vitamin C: 80 mg; Vitamin K: 122 mcg; ½ CARBS

Lentil, Brown Rice, and Mushroom Pilaf GF DF V

Protein and folate promote your baby's cell, nervous system, and muscle development, while fiber keeps your digestion on track.

EARTHY and delicious, this lentil, brown rice, and mushroom casserole packs a healthy punch. For a more intense mushroom flavor, mushroom broth can be used in place of vegetable stock. Vegetarians or vegans who need more protein can add cubed tofu in Step 2 with the lentils. Don't have brown rice? Use long- or medium-grain white rice and reduce the cooking time to about one hour. Also, feel free to mix the grains, using half rice and half quinoa. Top with lots of nutrient-dense nuts and seeds, and/or Parmesan cheese, if you can eat dairy. This pilaf keeps for three days refrigerated.

SERVES 5

3 tablespoons olive oil
1 onion, chopped
1 garlic clove, minced
8 ounces cremini or button mushrooms, sliced
1 red bell pepper, cored, seeded, and quartered
1 teaspoon dried thyme
1 teaspoon dried oregano
¾ cup dried green lentils, picked over and rinsed
1 cup uncooked brown rice
1 teaspoon salt
5 cups vegetable stock

- Preheat the oven to 350°F.
- Heat the olive oil in a large skillet over medium-high heat. Add the onion and sauté for 3 minutes. Add the garlic, mushrooms, bell pepper, thyme, and oregano and sauté for 1 minute more. Add the lentils and rice and sauté for 1 minute. Add the salt and stock and bring to a boil.
- Carefully transfer the contents of the skillet to an 8 x 8 x 2-inch Pyrex baking dish. Bake for 2 hours, or until the rice and lentils in the center of the casserole are soft and the liquid is absorbed, covering the dish with parchment paper or foil during the last 30 minutes of baking. Serve hot.

Meal ideas

- Protein, such as meat, poultry, seafood, eggs, dairy, or plant-based
- Green salad or vegetable (see Awesome Homemade Salad Dressings, page 214)
- Reduced-fat milk or yogurt
- Fresh fruit

Meal ideas and tips for diabetes

- Protein, such as meat, poultry, seafood, eggs, dairy, or plant-based
- Green salad or nonstarchy vegetable (above)
- Reduced-fat milk or unsweetened reduced-fat yogurt, 1 CARB

1 cup pilaf: Calories: 206 cals; Protein: 11 g; Carbohydrates: 30 g; Fat: 5 g; Fiber: 9 g; Sodium: 879 mg; Folate: 110 mcg; 2 CARBS

Southern-Style Sweet Potato Casserole

Vitamin A fosters your baby's bone development.

THIS sweet potato casserole is a guaranteed pleaser, particularly during the holidays. It's been a staple on many Thanksgiving tables since the first edition of this book. Some folks have been known to have the leftovers for breakfast! In a hurry? Canned sweet potatoes in light syrup are a fine substitute. Drain and proceed with Step 3. The filling can be prepared up to one day in advance; cover and refrigerate. The nut crumb topping can be made two to five days in advance, but place it on the casserole just before baking. Gluten-free? Use your favorite gluten-free flour. Lactose intolerant? Use almond milk.

SERVES 6

Cooking spray or butter for baking dish

SWEET POTATO FILLING

2 pounds red sweet potatoes (about 3 medium), peeled and cut into large pieces of equal size (4 cups)

½ cup whole milk

2 tablespoons unsalted butter

2 tablespoons light brown sugar

1 large egg

½ teaspoon ground cinnamon, cloves, or allspice, or a mixture

¼ teaspoon salt

- Preheat the oven to 375°F. Spray an 8 x 8 x 2-inch baking dish or a 9-inch pie pan with cooking spray or butter.
- Prepare the filling: Place the potatoes in a large pot and add just enough water to cover. Bring to a boil, then lower the heat and simmer for 20 to 25 minutes, or until the potatoes are soft. Drain.
- Place the hot potatoes in a large bowl. Beat them with an electric mixer on low speed to break them up, then increase the speed to medium and beat for 1 to 2 minutes, or until fairly smooth. Or you can mash them by hand. Add the remaining filling ingredients and mix on low speed (or by hand) until well blended and almost smooth, about 1 minute. Transfer the pureed potatoes to the prepared baking dish.

Meal ideas

- Protein, such as meat, poultry, seafood, eggs, dairy, or plant-based (Mustard-Tarragon Pork Tenderloin, page 195)
- Green salad or vegetable
- Reduced-fat milk or yogurt
- Fresh fruit

One eighth of the casserole without the marshmallows: Calories: 227 cals; Protein: 3 g; Carbohydrates: 26 g; Fat: 12 g; Fiber: 3 g; Sodium: 128 mg; Vitamin A: 9,718 IU; Copper: 0.2 mg; Manganese: 0.5 mg; 2 CARBS

(continued)

NUT CRUMB TOPPING (OPTIONAL)

¼ cup all-purpose flour

⅓ cup loosely packed brown sugar

3 tablespoons unsalted butter

½ cup pecans

Mini marshmallows (optional)

- Prepare the nut crumb topping, if using: Combine the flour and brown sugar in a small bowl. Using a dull knife (such as a table knife) or your fingers, work in the butter until the dough has a crumblike consistency. Mix in the pecans.
- Distribute the topping evenly over the sweet potato casserole. Bake for 45 minutes, or until the casserole is heated through and the topping has set. If the topping has not set after 45 minutes, place the casserole under the broiler for a minute or two. Remove from the oven and serve immediately.
- If using the marshmallows, cover the top of the baked casserole with mini marshmallows or large ones cut in half. Place the casserole under the broiler for a few seconds. Watch carefully to avoid burning the marshmallows.

Meal ideas and tips for diabetes

- Reduce your portion size, if necessary.
- Do not use the nut crumb or marshmallow topping.
- Protein, such as meat, poultry, seafood, eggs, dairy, or plant-based (Mustard-Tarragon Pork Tenderloin, page 195)
- Green salad or nonstarchy vegetable
- Reduced-fat milk or unsweetened reduced-fat yogurt, 1 CARB

Tilapia Mediterranean Style

Protein, vitamins A, C, D, and K, and B vitamins help create a healthy baby and mom!

A beautiful, simple, and supremely healthy Mediterranean-inspired dish that works well with just about any kind of fish, including red snapper, sole, or cod. This recipe can be cut in half to serve two people. This dish keeps for two days refrigerated. It does not freeze well.

SERVES 4

2 tablespoons olive oil
1 garlic clove, minced
1 cup pitted kalamata olives
    or other brine-cured black
    olives, chopped
15 ounces cherry tomatoes
    (about 3 cups), halved
⅓ cup chopped fresh parsley
¼ cup chopped fresh basil
2 tablespoons freshly
    squeezed lemon juice
Salt and freshly ground black
    pepper
About 16 ounces tilapia fillets
    (4 fillets)

- Heat 1 tablespoon of the olive oil in a large skillet over medium-high heat. Add the garlic and sauté for 30 seconds. Add the olives, cherry tomatoes, parsley, basil, and lemon juice and cook for 2 minutes, or until the cherry tomatoes are soft and their skin wrinkled. Adjust the seasoning, transfer to a heatproof bowl, cover, and set aside. (Do not rinse the skillet.)

- Have a serving platter ready. Heat the remaining tablespoon of olive oil in the skillet over medium-high heat. Add half of the fish, season the fish with salt and pepper, and cook for 3 minutes on each side, turning once, or until cooked through. Transfer the cooked fish to the serving platter. Repeat this procedure with the remaining fish, making sure to reheat the skillet before adding the second batch of fish.

- Ladle the sauce over the fish and serve immediately.

Meal ideas

- Green salad or vegetable (Greek-Style Broccoli, page 248)
- Whole grain or starch
- Reduced-fat milk or yogurt
- Fresh fruit

Meal ideas and tips for diabetes

- Green salad or nonstarchy vegetable (above)
- Whole grain or starch, 1 CARB
- Reduced-fat milk or unsweetened reduced-fat yogurt, 1 CARB

1 tilapia fillet: Calories: 236 cals; Protein: 25 g; Carbohydrates: 8 g; Fat: 13 g; Fiber: 3 g; Sodium: 315 mg; Vitamin A: 1,720 IU; Vitamin C: 28 mg; Vitamin D: 141 mg; Vitamin K: 90 mcg; B$_{12}$: 2 mcg; Niacin: 5 mg; Copper: 0.2 mg; ½ CARB

Lemon-Herb Grilled Chicken

Protein and B vitamins enhance your baby's cell, nervous system, and muscle development.

GRILLED chicken topped with chopped herbs, olives, and capers, and a squeeze of lemon is always a hit. Use this wonderful marinade for seafood, too. Leftover grilled chicken is fantastic in salads, sandwiches, or anything else.

SERVES 6

MARINADE

2 tablespoons olive oil
2 tablespoons minced fresh
  herbs, such as thyme,
  tarragon, basil, and/or
  parsley
2 tablespoons thinly sliced
  fresh chive or scallion
Grated zest of 1 lemon
Juice of 1 lemon
1 garlic clove, minced
1 teaspoon sugar
1 teaspoon salt
¼ teaspoon red pepper flakes
2 pounds skinless, bone-in
  chicken parts

OPTIONAL GARNISHES

Lemon wedges
Chopped fresh parsley, dill or
  any other herbs
Chopped pitted olives
Jarred jalapeño peppers
Capers

- Marinate the chicken: Combine all the marinade ingredients in a bowl and mix until well blended.
- Prick holes in the chicken with a fork to allow the marinade to penetrate the meat or score the meaty part of the chicken with a sharp knife, about ¼ inch deep (scoring it will also speed up the grilling time). Marinate for at least 3 hours, and up to 24.
- When ready to cook, preheat the grill. Grill the chicken over medium-high heat for 35 to 30 minutes, or until nicely browned and cooked through. Check for doneness by cutting into the meat. Turn and move the chicken around on the grill as necessary to promote even cooking and to avoid scorching.
- Place the cooked chicken in a serving bowl, and garnish as you wish.

Meal ideas

- Whole grain or starch
- Green salad or vegetable (Grilled or Roasted Vegetables, page 246)
- Reduced-fat milk or yogurt
- Fresh fruit

Meal ideas and tips for diabetes

- Whole grain or starch, 1 CARB
- Green salad or nonstarchy vegetable (above)
- Reduced-fat milk or unsweetened reduced-fat yogurt, 1 CARB

4 ounces chicken (no toppings): Calories: 163 cals; Protein: 31 g; Carbohydrates: 0 g; Fat: 5 g; Fiber: 0 g; Sodium: 262 mg; B_6: 1 mg; Niacin: 11 mg; Phosphorus: 299 mg; Selenium: 40 mcg; 0 CARBS

Asian-Style Beef and Bok Choy

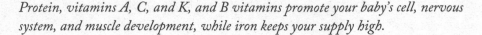

Protein, vitamins A, C, and K, and B vitamins promote your baby's cell, nervous system, and muscle development, while iron keeps your supply high.

A great dish for beef lovers. You can substitute a pound of chicken, if red meat is not your thing. In keeping with the Asian theme, serve over udon noodles or brown rice. Gluten-free? Be sure to choose gluten-free brands of soy sauce or tamari, as well as noodles. Leftovers keep for three days refrigerated.

SERVES 4

1 pound top sirloin steak, thinly sliced against the grain into ¼-inch thick slices

3 tablespoons cornstarch

2 tablespoons canola oil

1 large garlic clove, minced

2 tablespoons minced fresh ginger

2 cups sliced baby bok choy, both stems and leaves

¼ cup light soy sauce or wheat-free tamari (for gluten-free)

½ cup pure maple syrup

3 green onions, sliced

½ cup cashews

- Place the beef in a bowl and sprinkle the cornstarch over the meat. Mix to coat the meat (don't worry if some of the pieces are not coated). Have ready a large plate.
- Heat 1 tablespoon of the oil in a large skillet or wok over high heat. Working in batches, sear the one third of the meat, turning only once. When browned, after 3 to 4 minutes, transfer it to the plate.
- Reheat the skillet and finish cooking the rest of the meat the same way. Once all of the meat is cooked, reheat the empty skillet over medium high heat. Add the garlic and ginger and sauté for 1 minute.
- Add the bok choy and cook for 2 minutes, stirring occasionally. Add the soy sauce and maple syrup and bring to a boil.
- Add the beef back to the skillet along with the green onions and cashews and return the heat to a simmer. Cook until the sauce thickens a bit. Remove from the heat and serve.

Meal ideas

- Whole grain or starch (Easy Rice and Green Lentil Side Dish, page 89)
- Reduced-fat milk or yogurt
- Fresh fruit with vitamin C

Meal ideas and tips for diabetes

- Whole grain or starch, 1 CARB

One quarter of the beef dish: Calories: 440 cals; Protein: 30 g; Carbohydrates: 40 g; Fat: 19 g; Fiber: 1 g; Sodium: 747 mg; Vitamin A: 1,677 IU; Vitamin C: 18 mg; Vitamin K: 50 mcg; Riboflavin: 0.5 mg; Copper: 0.3 mg; Iron: 5 mg; Manganese: 2 mg; 2½ CARBS

Protein-Packed Burritos

Protein, vitamins A and K, B vitamins, and folate optimize your baby's cell, nervous system, and muscle development, while iron keeps your supply high and fiber aids digestion.

BRING on these nutrient-dense burritos! Add your favorite ingredients, and serve with extra salsa, guacamole (page 135), sliced lettuce, and cheese. Going meatless or vegan? Instead of the chicken, use one 15-ounce package (drained weight) extra-firm tofu, cut into ½-inch cubes. Cook it in step 2. Wrap these burritos for a meal on the go. Or skip the tortillas entirely and turn this dish into an amazing salad. The filling can be made up to two days in advance. Reheat in a microwave oven before serving.

MAKES 6 BURRITOS

1½ tablespoons olive oil
1 small onion, chopped
1 small garlic clove, minced
1½ teaspoons roasted ground cumin
1½ teaspoons chili powder, or to taste
1½ teaspoons dried oregano
10 ounces chicken breast, cut into cubes
1 cup canned black beans, drained and rinsed
4 large burrito-size (8-inch) tortillas
1½ cups grated Cheddar cheese (about 6 ounces), Monterey Jack, or a mixture
⅓ cup chopped fresh cilantro
3 cups thinly sliced romaine lettuce
½ cup tomato salsa

- Heat the olive oil in a large skillet over medium-high heat. Add the onion and sauté for 3 minutes, or until light golden. Add the garlic, cumin, chili powder, and oregano and sauté for 30 seconds longer.
- Add the chicken and sauté for 5 minutes. Add the beans and sauté until heated through, about 5 minutes more. Check to make sure the chicken is fully cooked. Cover to keep warm and set aside.
- Assemble the burritos: Heat a large skillet over medium-high heat. Place a tortilla in the skillet and heat for 30 seconds on each side, or just until heated but not crisp (you need to be able to roll it). Place the tortilla on a work surface. Add ⅔ cup of the filling on the bottom third of the tortilla, and top with some of the cheese, cilantro, and lettuce. Make sure that the filling is neatly stacked and compressed, then fold the bottom edge over the filling, tuck in the sides, and roll up. Repeat with the remaining ingredients. Serve with salsa.

Meal ideas

- Green salad or vegetable (Everyone's Favorite Caesar Salad, page 84)
- Reduced-fat milk or yogurt

Meal ideas and tips for diabetes

- Skip the tortilla and serve on top of a salad, if necessary.
- Green salad or nonstarchy vegetable

1 burrito: Calories: 520 cals; Protein: 30 g; Carbohydrates: 41 g; Fat: 26 g; Fiber: 5 g; Sodium: 1,001 mg; Vitamin A: 3,630 IU; Vitamin K: 44 mcg; B_6: 0.5 mg; B_{12}: 0.5 mcg; Niacin: 14 mg; Folate: 100 mcg; Copper: 0.2 mg; Phosphorus: 344 mg; Selenium: 21 mcg; 3 CARBS

Apple-Blueberry Crisp

B vitamins and folate promote your baby's cell, brain, and nervous system development.

WARM from the oven, topped with a scoop of frozen yogurt, ice cream, or whipped cream, nothing beats this crisp for a satisfying dessert (or breakfast, yes, readers and their families can't get enough of it). You can also use frozen blueberries instead of fresh. Indulge and enjoy! You deserve it.

MAKES ONE 9-INCH CRISP; SERVES 8

APPLE-BLUEBERRY FILLING

4 large Granny Smith apples (about 1¾ pounds), peeled, cored, and sliced
1 dry pint fresh blueberries (2 cups)
½ cup light brown or granulated sugar
2 teaspoons ground cinnamon
2 tablespoons all-purpose flour or cornstarch

GRANOLA TOPPING

½ cup all-purpose flour
½ cup light brown sugar
6 tablespoons cold unsalted butter, cut into pieces
1½ cups granola without raisins or fruit

- Preheat the oven to 375°F. Have ready an 8- or 9-inch baking dish.
- Prepare the filling: Combine all the filling ingredients in a large bowl and mix until well blended. Transfer the filling to the baking dish and set aside.
- Prepare the granola topping: Combine the flour and brown sugar in a bowl. Add the butter and, using your fingers, rub the mixture until it resembles coarse meal. Add the granola and continue to mix until the granola is incorporated and the topping holds together in small clumps.
- Distribute the topping evenly over the filling. Bake for about 45 minutes, or until the apples are tender when pierced with the tip of a knife and the juices are bubbling. Remove the crisp from the oven and allow to cool slightly before serving.

Tips for diabetes
- Reduce your portion size, or skip this recipe.

One eighth apple-blueberry crisp: Calories: 330 cals; Protein: 3 g; Carbohydrates: 59 g; Fat: 10 g; Fiber: 5 g; Sodium: 55 mg; B_6: 0.8 mg; B_{12}: 2 mcg; Thiamine: 0.3 mg; Folate: 173 mcg; Copper: 0.2 mg; 4 CARBS

MONTH 8

Growth and Immune System Development

Weeks 32 Through 35

You're almost there. This is a big month for your baby's growth. You may find that you're eating a lot more to keep up with your baby's development and rapid growth. He or she is gaining as much as ½ pound per week. This is all good news, though you may be more focused on the pain in your lower back or sides, swollen ankles, indigestion, and expanding belly! At Week 32, your baby is about 16 inches long and weighs about 3.75 pounds. Think of a large cantaloupe.

YOUR BABY'S DEVELOPMENT

- In Week 32, your baby is swallowing and sucking. Kicking is regular. His or her skin is less transparent. The brain continues to develop rapidly throughout this month.
- In Week 33, your baby's immune system continues to mature. Bones are growing at a fast rate.
- In Week 34, the slippery coating of vernix is getting thicker.
- In Week 35, most babies are in a head-down position to get ready for birth.

CHANGES IN YOUR BODY

You might be feeling more energy, and your baby might, too, issuing more aggressive kicks, especially after you consume foods or beverages with sugar and/or caffeine. Some moms feel achiness in their lower abdomen or sides as the baby gets bigger. And some experience Braxton Hicks contractions. The usual gastrointestinal discomforts may be present. Skin issues from discoloration to itching and stretch marks may appear now or get more intense if you already had them. Difficulty sleeping is common, and some women experience leg cramps, especially at night. Shortness of breath is common, too, as well as a quicker pulse. Your breasts are getting ready to go to work; they may start leaking colostrum.

IDEAL NUTRITION

Your nutrition focus is foods to enhance your baby's brain and bone development, blood volume, and immunity. The following nutrients will help achieve this.

- B vitamins: cell division, brain formation, nervous system development
- Calcium: bones and teeth
- Copper: iron utilization
- Iron: maternal blood volume
- Magnesium: heart functioning, blood glucose regulation, blood pressure control
- Manganese: bone development, thyroid, blood glucose regulation, nervous system
- Omega-3s: brain and eye development
- Phosphorus: bone development
- Protein: supports fetal muscle growth
- Selenium: cell growth and immunity
- Vitamin A: cell formation, bones, teeth, central nervous system, vision
- Vitamin C: iron absorption, healthy teeth and gums, immunity
- Vitamin D: calcium absorption
- Vitamin E: cell structure and immunity
- Vitamin K: bone mineralization
- Zinc: cell structure and immunity

OPTIMAL FOODS FOR MONTH 8

PROTEIN	DAIRY	GRAINS/ LEGUMES	VEGETABLES	FRUITS	FATS/OTHER
Eggs	Cheese	All-bran cereal and other fortified breakfast cereals	Artichokes	Bananas	Brewer's or nutritional yeast
Meats	Enriched plant-based milks (rice soy, and almond)	Beans: soy, black, navy, pinto, kidney, white, great northern, black-eye, pink, cranberry, Lima, and cannellini	Asparagus	Cantaloupe	Olive oil
Nuts: almonds, cashews, pistachios, Brazil nuts, walnuts, and nut butters	Fortified dairy milk	Chickpeas	Avocados	Citrus fruits and juices: oranges, tangerines, grapefruit, lemonade	Omega-3s
Pork	Fortified orange juice and other juices	Corn and flour tortillas	Baked potato with skin on and all other potatoes	Dried apricots and figs	Molasses, blackstrap
Poultry	Yogurt	Cream of Wheat	Beets	Guava	Seaweed, kelp, spirulina
Seafood (fish and shellfish): salmon (wild and Atlantic), tuna, mackerel, herring, sardines in oil, halibut, cod, catfish, canned oysters		Edamame	Broccoli and broccoli rabe	Kiwi	
Seeds: sunflower, pumpkin, chia, hemp seed, and flaxseed		Folic acid–fortified products	Brussels sprouts	Lychee	
Tahini		Lentils	Butternut squash	Mangoes	
Tofu and tempeh		Oatmeal	Cabbage	Papaya	
		Peanuts	Carrots	Prune juice	
		Wheat germ	Cauliflower	Pineapple	
		Whole grains: quinoa, barley, brown rice, bulgur, and whole wheat couscous	Dark, leafy greens: kale, collards, mustard, Swiss chard, bok choy, and turnip greens	Raspberries	
			Hearts of palm	Strawberries	
			Mushrooms		
			Pumpkin		
			Red bell peppers		
			Romaine lettuce		
			Snow peas		
			Spinach		
			Sweet potatoes		
			Tomatoes and tomato juice		

RECIPES FOR MONTH 8

Omega-Charged Chia Juice

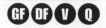

Vitamin C, iron, and fiber foster great health for mom and baby!

YOU'VE probably noticed those superhealthy, superexpensive chia drinks in the grocery store. The truth is, you don't need to spend your money on fancy bottled drinks, when you can make them at home in no time, for a fraction of the price. Here are two supersimple recipes to get you started on your chia adventure. Feel free to adjust the measurements— use more or less juice and chia seeds, or branch off into other beverages, such as almond milk, coconut water, or anything else. Chia is an excellent way to keep your digestion on track. These drinks can be refrigerated for up to one week.

BASIC SINGLE SERVING (MAKES 1 CUP)

½ cup fruit juice of your choice
2 tablespoons chia seeds

- Mix together ½ cup of water, the fruit juice, and the chia seeds in a large glass or container and let the seeds gel in the in fridge for at least 30 minutes.

Tip for diabetes
- Reduce your portion size to ½ cup for 1 CARB.

BASIC PITCHER (MAKES 4 CUPS)

2 cups water
2 cups fruit juice of your choice
½ cup chia seeds

- Whisk together 2 cups of water, the fruit juice, and the chia seeds in a large pitcher. Let sit for 15 minutes and mix again. This will prevent the seeds from gumming together in one big clump. Whisk again, if needed. Once the seeds are well separated and suspended in the juice, cover and refrigerate until cool, 2 to 3 hours.

1 cup chia juice (made with cranberry apple juice): Calories: 237 cals; Protein: 6 g; Carbohydrates: 31 g; Fat: 10 g; Fiber: 10 g; Sodium: 8 mg; Vitamin C: 51 mg; Magnesium: 97 mg; Iron: 4 mg; 2 CARBS

Ham and Egg Cups

Protein and B vitamins enhance your baby's cell, brain, nervous system, and muscle development.

THIS new recipe won the taste buds of our recipe testers. If you have fresh herbs, by all means add them. Tomatoes and green onions are used here because they don't require advance cooking. You can use spinach, mushrooms, kale, or broccoli, but you will need to sauté such vegetables before adding them to the cups. You can store the cooked egg cups in the fridge and reheat them in a microwave oven. They are great, hot or cold, sandwiched in between hearty bread, English muffins, rolled up in a tortilla, or enveloped in a pita pouch (choose gluten-free options, if necessary).

SERVES 6

Cooking spray or olive oil
6 (4-inch) round thin slices deli-style ham
1 cup chopped tomatoes, drained and seeded
⅓ cup thinly sliced green onion
1 teaspoon dried basil or oregano, or ⅓ cup chopped fresh herbs (any kind)
1 cup grated Cheddar or Parmesan cheese
Salt and freshly ground black pepper
7 large eggs, lightly beaten

- Preheat the oven to 350°F. Coat each well of a standard-size six-well muffin pan with cooking spray or olive oil. Line each well with one slice of ham, pressing it into the bottom and up the sides. The slices will rise above the rims, which is good.

- Evenly divide the tomatoes, green onion, basil, and cheese among the wells. Sprinkle each with salt and pepper. Divide the beaten egg evenly among the six prepared wells.

- Bake for 20 to 25 minutes, or until the eggs are cooked through. If the top of the eggs need more cooking after 25 minutes, switch to broiling on HIGH for a few minutes to finish the cooking process. Remove from the oven and serve.

Meal ideas

- Whole wheat bread, roll, or starch (Spiced-Up Hash Browns, page 263)
- Reduced-fat milk or yogurt
- Fresh fruit

Meal ideas and tips for diabetes

- Whole wheat bread, roll, or starch (above), 1 CARB
- Reduced-fat milk or unsweetened reduced-fat yogurt, 1 CARB

1 egg cup: Calories: 221 cals; Protein: 15 g; Carbohydrates: 3 g; Fat: 16 g; Fiber: 0 g; Sodium: 470 mg; B_{12}: 0.9 mcg; Riboflavin: 0.3 mg; Selenium: 27 mcg; 0 CARBS

Spiced-Up Hash Browns

Vitamins C and K, B vitamins, and fiber optimize your baby's cell, brain, and nervous system development and your digestion.

DON'T be surprised if you eat these hash browns for breakfast, lunch, and dinner (maybe a snack, too). The high starch content of Yukon gold or russet potatoes will produce softer, slightly mushy hash browns, whereas waxier potatoes, such as new potatoes, will result in a bouncier texture. You can swap out the black beans for your favorite variety of beans.

SERVES 5

4 cups skin-on diced potatoes (about 1¼ pounds)
2 tablespoons olive oil
1 medium-size onion, chopped
1 garlic clove, minced, or ½ teaspoon garlic powder
1 teaspoon regular or smoked paprika
Pinch of cayenne pepper
1 teaspoon dried oregano or Italian seasoning
1 cup canned black beans, drained and rinsed
3 tablespoons chopped fresh flat-leaf parsley (optional)

- Bring a medium-size saucepan of water to a rolling boil. Add the potatoes and cook for 5 to 7 minutes, or until al dente. Do not overcook; the potatoes will be sautéed later. Drain and set aside.

- In a large skillet, heat the olive oil over medium-high heat. Add the onion and sauté, stirring occasionally, until light golden, 3 to 4 minutes. Add the garlic, paprika, cayenne, oregano, and potatoes, increase the heat to high, and cook until the potatoes are light golden, 10 to 15 minutes. If desired, smash some of the potatoes with a fork to break them up. Add the black beans, stirring to heat evenly. Adjust the seasoning and garnish with the parsley, if using.

Meal ideas

- Protein, such as meat, poultry, seafood, eggs, dairy, or plant-based (Spinach and Cheese Omelet for One, page 159)
- Reduced-fat milk or yogurt
- Fresh fruit

Meal ideas and tips for diabetes

- Protein, such as meat, poultry, seafood, eggs, dairy, or plant-based (above)
- Reduced-fat milk or unsweetened reduced-fat yogurt 1 CARB

One fifth of the hash browns: Calories: 214 cals; Protein: 6 g; Carbohydrates: 36 g; Fat: 6 g; Fiber: 5 g; Sodium: 73 mg; Vitamin C: 22 mg; Vitamin K: 32 mcg; B_6: 0.4 mg; Copper: 0.3 mg; 2 CARBS

No-Brainer Banana Vegan Pancakes

GF **DF** **V** **Q**

Protein and B vitamins boost your baby's cell, brain, and nervous system development, and iron adds to your iron stores, while fiber keeps your digestion running smoothly.

NOT just for vegans—this awesome recipe will make anyone happy. Serve these pancakes with coconut flakes, berries, nuts, chia seeds, and maple syrup. Any leftover pancakes should be covered and refrigerated, or frozen with layers of parchment paper between each pancake. Reheat them in an ungreased skillet just until hot, one to two minutes per pancake. Don't use the microwave, which will make the pancakes unpleasantly rubbery. Add 2 to 3 tablespoons of ground flaxseeds to the batter for a nutrition boost. See "How to Make Oat Flour," page 265, for instructions on making and storing oat flour.

MAKES ABOUT NINE 5-INCH PANCAKES

1 cup unsweetened almond or soy milk
1 tablespoon cider vinegar
1½ cups quick cooking or old-fashioned oats (check label for gluten-free)
1 tablespoon baking powder
2 tablespoons sugar
2 ripe bananas
Pinch of salt
½ teaspoon pure vanilla extract
2 tablespoons coconut or canola oil

- Combine the milk and cider vinegar in a small bowl to make "buttermilk"; let sit for 10 minutes.
- Place the oats in a blender and process to a flourlike consistency. Add the "buttermilk" mixture and all the remaining ingredients, except the coconut oil, and process for a minute or two. Scrape down the sides of the blender and continue to process until smooth and thick.
- Heat a medium-size skillet over medium to medium-high heat until hot. Using a heatproof brush, lightly brush the skillet with the coconut oil. Add a scant ⅓ cup of the batter and immediately swirl the batter to form a pancake. Cook until the surface bubbles and sets and the underside is golden brown, about 1 minute. Flip the pancake with a wide spatula and cook for 1 minute more, or until cooked through. Repeat this procedure with the remaining batter, lightly oiling the skillet as needed. You can keep the pancakes warm in a low oven.

Meal ideas
- Reduced-fat milk or yogurt (Pineapple-Banana-Calcium Smoothie, page 207)
- Fresh fruit

Meal ideas and tips for diabetes
- Reduce your portion size, or skip this recipe.
- Use a low-sugar jam (such as Polaner All Fruit; 2 teaspoons are FREE).
- Protein, such as natural nut butter or eggs

3 pancakes: Calories: 422 cals; Protein: 15 g; Carbohydrates: 79 g; Fat: 7 g; Fiber: 10 g; Sodium: 545 mg; Niacin: 4 mg; B$_6$: 0.4 mg; Thiamine: 0.7 mg; Copper: 1 mg; Iron: 4 mg; Magnesium: 166 mg; Manganese: 4 mg; Phosphorus: 434 mg; Selenium: 21 mcg; Zinc: 3 mg; 5 CARBS

KITCHEN WISDOM: HOW TO MAKE OAT FLOUR

TODAY, more than ever, whole grains are available in wonderful flours—you'll find millet flour, teff flour, buckwheat flour, quinoa flour, and the list goes on. Oat flour, which you can make at home, is excellent in waffles, pancakes, muffins, cookies, and other baked goods. To make your own, blend old-fashioned rolled or quick-cooking oats in a food processor or blender until they are ground to a fine powder. Any leftover flour (not used in a recipe) can be stored in an airtight bag for later use. Making a large batch is advisable so you can keep it in your pantry. If prefer to buy oat flour, the following are good brands: Arrowhead Mills, Bob's Red Mill, Gold Medal, Pillsbury, and King Arthur.

Best-Ever Bruschetta

Protein, vitamin A, and B vitamins promote your baby's cell, brain, nervous system, bone, and muscle development.

WHAT makes this the best-ever bruschetta? A layer of Parmesan cheese, melted under the broiler, is the secret to keeping the toast from getting soggy. Feeling adventurous? Go beyond traditional tomatoes and basil and add chopped black or green olives, marinated artichoke hearts, or jarred roasted red bell peppers. Vegan? Skip the cheese. Gluten-free? Choose a gluten-free bread or use the topping on gluten-free crackers. These delicious toasts are great as a partner to a salad, soup, or as a snack. The topping will keep for two days refrigerated.

MAKES 4 SLICES

TOPPING

2 large or 3 medium-size tomatoes, diced and drained in a sieve

2 teaspoons cider or balsamic vinegar, or to taste

½ teaspoon minced garlic, or a sprinkle of garlic powder

½ teaspoon Italian seasoning, or to taste

A handful of fresh basil leaves, chopped

Salt and freshly ground black pepper

BREAD

4 slices whole-grain bread, preferably from a baguette or small country-style loaf

¼ cup grated Parmesan cheese

- Prepare the topping: Combine all the topping ingredients in a bowl and gently mix. Adjust the seasoning and set aside.
- Prepare the bruschetta: Preheat the broiler or toaster oven to HIGH. Lightly toast the bread on both sides. Distribute the grated Parmesan cheese evenly over the bread slices and then broil again until the cheese melts and begins to bubble. Transfer the bread to a serving plate and top with the tomato topping. Serve promptly.

Meal ideas

- Protein, such as meat, poultry, seafood, eggs, dairy, or plant-based
- Green salad or vegetable (Creamy Asparagus Artichoke Soup, page 136)
- Reduced-fat milk or yogurt
- Fruit

Meal ideas and tips for diabetes

- Protein, such as meat, poultry, seafood, eggs, dairy, or plant-based
- Green salad or nonstarchy vegetable (Great Green Broccoli-Spinach Soup, page 184)
- Reduced-fat milk or unsweetened reduced-fat yogurt, 1 CARB

2 slices bruschetta: Calories: 201 cals; Protein: 11 g; Carbohydrates: 28 g; Fat: 5 g; Fiber: 5 g; Sodium: 384 mg; Vitamin A: 1,042 IU; Niacin: 5 mg; Copper: 0.2 mg; Manganese: 1 mg; Selenium: 21 mcg; 2 CARBS

Beef, Barley, and Vegetable Soup

Protein, vitamins A and K, and B vitamins foster your baby's cell, brain, nervous system, bone, and muscle development.

THIS hearty soup is sure to satisfy your growing appetite. Any vegetables, from potatoes and turnips to broccoli and spinach, can be added in place of the beef to make this a rich vegetarian soup. Slow cooker/Instant Pot instructions follow. Keeps refrigerated for up to three days, or freeze for up to one month.

SERVES 8; MAKES ABOUT 8 CUPS

2 tablespoons olive oil
1 medium-size onion, diced
3 cups sliced carrot
½ cup uncooked pearl barley, rinsed under hot water
1¼ pounds bone-in beef shank
1 (14.5-ounce) can diced tomatoes (do not drain), or 1½ cups peeled and diced fresh tomatoes
8 cups stock, plus more as needed
1 zucchini, halved lengthwise and sliced
8 ounces mushrooms, sliced (2 cups)
Salt and freshly ground black pepper, to taste
¼ cup chopped fresh parsley, for garnish (optional)

- Heat the olive oil in a 6-quart saucepan over medium-high heat. Add the onion and sauté for 3 minutes. Add the carrot and barley and sauté for 3 minutes. Add the beef, tomatoes, and stock and bring to a boil. Lower the heat and simmer, uncovered, for 20 minutes.

- Add the zucchini and mushrooms and simmer for about 25 minutes longer, or until the barley and meat are tender.

- Remove the shank from the soup, and when it is cool enough to handle, remove the meat from the bone. Cut the meat into small pieces and return it to the soup.

- Add more canned stock or water to thin the soup, if desired, and adjust the seasoning and heat through before serving. Garnish with the parsley, if desired, and serve immediately.

Meal ideas

- Green salad or vegetable (Easy Cheese-y Toast, page 243)
- Reduced-fat milk or yogurt
- Fruit

Meal ideas and tips for diabetes

- Green salad or nonstarchy vegetable
- Reduced-fat milk or unsweetened reduced-fat yogurt, 1 CARB

(continues)

1 cup beef barley soup: Calories: 239 cals; Protein: 20 g; Carbohydrates: 19 g; Fat: 10 g; Fiber: 4 g; Sodium: 549 mg; Vitamin A: 8,190 IU; Vitamin K: 44 mcg; B_6: 0.6 mg; B_{12}: 2 mcg; Niacin: 8 mg; Riboflavin: 0.5 mg; Thiamine: 0.3 mg; Copper: 0.4 mg; Phosphorus: 272 mg; Selenium: 19 mcg; Zinc: 5 mg; 1½ CARBS

Beef, Barley, and Vegetable Soup (continued)

SLOW COOKER OR INSTANT POT INSTRUCTIONS:

- Use 6 cups of stock instead of 8.
- Drain the diced tomatoes.
- Using a large skillet instead of a saucepan, or your Instant Pot, sauté the onion as directed in Step 1. Add the carrots and barley and sauté for 3 minutes.
- Transfer the contents of the skillet to the slow cooker, then add the beef shank, drained diced tomatoes, stock, and zucchini. Cover and cook on HIGH for 6 hours. Finish the soup as directed in Steps 3 and 4.

Beets with Goat Cheese and Greens

Protein, vitamins A, E, and K, and folate boost your baby's cell, brain, nervous system, bone, and muscle development.

LOVE beets? This one's for you, healthy mama! The recipe calls for packaged or jarred cooked beets (such as Love Beets) found in the produce section of many grocery stores. Toasting the walnuts or pecans is optional, but it greatly enhances their flavor. Baby arugula, kale, spinach, or romaine are all smart choices. If you have fresh dill on hand, throw some in, too. Use only pasteurized goat cheese, or swap out for your favorite cheese (pasteurized feta is great).

SERVES 2

1 tablespoon cider vinegar
1 teaspoon Dijon mustard
¼ cup olive oil
5 cups baby greens, such as arugula or mâche
1 cup sliced store-bought cooked beets
½ cup pasteurized goat cheese, broken into small chunks
⅓ cup chopped walnuts or pecans, toasted
Salt and freshly ground black pepper

- Stir together the vinegar and Dijon in a small bowl, then whisk in the olive oil. Set aside.
- Arrange the baby greens in a serving bowl or on a platter. Place the beets on top of the greens. Drizzle the Dijon mixture evenly over the top, then garnish with the goat cheese and walnuts. Sprinkle with salt and pepper to taste and serve immediately.

Meal ideas

- Protein, such as meat, poultry, seafood, eggs, dairy, or plant-based (Spaghetti with Herbed Tofu Balls, page 273)
- Reduced-fat milk or yogurt
- Fruit with vitamin C

Meal ideas and tips for diabetes

- Protein, such as meat, poultry, seafood, eggs, dairy, or plant-based (Mustard-Tarragon Pork Tenderloin, page 195)
- Reduced-fat milk or unsweetened reduced-fat yogurt, 1 CARB

Half of the beet salad: Calories: 497 cals; Protein: 11 g; Carbohydrates: 15 g; Fat: 46 g; Fiber: 5 g; Sodium: 325 mg; Vitamin A: 1,602 IU; Vitamin E: 4 mg; Vitamin K: 132 mcg; Folate: 155 mcg; Copper: 0.7 mg; Manganese: 1 mg; 1 CARB

Nutty Baked Acorn Squash

Vitamin E and B vitamins foster your baby's cell, brain, and nervous system development.

MAKE your squash more nutty and nutritious. A drizzle of honey or maple syrup adds a sweet touch. Quinoa or any whole grain is a great complementary side dish.

SERVES 5

1 acorn squash
(about 2 pounds), sliced in half and seeded
2 tablespoons olive oil
2 tablespoons light brown sugar
2 teaspoons ground cinnamon, cloves, or allspice, or a mixture
½ cup chopped pecans or sliced almonds
½ cup pumpkin seeds
¼ cup sunflower seeds
Salt and freshly ground black pepper
3 tablespoons pure maple syrup or honey, for drizzling (use maple if vegan)
⅓ cup pomegranate seeds, for garnish (optional)

- Preheat the oven to 375°F. Line a rimmed baking sheet with parchment paper or foil; set aside.
- Position one squash half, cut side down, on a chopping board and slice it into 2-inch-thick semicircles. Transfer the pieces to a large bowl and repeat with the remaining squash half. Add the olive oil, brown sugar, and cinnamon to the bowl and mix until the squash is coated. Transfer the squash to the prepared baking sheet, arranging the pieces in a single layer. Bake for 20 minutes.
- Remove from the oven. Sprinkle the nuts and seeds on top. Continue to bake for 15 minutes, or until the squash is tender. Check for doneness by piercing the squash with the tip of a knife. Transfer to a serving dish. Season with salt and pepper to taste and drizzle with the maple syrup. Garnish with the pomegranate seeds, if using.

Meal ideas

- Protein, such as meat, poultry, seafood, eggs, dairy, or plant-based (Slow-Cooked Ginger-Garlic Chicken, page 277)
- Whole grain or starch
- Green salad or vegetable
- Reduced-fat milk or yogurt
- Fruit with vitamin C

Meal ideas and tips for diabetes

- Protein, such as meat, poultry, seafood, eggs, dairy, or plant-based (above)
- Green salad or nonstarchy vegetable
- Reduced-fat milk or unsweetened reduced-fat yogurt, 1 CARB

One fifth of the squash: Calories: 326 cals; Protein: 8 g; Carbohydrates: 28 g; Fat: 23 g; Fiber: 6 g; Sodium: 201 mg; Vitamin E: 4 mg; Niacin: 4 mg; Thiamine: 0.4 mg; Copper: 0.5 mg; Magnesium: 155 mg; Manganese: 2 mg; Phosphorus: 282 mg; Zinc: 2 mg; 2 CARBS

Cauliflower-Broccoli Rice

Vitamins C, E, and K and folate optimize your baby's cell, brain, and nervous system development.

AN awesome vitamin-filled alternative to rice, with zero carbs (created, in part, for our wonderful moms managing diabetes during pregnancy). This side dish goes with everything, and it's simple to make—but you do need a food processor, unless you can find ready-cut cauliflower rice in your produce section. The term *chopped-up* in the ingredients list refers to large bits of cauliflower and broccoli, about the size of granola. Gluten-free? Use gluten-free bread to make the crumbs or omit them. If seeds are not your thing, skip them, or add pine nuts or any other nuts instead.

MAKES ABOUT 6 CUPS

6 tablespoons olive oil
1 cup "crumbled" bread crumbs (from 2 slices of dairy-free white bread, ideally slightly stale)
3½ cups chopped-up cauliflower florets (from about 1 pound of florets; see headnote)
3 cups chopped-up broccoli florets (from about 12 ounces of florets; see headnote)
1 garlic clove, minced
Zest and juice of 1 lemon
¼ cup sunflower seeds
Salt and freshly ground black pepper
¼ chopped fresh parsley

• Heat 3 tablespoons of the olive oil in a very large skillet over medium-high heat. Add the bread crumbs and sauté, stirring occasionally, for 2 minutes, or until golden brown. Transfer to a bowl; set aside. Do not rinse the skillet.

• Return the skillet to medium-high heat. Add the remaining 3 tablespoons of olive oil. When hot, add the cauliflower and broccoli and sauté, stirring occasionally, for 6 minutes, or until al dente and slightly golden. Push to one side, add the garlic, lemon zest and juice, and sunflower seeds, and sauté for 1 minute. Then, mix together the contents of the skillet, add salt and pepper to taste, and sauté for one more minute.

• Transfer to a large serving dish. Sprinkle with the bread crumbs and parsley and serve.

Meal ideas

• Protein, such as meat, poultry, seafood, eggs, dairy, or plant-based (Steak on the Grill, page 279)
• Green salad
• Reduced-fat milk or yogurt
• Fresh fruit

Meal ideas and tips for diabetes

• Protein, such as meat, poultry, seafood, eggs, dairy, or plant-based (above)
• Green salad
• Reduced-fat milk or unsweetened reduced-fat yogurt, 1 CARB

1 cup cauliflower rice: Calories: 213 cals; Protein: 5 g; Carbohydrates: 12 g; Fat: 17 g; Fiber: 3 g; Sodium: 90 mg; Vitamin C: 72 mg; Vitamin E: 5 mg; Vitamin K: 105 mcg; Folate: 99 mcg; Copper: 0.3 mg; 1 CARB

Couscous Salad with Chickpeas and Artichokes

DF V Q

Vitamins A, C, and folate promote your baby's cell, brain, and nervous system development.

THIS couscous salad is quick and easy, despite the long list of ingredients. Add what you want and make substitutions. For this salad, any small-grained pasta (such as orzo or acini di pepe) or quinoa can be used in place of the couscous. Short on time? Pick up your favorite ready-cut vegetables, such as grated carrots, bell peppers, zucchini, broccoli florets, cucumbers, tomatoes, or chickpeas, from a salad bar. Need more protein? Add cooked chicken, shrimp, hard-boiled eggs, cheese, or tofu (to keep it vegan) to this salad. Gluten-free? Use an equal amount of brown rice or quinoa in place of the couscous. Leftovers keep refrigerated for three days.

SERVES 6; MAKES ABOUT 5 CUPS

3 tablespoons cider vinegar
1 teaspoon Dijon mustard
¼ cup olive oil
2 medium-size tomatoes, diced, or 12 cherry or grape tomatoes, halved
1 cup diced red bell pepper
⅔ cup chickpeas (1 [7¾-ounce] can)
⅔ cup canned or jarred artichoke hearts, quartered
½ cup olives (any kind)
¼ cup pine nuts or your favorite nuts, toasted
3 cups cooked couscous (from about 1 cup uncooked)
Freshly squeezed lemon juice
Salt and freshly ground black pepper

- In a small bowl, stir together the vinegar and Dijon until well blended. Add the olive oil, mix well, and set aside.
- Add the tomatoes, bell pepper, chickpeas, artichoke hearts, olives, and pine nuts to the couscous, then add the Dijon mixture and mix gently until all the ingredients are well combined. Add lemon juice to taste, adjust the seasoning, and serve.

Meal ideas

- Protein, such as meat, poultry, seafood, eggs, dairy, or plant-based (Mustard-Tarragon Pork Tenderloin, page 195)
- Reduced-fat milk or yogurt
- Fruit with vitamin C

Meal ideas and tips for diabetes

- Protein, such as meat, poultry, seafood, eggs, dairy, or plant-based (above)
- Reduced-fat milk or unsweetened reduced-fat yogurt, 1 CARB

¾ cup couscous salad: Calories: 276 cals; Protein: 7 g; Carbohydrates: 30 g; Fat: 15 g; Fiber: 5 g; Sodium: 339 mg; Vitamin A: 1,173 IU mg; Vitamin C: 40 mg; Folate: 79 mcg; Copper: 0.3 mg; Manganese: 1 mg; Selenium: 22 mcg; 2 CARBS

Spaghetti with Herbed Tofu Balls

Protein, calcium, vitamins A and C, and folate enhance your baby's cell, brain, bone, and nervous system development, plus fiber for your digestion and iron for your supply.

A fabulous vegetarian twist on real meatballs that will satisfy meat lovers as well. No time? Use your favorite store-bought spaghetti sauce and fresh pasta. Gluten-free? Serve these meatballs on top of your favorite gluten-free grain. You can jazz up our simple tomato sauce by adding onions, mushrooms, or red bell pepper. Add any fresh herbs at the last minute. The tofu balls will keep refrigerated for up to five days. They do not freeze well.

SERVES 4 (MAKES ABOUT 25 TOFU BALLS AND ABOUT 3½ CUPS TOMATO SAUCE)

12 to 16 ounces enriched thin spaghetti or linguine
1½ teaspoons olive oil

HERBED TOFU BALLS

1 (15-ounce) package (drained weight) extra-firm tofu, drained, finely crumbled (use your hands or a fork), and blotted with paper towels
½ cup plain or seasoned bread crumbs
⅓ cup finely grated Parmesan cheese
3 large eggs, lightly beaten
¼ cup chopped fresh cilantro
¼ cup chopped fresh parsley
½ cup thinly sliced scallion
½ teaspoon salt
Freshly ground black pepper
1 tablespoon olive oil

- Cook the pasta according to the package directions; drain and return to the pot. Add the olive oil, stir, cover, and set aside in a warm place.
- Prepare the herbed tofu balls: Combine all the tofu ball ingredients, except the oil, in a bowl and mix until well blended. Using a rounded measuring tablespoon, scoop out mounds of the tofu mixture and place on two large plates, then form each portion into a ball.
- Heat the olive oil in a large skillet over medium-high heat. Add half of the tofu balls and sauté, turning several times, for about 7 minutes, or until light golden brown and heated through. Repeat with the remaining tofu balls. Transfer the tofu balls to a clean plate lined with a paper towel. Cover to keep warm. Do not rinse the skillet.

Meal ideas

- Green salad or vegetable (Asian-Inspired Spinach Salad, page 186)
- Reduced-fat milk or yogurt
- Fruit with vitamin C

Meal ideas and tips for diabetes

- Reduce the amount of pasta, and ideally use whole wheat pasta, 1 CARB
- Green salad or nonstarchy vegetable (Greek-Style Broccoli, page 248)

(continues)

5 tofu balls: Calories: 207 cals; Protein: 17 g; Carbohydrates: 12 g; Fat: 10 g; Fiber: 0.7 g; Sodium: 467 mg; Calcium: 188 mg; 1 CARB

1¼ cups cooked spaghetti with ¾ cup sauce: Calories: 355 cals; Protein: 12 g; Carbohydrates: 64 g; Fat: 7 g; Fiber: 7 g; Sodium: 555 mg; Vitamin A: 14,445 IU; Vitamin C: 18 mg; Folate: 148 mcg; Iron: 5 mg; 4 CARBS

Spaghetti with Herbed Tofu Balls (continued)

TOMATO SAUCE

1 tablespoon olive oil
1 garlic clove, minced
1 teaspoon dried oregano
1 teaspoon Italian seasoning
1 (28-ounce) can crushed
   tomatoes

Additional chopped fresh
   cilantro and parsley, for
   garnish (optional)
Grated Parmesan cheese,
   for serving

- Prepare the tomato sauce: Heat the olive oil in the same skillet over medium heat. Add the garlic, oregano, and Italian seasoning and cook for 30 seconds. Add the crushed tomatoes, stir, and simmer for 10 minutes, or until slightly thickened. Adjust the seasoning before serving.

- To serve, place some of the pasta in a bowl, top with some of the tofu balls, and cover with sauce and chopped fresh herbs. Serve with Parmesan cheese.

Baked Salmon and Broccoli Rabe with Scallion-Ginger Sauce

Protein, vitamins A, C, D, E, and K, B vitamins, and omega-3 DHA optimize your baby's cell and brain development, and boost your immunity.

PACKED with vitamins—if you love salmon, you'll keep coming back to this recipe! No broccoli rabe? Use regular broccoli or your favorite veggie instead. Serve this salmon with soba noodles, brown rice, or quinoa, tossed with a bit of toasted sesame oil and garnished with chopped fresh cilantro.

SERVES 4

SCALLION-GINGER SAUCE (MAKES ABOUT ¾ CUP)

½ cup warm water

2 tablespoons light soy sauce or wheat-free tamari (for gluten-free)

1 tablespoon seasoned rice vinegar

3 tablespoons light brown sugar

1 teaspoon cornstarch

1 tablespoon olive oil

1 cup thinly sliced scallion

2 tablespoons minced fresh ginger

1 tablespoon minced green chile pepper (optional)

- Prepare the sauce: In a small bowl, stir together the warm water, soy sauce, rice vinegar, brown sugar, and cornstarch; set aside. In a small skillet, heat the olive oil over medium heat. Add the scallion, ginger, and green chile pepper, if using, and sauté for 2 minutes. Add the brown sugar mixture and cook, stirring occasionally, until the sauce begins to thicken, about 3 minutes, then set aside.

- Center an oven rack and preheat the oven to 400°F. Line a rimmed baking sheet with parchment paper or foil and spray with cooking spray.

Meal ideas

- Whole grain or starch (Easy Rice and Green Lentil Side Dish, page 89)
- Green salad or vegetable
- Reduced-fat milk or yogurt
- Fresh fruit

(continues)

One quarter of the salmon dish (4 ounces salmon): Calories: 324 cals; Protein: 26 g; Carbohydrates: 12 g; Fat: 19 g; Fiber: 2 g; Sodium: 653 mg; Vitamin A: 1,855 IU; Vitamin C: 19 mg; Vitamin D: 500 IU; Vitamin E: 6 mg; Vitamin K: 161 mcg; B_6: 0.9 mg; B_{12}: 4 mcg; Niacin: 11 mg; Thiamine: 0.3; Riboflavin: 0.3 mg; Phosphorus: 332 mg; Manganese: 0.3 mg; Omega-3 DHA: 1.2 g; 1 CARB

Cooking spray

4 center-cut salmon fillets (about 4 ounces each), rinsed and patted with paper towels

8 ounces broccoli rabe, ends trimmed and stalks cut in half

- Line up the salmon, skin side down, on the prepared baking sheet. Arrange the broccoli rabe in a single layer next to the salmon, but not touching it. Bake for 15 to 20 minutes, depending on the thickness of the salmon, until the fish is cooked through when flaked with the tip of a knife in the thickest part of the flesh. (There is no need to turn the fish.)

- Meanwhile, rewarm the sauce over low heat. Arrange the salmon and broccoli rabe on a platter and spoon the sauce over it. Serve promptly.

Meal ideas and tips for diabetes

- Whole grain or starch, 1 CARB
- Green salad or nonstarchy vegetable
- Reduced-fat milk or unsweetened reduced-fat yogurt, 1 CARB

Slow-Cooked Ginger-Garlic Chicken   **DF** **LC**

Protein, vitamin K, and B vitamins foster your baby's cell, brain, nervous system, and muscle development, and fiber supports your healthy digestion.

WHO does not love to come home to a delicious slow-cooked meal ready to eat? This recipe calls for a whole chicken, but feel free to use 2 pounds of bone-in chicken parts. To save time, chop up the garlic and ginger in a mini food processor. Use your favorite vegetables. Green beans, snow peas, carrots, shiitake mushrooms, and broccoli rabe are all great options. Brown rice, quinoa, or any whole grain is the perfect pairing for the chicken and sauce.

SERVES 5

¼ cup packed light brown sugar

3 tablespoons minced fresh ginger

3 large garlic cloves, smashed and peeled

3 tablespoons light soy sauce or tamari

2 tablespoons fresh lemon or lime juice

4 scallions, trimmed and cut into thirds or quarters

5 sprigs fresh cilantro

¼ teaspoon red pepper flakes, or to taste (optional)

1 (2½-pound) chicken, rinsed and all visible fat trimmed

2 tablespoons cornstarch

- Combine all the stew ingredients, except the chicken and cornstarch, in an Instant Pot or slow cooker and mix well. Add the chicken and turn to coat. Position the chicken breast side up, and make sure some of the seasonings coat the top of the chicken. Cover and cook on LOW for 2 hours, or on HIGH for 1½ hours. Then turn the chicken over, so the breast side is down, and cook on low for 2 hours longer, or on HIGH for 45 minutes, or until the juices run clear when the thick part of the thigh is pierced with the tip of a knife. (Note: The cooking time will depend on your slow cooker and the size of the chicken. If you don't turn the chicken, it's not a big deal.)

- Alternatively, to braise the chicken in the oven, preheat the oven to 250°F. Place all the chicken stew ingredients, except the cornstarch, in a lidded, ovenproof casserole dish and cook for 2 to 3 hours, until the chicken is done when tested as above.

Meal ideas

- Whole grain or starch (Loaded Sesame Noodles, page 292)
- Green salad or vegetable
- Reduced-fat milk or yogurt
- Fruit

Meal ideas and tips for diabetes

- Whole grain or starch, 1 CARB
- Green salad or nonstarchy vegetable
- Reduced-fat milk or unsweetened reduced-fat yogurt, 1 CARB

(continues)

One fifth of the chicken and vegetables: Calories: 229 cals; Protein: 28 g; Carbohydrates: 13 g; Fat: 7 g; Fiber: 1 g; Sodium: 472 mg; Vitamin K: 30 mcg; B$_6$: 0.5 mg; Niacin: 14 mg; Selenium: 21 mcg; 1 CARB

- Once the chicken is cooked, carefully transfer it to a chopping board. Strain the cooking liquid into a small saucepan. Skim any fat off the sauce. Dissolve 2 teaspoons of the cornstarch in 3 tablespoons of water, add the mixture to the saucepan, and cook over medium heat, stirring, for 4 to 5 minutes, until the sauce is thickened to the desired consistency. Serve the chicken with the sauce.

Steak on the Grill

DF **LC**

Protein and B vitamins enhance your baby's cell, brain, nervous system, and muscle development.

QUICK and easy is the name of the game here. If you're short on time, buy a good dry rub from the grocery store or off the Internet (hint: Williams-Sonoma has some great rubs). Leftover rub will keep covered in the refrigerator for up to two weeks. Use it on poultry, fish, or anything else.

SERVES 2
MAKES ENOUGH FOR UP TO 2 POUNDS STEAK

RUB

1 tablespoon chili powder

1 teaspoon roasted ground cumin

1 teaspoon freshly ground black pepper

½ teaspoon sugar

1 teaspoon garlic powder

2 teaspoons Worcestershire sauce

8 ounces rib-eye steak

- Prepare the rub: Combine all the rub ingredients in a small bowl and mix until well blended.
- Place the steaks in a large bowl. Using the back of a spoon, smear the rub over the surface of the meat. Prick them with a fork to allow the marinade to penetrate the meat. Cover and refrigerate for ideally 2 hours, or up to 12, before cooking.
- Cook the steaks to the well-done stage on the grill or under a broiler. The timing will depend on the size and thickness of your steak.

Meal ideas

- Whole grain or starch (Mexican-Style Rice and Beans, page 220)
- Green salad or vegetable
- Reduced-fat milk or yogurt
- Fruit with vitamin C

Meal ideas and tips for diabetes

- Whole grain or starch (above), 1 CARB
- Green salad or nonstarchy vegetable
- Reduced-fat milk or unsweetened reduced-fat yogurt, 1 CARB

One 4-ounce steak: Calories: 220 cals; Protein: 21 g; Carbohydrates: 0 g; Fat: 15 g; Fiber: 0 g; Sodium: 73 mg; B$_{12}$: 3 mg; Zinc: 8 mg; Selenium: 27 mcg; 0 CARBS

Chunky Apple and Apricot Sauce

Great fiber for your digestion.

A chunky applesauce topped with nuts and seeds is lovely on top of waffles, French toast, or pancakes. Add it to oatmeal or cold cereal. Make a parfait with plain Greek yogurt. Serve it with pork chops or pork tenderloin. The apples are left unpeeled to save time and to add fiber. This applesauce keeps for three days refrigerated, and it can be frozen for up to one month.

SERVES 6; MAKES ABOUT 4 CUPS

6 large apples (about 1½ pounds), cored and diced
1 cup water or apple juice
½ cup dried apricots (about 10 pieces)
⅓ cup dried cranberries
1 teaspoon ground cinnamon, or 1 cinnamon stick
⅓ cup sugar, pure maple syrup or honey, or to taste (skip honey if vegan)
½ cup chopped walnuts, for garnish
⅓ cup pumpkin seeds, for garnish

- Combine the apples, water or apple juice, dried apricots, dried cranberries, and cinnamon in a medium-size saucepan. Bring to a boil. Lower the heat and simmer, stirring occasionally, for 10 to 15 minutes, or until the fruit is soft.
- Remove the saucepan from the heat, stir in the sugar, let cool, then puree the mixture in a blender or food processor to your desired consistency, making it as smooth or chunky as you like. Garnish with the chopped walnuts and pumpkin seeds.

Tip for diabetes
- Reduce your portion size, or skip this recipe.

⅔ cup applesauce: Calories: 290 cals; Protein: 5 g; Carbohydrates: 51 g; Fat: 11 g; Fiber: 7 g; Sodium: 4 mg; Copper: 0.3 mg; Manganese: 0.7 mg; 3 CARBS

KITCHEN WISDOM: HOW TO TOAST AND FREEZE NUTS

TOASTING certain varieties of nuts, such as walnuts and pecans, can add to their flavor. Having pretoasted nuts in the freezer is a real bonus, especially when you're in a hurry. There are a couple of ways to toast nuts. Preheat the oven to 300°F. Spread them in a single layer (it's okay if they overlap a bit) on a baking sheet and bake for 10 minutes. Stir and bake for 10 minutes more, or until they give off a nutty smell and are light golden. Watch carefully to prevent burning; some nuts may take less than 20 minutes. Transfer to a plate to cool. Or you can toast nuts in a dry skillet on the stovetop over low to medium heat. Stir them every now and then to prevent burning. The timing will depend on how high your heat is. Once they are completely cooled, store them in an airtight container in the freezer.

Dreamy Chia Pudding with Berries

B vitamins enhance your baby's cell development, and fiber promotes your digestion.

CHIA seeds and coconut milk make a dreamy combo. Feel free to change the ingredients and flavors by adding bananas, nuts, seeds, dried fruit, orange zest, vanilla extract, chocolate shavings (vegan if necessary), and using almond or vanilla soy milk in place of coconut. Storing in a small mason jar is ideal, especially if you plan to eat this pudding on the go. This pudding will keep for three days refrigerated.

SERVES 4

2 cups light coconut milk
1 teaspoon pure vanilla extract
¼ cup pure maple syrup
¼ teaspoon ground cinnamon
½ cup chia seeds
1 cup fresh raspberries or
    blueberries, for topping
Coconut shaving or shredded
    coconut, for garnish

- Heat the coconut milk in a small saucepan over medium heat or place it in a measuring cup and use a microwave. Add the vanilla, maple syrup, cinnamon, and chia seeds and stir constantly to make sure the chia seeds don't clump together. Remove from the heat. Let the mixture rest for 5 minutes and stir again. Adjust the flavors.
- Divide the warm mixture among four jars or small bowls. Cover and refrigerate for 3 hours. Top with the berries and coconut.

Tips for diabetes
- Reduce or skip the maple syrup.
- Reduce your portion size, or skip this recipe.

½ cup chia pudding: Calories: 288 cals; Protein: 7 g; Carbohydrates: 34 g; Fat: 16 g; Fiber: 13 g; Sodium: 30 mg; Niacin: 2 mg; Riboflavin: 0.3 mg; Copper: 0.3 mg; Phosphorus: 258 mg: Magnesium: 109 mg; Manganese: 1 mg; Selenium: 16 mcg; 2 CARBS

Getting Ready for Birth and Beyond

Weeks 36 Through 40

Finally, you are weeks, maybe even days, away from delivery. Confetti, please! At Week 37, your baby is considered full term. So, you made it, mama! But we'll wait for the big day to formally congratulate you. Just keep in mind, fewer than 5 percent of babies are born on their due date. By Week 36, your baby is the size of a large honeydew melon and weighs about 6 pounds. At delivery, your beautiful baby will be about 20 inches and weigh somewhere around 7.5 pounds. One gorgeous healthy pumpkin.

YOUR BABY'S DEVELOPMENT

- In Week 36, your baby's senses are well developed. All of his or her body parts are sensitive to hot and cold, and to pressure.
- In Week 37, your baby continues to get ready to breathe by inhaling amniotic fluid.
- In Week 38, your baby's organs and systems continue maturing while fat and muscles build.
- In Week 39, your baby is having a dress rehearsal. You should have your birth plan mapped out by now.
- In Week 40, it's showtime! You'll be meeting your beautiful baby soon.

CHANGES IN YOUR BODY

All the same symptoms as you may have experienced in Month 8, only more intense. Some moms will experience "lightening," when the baby "drops" and breathing gets easier. You may feel increased fatigue or you may have more energy from nesting syndrome. Your baby is doing more squirming and less kicking because there's less room. Your cervix is getting dilated. It's weeks or days before your water breaks and the mucus plug falls out. Or not. Sometimes, this has to be induced.

IDEAL NUTRITION

Your nutrition focus is foods to enhance your baby's brain and bone development, blood volume, immunity, and delivery. The following nutrients will help achieve this.

- B vitamins: cell division, brain formation, nervous system development
- Calcium: bones and teeth
- Copper: iron utilization
- Iron: maternal blood volume
- Magnesium: heart functioning, blood glucose regulation, blood pressure control
- Manganese: bone development, thyroid, blood glucose regulation, nervous system
- Omega-3s: brain and eye development
- Phosphorus: bone development
- Protein: supports fetal muscle growth
- Selenium: cell structure and immunity
- Vitamin A: cell formation, bones, teeth, central nervous system, vision
- Vitamin C: iron absorption and immunity, healthy gums and teeth
- Vitamin D: calcium absorption
- Vitamin E: cell structure and immunity
- Vitamin K: bone mineralization
- Zinc: cell structure, immunity, and wound healing

OPTIMAL FOODS FOR MONTH 9

PROTEIN	DAIRY	GRAINS/ LEGUMES	VEGETABLES	FRUITS	FATS/OTHER
Eggs	Cheese	All-bran cereal and other fortified breakfast cereals	Artichokes	Bananas	Brewer's or nutritional yeast
Meats	Enriched plant-based milks (rice soy, and almond)	Beans: soy, black, navy, pinto, kidney, white, great northern, black-eyed, pink, cranberry, Lima, and cannellini	Asparagus	Cantaloupe	Olive oil
Nuts: almonds, cashews, pistachios, Brazil nuts, walnuts and nut butters	Fortified dairy milk		Avocados	Citrus fruits and juices: oranges, tangerines, grapefruit, lemonade	Omega-3s
Pork	Fortified orange juice and other juices		Baked potato with skin on and all other potatoes		Molasses, blackstrap
Poultry	Yogurt	Chickpeas	Beets	Dried apricots and figs	Seaweed, kelp, spirulina
Seafood (fish and shellfish): salmon (wild and Atlantic), tuna, mackerel, herring, sardines in oil, halibut, cod, catfish, canned oysters		Corn and flour tortillas	Broccoli and broccoli rabe	Guava	
		Cream of Wheat	Brussels sprouts	Kiwi	
		Edamame	Butternut squash	Lychee	
		Folic acid–fortified products	Cabbage	Mangoes	
Seeds: sunflower, pumpkin, chia, hemp seed, and flaxseed		Lentils	Carrots	Papaya	
		Oatmeal	Cauliflower	Prune juice	
Tahini		Peanuts	Dark, leafy greens: kale, collards, mustard, Swiss chard, bok choy, and turnip greens	Pineapple	
Tofu and tempeh		Wheat germ		Raspberries	
		Whole grains: quinoa, barley, brown rice, bulgur, and whole wheat couscous	Hearts of palm	Strawberries	
			Mushrooms		
			Pumpkin		
			Red bell pepper		
			Romaine lettuce		
			Snow peas		
			Spinach		
			Sweet potatoes		
			Tomatoes and tomato juice		

RECIPES FOR MONTH 9

Berry-Peach-Flax Smoothie

Vitamin C and the B vitamins enhance your baby's cell, brain, and nervous system development and vitamin C boosts your immunity.

SMOOTHIES are just plain fun and nutritious. Lactose intolerant or vegan? No worries. Soy or coconut yogurt can be used. For a protein boost, add your favorite protein powder. To sweeten, add a little bit of sugar, agave nectar, or honey. Use water or juice to adjust the consistency. Smoothies can last for a day in the fridge and can be frozen for one month. Mix well before serving.

MAKES 2 CUPS

¾ cup plain yogurt
⅔ cup sliced fresh, canned, or
   frozen peaches
½ cup fresh or frozen
   raspberries or strawberries
⅓ cup orange juice or water
2 tablespoons ground
   flaxseeds
Ice cubes

- Place all the ingredients in a blender and process until smooth. Serve over ice.

Tips for diabetes
- Reduce your portion size, or skip this recipe.

1 cup berry-peach-flax smoothie: Calories: 156 cals; Protein: 7 g; Carbohydrates: 25 g; Fat: 4 g; Fiber: 5 g; Sodium: 68 mg; B$_{12}$: 0.5 mcg; Vitamin C: 31 mg; 2 CARBS

Perfect Popovers

Protein and B vitamins enhance your baby's cell, brain, nervous system, and muscle development.

HIGH and mighty, these popovers are best eaten warm straight from the oven with your favorite jam. Don't have whole wheat flour? No sweat. Use a total of 1 cup of all-purpose. Gluten-free? Use an equal amount of all-purpose gluten-free flour. To freeze, let cool completely, then place the popovers in a resealable plastic bag and freeze. To reheat, place the popovers in a preheated 350°F oven for about ten minutes. Do not microwave, as they will get soggy.

MAKES 6 LARGE POPOVERS

½ cup whole wheat flour
½ cup all-purpose flour
1 cup milk
2 large eggs
1 large egg white
2 tablespoons canola oil or melted unsalted butter
½ teaspoon salt
Cooking spray

- Preheat the oven to 450°F. Have ready a six-well popover pan.
- In a large mixing bowl, mix together the whole wheat and all-purpose flours. Add the remaining ingredients, except the cooking spray, and beat with an electric mixer on high speed for 30 seconds. Scrape down the sides of the bowl and beat for 15 seconds more. (Note: Don't be concerned if you see tiny lumps of flour. Mash any big lumps against the side of the bowl with the back of a spatula.)
- Preheat the popover pan in the oven for 2 minutes, then remove it and spray with cooking oil. Divide the batter evenly among the popover wells.
- Bake for 20 minutes, then lower the heat to 350°F and bake for 20 more minutes, or until golden brown and puffed. Remove the popovers from the oven and serve immediately.

Meal ideas

- Protein, such as meat, poultry, seafood, eggs, dairy, or plant-based
- Reduced-fat milk or yogurt (Berry-Peach-Flax Smoothie, page 287)
- Fruit

Meal ideas and tips for diabetes

- Reduce your portion size, if necessary.
- Use a low-sugar jam (such as Polaner All Fruit; 2 teaspoons are FREE).
- Protein, such as meat, poultry, seafood, eggs, dairy, or plant-based
- Reduced-fat milk or unsweetened reduced-fat yogurt, 1 CARB

2 popovers: Calories: 287 cals; Protein: 13 g; Carbohydrates: 35 g; Fat: 11 g; Fiber: 3 g; Sodium: 489 g; B_{12}: 0.7 mcg; Niacin: 5 mg; Thiamine: 0.3 mg; Riboflavin: 0.5 mg; Manganese: 1 mg; Selenium: 35 mcg; 2 CARBS

Gazpacho (Without the Gas)

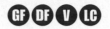

Vitamins A and C optimize your baby's cell and bone development and boost your immunity.

GAZPACHO is loaded with vitamins, but sometimes those raw onions, garlic, cucumbers, tomatoes, and peppers can leave you burping or gassy. To prevent this, briefly cooking the ingredients before blending can help. Jarred or fresh jalapeños and sun-dried tomatoes add a wonderful layer of flavor, but you can skip them. Include whatever works best for you. Cover and refrigerate leftovers for up to three days.

SERVES 4

1 tablespoon olive oil
1 small sweet onion, chopped
1 garlic clove, minced
2 tablespoons thinly sliced jalapeño peppers, or to taste (optional)
¼ cup sun-dried tomatoes in oil, drained (about 3 pieces)
1¼ pounds ripe tomatoes, diced (4 cups)
1 cup diced seedless cucumber
1 cup water or vegetable stock
¼ teaspoon salt, or to taste
Freshly ground black pepper or hot sauce
3 tablespoons chopped fresh cilantro, dill, or chervil

- In a medium-size saucepan, heat the olive oil over medium heat. Add the onion and cook, stirring occasionally, for 3 minutes. Add the garlic, jalapeños, if using, and sun-dried tomatoes and sauté for 1 minute. Add the remaining ingredients, except the fresh herbs, stir, and bring to the point just before boiling. Remove from the heat and let cool.

- In a blender or food processor or using a handheld immersion blender, puree the gazpacho to your desired consistency, smooth or chunky. Adjust the seasoning and refrigerate until well chilled. Garnish with the fresh herbs before serving.

Meal ideas

- Protein, such as meat, poultry, seafood, eggs, dairy, or plant-based
- Whole grain or starch (Black Bean, Mushroom, and Spinach Quesadillas, page 293)
- Reduced-fat milk or yogurt
- Fruit

Meal ideas and tips for diabetes

- Protein, such as meat, poultry, seafood, eggs, dairy, or plant-based
- Whole grain or starch (above), 1 CARB
- Reduced-fat milk or unsweetened reduced-fat yogurt, 1 CARB

1 cup gazpacho (made with water): Calories: 90 cals; Protein: 2 g; Carbohydrates: 12 g; Fat: 5 g; Fiber: 3 g; Sodium: 29 mg; Vitamin A: 1,666 IU; Vitamin C: 34 mg; 1 CARB

Healthy Hummus

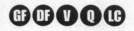

Protein and B vitamins promote your baby's cell, brain, nervous system, and muscle development.

HUMMUS is a wonderful addition to anyone's diet, especially a pregnant woman's. Eat it with toasted whole wheat pita bread, whole wheat crackers, or sliced fresh vegetables (to keep it vegan). You can toss in some jarred red peppers to create a delicious red hummus, or roasted garlic cloves for an intense garlicky hummus. Sprinkle with your favorite seeds for an extra dose of nutrients. This dip keeps for three days refrigerated.

MAKES ABOUT 2 CUPS

1 (15-ounce) can chickpeas (about 1¾ cups), drained and rinsed
1 small garlic clove, minced
2 tablespoons freshly squeezed lemon juice, or to taste
3 tablespoons olive oil
1 tablespoon tahini
A few drops of Tabasco sauce or your favorite hot sauce (optional)
Salt
¼ cup sunflower seeds, for garnish

- Combine all the ingredients, except the sunflower seeds, in the bowl of a food processor or blender and process until completely smooth, scraping down the sides of the bowl as needed and adding 2 to 3 tablespoons of water to achieve your desired consistency. Adjust the seasoning, garnish with the seeds, and serve; refrigerate leftovers.

½ **cup hummus:** Calories: 234 cals; Protein: 7 g; Carbohydrates: 17 g; Fat: 16 g; Fiber: 6 g; Sodium: 440 mg; B$_6$ 0.6 mg; Copper: 0.3 mg; Manganese: 1 mg; 1 CARB

Favorite Broccoli Slaw

Protein, vitamins C, E, and K, B vitamins, and folate foster your baby's cell, brain, nervous system, bones, and muscle development, plus all these nutrients are excellent for you.

YOU'RE gonna love it! Colorful, cheerful, crunchy, and supremely healthy, this broccoli salad marries well with just about everything. No time? Use a good-quality bottled dressing. For more protein, toss in edamame, canned beans, or sautéed tofu. And nonvegan moms can add any of those ingredients, plus cheese or cooked chicken. This slaw is best consumed on the day it is made. It keeps for three days refrigerated.

MAKES 4¼ CUPS

SLAW

1 (12-ounce) package broccoli slaw (about 4 cups)
⅓ cup sunflower seeds
⅓ cup pumpkin seeds
⅓ cup chopped walnuts, toasted
⅓ cup dried cranberries

DRESSING

2 tablespoons cider vinegar
1 tablespoon Dijon mustard
1 tablespoon pure maple syrup or honey (use syrup if vegan)
¼ cup olive or canola oil
1 garlic clove, minced
Juice of ½ lemon, or to taste
Pinch of salt

- Prepare the slaw: Combine the slaw ingredients in a large bowl and set aside.
- Prepare the dressing: In a small bowl, combine all the dressing ingredients and whisk until well blended.
- Pour the dressing over the salad and toss gently until all the slaw ingredients are lightly coated. Allow to rest for 15 minutes before serving, so the flavors can develop.

Meal ideas

- Protein, such as meat, poultry, seafood, eggs, dairy, or plant-based (Baked or Fried Chicken Tenders, page 300)
- Whole grain or starch
- Reduced-fat milk or yogurt
- Fresh fruit

Meal ideas and tips for diabetes

- Protein, such as meat, poultry, seafood, eggs, dairy, or plant-based (above)
- Whole grain or starch, 1 CARB
- Reduced-fat milk or unsweetened reduced-fat yogurt, 1 CARB

1 cup slaw: Calories: 399 cals; Protein: 10 g; Carbohydrates: 24 g; Fat: 32 g; Fiber: 5 g; Sodium: 122 mg; Vitamin C: 80 mg; Vitamin E: 7 mg; Vitamin K: 96 mcg; B_6: 0.4 mg; Thiamine: 0.3 mg; Niacin: 5 mg; Folate: 98 mcg; Phosphorus: 312 mg; Magnesium: 141 mg; Manganese: 1 mg; Zinc: 2 mg; 2 CARBS

Loaded Sesame Noodles

Protein, vitamins A, C, and E, and B vitamins optimize your baby's cell, brain, nervous system, bone, and muscle development, plus all these nutrients are excellent for you.

A delicious salad popular with readers for years. This new version includes two protein options. Feel free to change the ingredients, including grated carrots, broccoli or cauliflower florets, zucchini slices, or edamame. Gluten-free? Use gluten-free noodles and wheat-free tamari. If you have toasted seeds on hand, add them as a garnish. This salad can be made a day ahead, but the spinach should be added just before serving. These noodles keep for three days refrigerated.

SERVES 5; MAKES ABOUT 5 CUPS

8 ounces dried udon or enriched linguine noodles

3 tablespoons toasted sesame oil

¼ cup light soy sauce or tamari, or to taste

1 tablespoon seasoned rice vinegar, or to taste

1 garlic clove, minced or ½ teaspoon garlic powder

1 cup seeded and sliced red bell pepper

2 cups packed baby spinach leaves or watercress leaves

⅓ cup pumpkin or sunflower seeds

PROTEIN OPTIONS

1½ cups cooked chicken breast, beef, shrimp, or 15 ounces sautéed extra-firm tofu

- Cook the noodles according to the package directions. Drain and place in a large bowl.
- Add the sesame oil, soy sauce, rice vinegar, and garlic to the noodles and toss to coat. Add the remaining ingredients, including your choice of protein options, and toss gently until well combined. Adjust the seasoning, adding more oil or vinegar as needed, and serve.

Meal ideas

- Reduced-fat milk or yogurt
- Fresh fruit (Refreshing Fruit Salad, page 130)

Meal ideas and tips for diabetes

- Reduced-fat milk or unsweetened reduced-fat yogurt, 1 CARB
- Fresh fruit, 1 CARB

1 heaping cup noodles with chicken: Calories: 302 cals; Protein: 19 g; Carbohydrates: 30 g; Fat: 13 g; Fiber: 5 g; Sodium: 552 mg; Vitamin A: 1,678 IU; Vitamin C: 35 mg; Vitamin E: 3 mg; B_6: 0.4 mg; Thiamine: 0.4 mg; Copper: 0.3 mg; Magnesium: 101 mg; Phosphorus: 293 mg; Selenium: 14 mcg; Zinc: 2 mg; 2 CARBS

1 heaping cup noodles with tofu: Calories: 300 cals; Protein: 15 g; Carbohydrates: 31 g; Fat: 15 g; Fiber: 6 g; Sodium: 528 mg; Vitamin A: 1,670 IU; Vitamin C: 35 mg; Vitamin E: 3 mg; Vitamin K: 49 mcg; Thiamine: 0.4 mg; Copper: 0.4 mg; Iron: 4 mg; Magnesium: 114 mg; Manganese: 0.8 mg; Phosphorus: 286 mg; Selenium: 13 mcg; Zinc: 3 mg; 2 CARBS

Black Bean, Mushroom, and Spinach Quesadillas

Q

Protein, vitamins A and K, B vitamins, and folate foster your baby's cell, brain, nervous system, bone, and muscle development, plus calcium keeps your bones strong and iron fortifies your stores.

SERVE these healthy quesadillas with salsa and guacamole (page 135) or simple avocado slices. Other ingredients to consider are olives, roasted red peppers, quick-cooked broccoli florets, asparagus tips, corn, or edamame. During pregnancy, avoid soft Mexican cheese, such as queso fresco and asadero.

MAKES THREE 6-INCH ROUND QUESADILLAS

1 tablespoon olive oil
1½ cups sliced mushrooms
4 cups packed baby spinach
½ cup canned black beans, drained and rinsed
2 tablespoons jarred jalapeño peppers (optional)
6 (6- to 8-inch) corn or wheat tortillas
1½ cups grated Cheddar cheese or Monterey Jack

FOR SERVING

Salsa
Avocado slices or guacamole

- In a large skillet, heat the olive oil over medium-high heat. Add the mushrooms and sauté, stirring occasionally, for 5 minutes. Add the spinach and continue to sauté for 2 minutes. Add the black beans and jalapeños, if using, and cook until warm. Remove the skillet from the heat and transfer the contents to a heatproof bowl. Rinse the skillet and wipe with paper towels.

- Return the skillet to medium-low heat and heat until hot. Place one tortilla in the skillet. Add one third of the cheese. Top with one third of the mushroom mixture, spreading it evenly over the cheese. Cover with a second tortilla. Press gently. When the cheese is melted and the filling sticks together (gently press to adhere), carefully flip the tortilla sandwich and cook until light golden, about 2 minutes. Watch carefully to prevent burning. Transfer to a serving plate.

- Using kitchen scissors or a knife, cut the quesadilla into quarters and serve with your favorite toppings.

Meal ideas

- Green salad (see Awesome Homemade Dressings, page 214)
- Fresh fruit

Meal ideas and tips for diabetes

- Reduce your portion size.
- Green salad (above)

1 quesadilla (made with 8-inch flour tortillas): Calories: 617 cals; Protein: 27 g; Carbohydrates: 62 g; Fat: 30 g; Fiber: 4 g; Sodium: 1,371 mg; Vitamin A: 4,259 IU; Vitamin K: 186 mcg; B₁₂: 0.6 mcg; Niacin: 8 mg; Riboflavin: 0.5 mg; Folate: 119 mcg; Calcium: 647 mcg; Copper: 0.2 mg; Iron: 4 mg; Phosphorus: 342 mg; Selenium: 21 mcg; Zinc: 3 mg; 4 CARBS

Okra and Tomatoes Greek Style

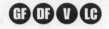

Vitamins A, C, and K optimize your baby's cell, brain, nervous system, bone, and muscle development, plus the vitamin C keeps you healthy.

OKRA is a nutritional powerhouse. When in season, fresh tender okra is delicious, but it's often hard to find. One 10-ounce package of sliced frozen okra, cooked according to the label, can be substituted for the fresh okra. Add your favorite vegetables, such as zucchini, artichoke hearts, or green beans, along with the okra—the more vegetables the merrier. This dish keeps for three days refrigerated.

SERVES 4; MAKES ABOUT 3 CUPS

1 tablespoon olive oil
½ cup chopped onion
1 garlic clove, minced
1 teaspoon Italian seasoning or dried oregano
10 ounces okra, ends trimmed, cut into ½-inch slices
1 (14.5-ounce) can diced tomatoes (do not drain)
1 teaspoon sugar
Salt and freshly ground black pepper

- Heat the olive oil in a large saucepan over medium-high heat. Add the onion and sauté for 3 minutes, or until light golden brown.
- Add the remaining ingredients and bring to a boil, then lower the heat, cover, and simmer gently for 30 to 35 minutes, or until the okra is tender. Adjust the seasoning and serve.

Meal ideas

- Protein, such as meat, poultry, seafood, eggs, dairy, or plant-based (Panfried Chicken with Tzatziki, page 118)
- Reduced-fat milk or yogurt
- Fruit

Meal ideas and tips for diabetes

- Protein, such as meat, poultry, seafood, eggs, dairy, or plant-based (above)
- Whole grain or starch, 1 CARB
- Reduced-fat milk or unsweetened reduced-fat yogurt, 1 CARB

¾ **cup okra and tomatoes:** Calories: 81 cals; Protein: 2 g; Carbohydrates: 12 g; Fat: 4 g; Fiber: 4 g; Sodium: 10 mg; Vitamin A: 1,164 IU; Vitamin C: 29 mg; Vitamin K: 31 mcg; Manganese: 0.7 mg; 1 CARB

Roasted Brussels Sprouts

GF **LC**

Vitamin C, K, and E foster your baby's cell, nervous system, and bone development, plus the vitamin C is great for you.

IF you're a fan of these mini-cabbages, you'll love them roasted. Sliced almonds can be substituted for the pine nuts. Dairy-free or vegan? Skip the Parmesan.

SERVES 4

12 ounces fresh Brussels sprouts, ends trimmed and loose or damaged outer leaves removed, cut in half (or quarters, if they are very large)

Salt and freshly ground black pepper

3 tablespoons olive oil

¼ cup toasted pine nuts

⅓ cup finely grated Parmesan cheese

Drizzle of balsamic vinegar (optional)

- Adjust an oven rack to the top section of the oven. Preheat the oven to 400°F. Line a rimmed baking sheet with parchment paper or foil.
- Place the Brussels sprouts on the prepared baking sheet, season with salt and pepper, and toss with the olive oil so the sprouts are well coated. Spread them out in a single layer. Roast for 15 minutes. Remove from the oven, stir, add the pine nuts, and continue to roast for 10 minutes. The sprouts should be nicely browned and crisp.
- Remove from the oven. Transfer to a serving bowl or plates. Sprinkle with the Parmesan and a light drizzle of balsamic, if using. Adjust the seasoning and serve.

Meal ideas

- Protein, such as meat, poultry, seafood, eggs, dairy, or plant-based (Grilled or Broiled Lamb Chops, page 228)
- Reduced-fat milk or yogurt
- Fruit

Meal ideas and tips for diabetes

- Protein, such as meat, poultry, seafood, eggs, dairy, or plant-based (above)
- Whole grain or starch, 1 CARB
- Reduced-fat milk or unsweetened reduced-fat yogurt, 1 CARB

1 cup Brussels sprouts: Calories: 112 cals; Protein: 6 g; Carbohydrates: 10 g; Fat: 18 g; Fiber: 4 g; Sodium: 141 mg; Vitamin C: 72 mg; Vitamin K: 161 mcg; Vitamin E: 3 mg; Copper: 0.2 mg; Manganese: 1 mg; 1 CARB

Best-Ever Vegetarian Lasagne

Protein, vitamins A, and C, and folate promote your baby's cell, brain, nervous system, and muscle development, plus the calcium, iron, and fiber are all excellent for you.

LASAGNE is a bit time consuming to make—but it's always worth it. To cut time, use frozen spinach, presliced mushrooms, and store-bought high-quality pasta sauce (you will need 4 cups of sauce). If adding tofu for extra protein, drain it well, then slice it into ½-inch slices. Line a large plate with a triple thickness of paper towels, place the tofu slices on the plate, then using a second bunch of paper towels, blot the tofu to remove excess water. Repeat for the remaining slices. Do not use the tofu if you plan to freeze the lasagne before baking.

The sauce can be made up to three days in advance, covered, and refrigerated. After completing Step 3, the lasagne can be wrapped with plastic wrap and refrigerated overnight, or the uncooked lasagna can be frozen for up to one month. To cook, place the frozen lasagne directly in the oven. The cooking time will increase by fifteen to twenty minutes.

SERVES 8

**TOMATO SAUCE
(MAKES ABOUT 4 CUPS)**

2 tablespoons olive oil
1 medium-size onion, chopped
1 garlic clove, minced
1 tablespoon dried basil or Italian seasoning
1 tablespoon dried oregano
1 (28-ounce) can crushed tomatoes
2 tablespoons chopped fresh basil, oregano, or dill, or a combination

- Prepare the sauce: Heat the olive oil in a large saucepan over medium-high heat. Add the onion and sauté for 3 minutes. Add the garlic, basil, and oregano and continue to sauté for 2 minutes. Add the crushed tomatoes, stir, and bring to a boil, then lower the heat and simmer, uncovered, for 10 minutes. Stir in the fresh herbs and remove from the heat. The sauce should yield 4 cups; if not, add water or tomato juice to make 4 cups. Set aside.

Meal ideas

- Green salad (Quick Romaine and Avocado Salad, page 109)
- Reduced-fat milk or yogurt
- Fresh fruit

Meal ideas and tips for diabetes

- Reduce your portion size, if necessary.
- Green salad (above)
- Fresh fruit, 1 CARB

One eighth of the lasagne: Calories: 371 cals; Protein: 24 g; Carbohydrates: 34 g; Fat: 16 g; Fiber: 7 g; Sodium: 526 mg; Vitamin A: 2,944 IU; Vitamin C: 19 mg; Folate: 83 mcg; Calcium: 480 mg; Iron: 5 mg; 2 CARBS

(continued)

VEGETABLE LASAGNE

1 tablespoon olive oil

1 pound mushrooms, thinly sliced

10 ounces baby spinach, or 10 ounces frozen chopped spinach, thawed and drained

Enough no-boil (oven-ready) lasagna noodles to fill a 9 x 13 x 2-inch pan

1 (15-ounce) package (drained weight) firm tofu, thinly sliced and pressed (optional)

4 cups shredded pasteurized mozzarella cheese (about 1 pound)

6 tablespoons grated Parmesan cheese (optional)

Cooking spray

- Prepare the vegetables for the lasagne: Heat the olive oil in a large skillet over medium-high heat. Add the mushrooms and sauté for 5 minutes. Using a slotted spoon, transfer the mushrooms to a bowl, leaving behind any juices in the skillet. If using fresh spinach, add it to the skillet, in batches if necessary, and sauté until just wilted, about 3 minutes. Add the spinach to the mushrooms and set aside. (If using frozen spinach, add it directly to the mushrooms.)

- Assemble the lasagne: Spread ¾ cup of the sauce over the bottom of an ungreased 9 x 13 x 2-inch pan. Place three or four no-boil lasagna noodles over the sauce (follow the instructions on your lasagna box—different brands require different preparation methods). Spread about one third of the spinach and mushrooms evenly over the noodles, followed by one third of the tofu slices, if using, ¾ cup of the sauce, 1 cup of the mozzarella cheese, and 2 tablespoons of the Parmesan, if using. Repeat the layering process of noodles, vegetables, tofu, sauce, and cheeses two more times. For the last layer, place three or four noodles on top of the cheese, then add the remaining sauce to cover the noodles and top with the remaining mozzarella cheese.

- To bake, adjust an oven rack to the middle position and preheat the oven to 375°F. Cover the pan with parchment paper or foil (lightly sprayed on its inner side with cooking spray) and bake for 45 minutes.

- Remove the paper or foil and bake for 15 minutes more, or until the top is nicely browned and a knife inserted into the middle of the lasagne indicates soft noodles. Remove the lasagne from the oven and let cool for 10 minutes before slicing.

Salmon with Artichoke-Olive Tapenade

GF **DF** **LC**

Protein, vitamins D and E, B vitamins, and omega-3 DHA foster your baby's cell, brain, and nervous system development, plus calcium absorption for you.

IF you like olives and artichokes, this tapenade will make you swoon! It's amazing on everything from pita chips to baked or broiled fish. Some of our readers make a double batch of tapenade just to have the leftovers. Instead of salmon, use halibut steaks or any other fish fillet or shellfish, meat, poultry, or tofu. The tapenade keeps refrigerated for three days.

SERVES 2

ARTICHOKE-OLIVE TAPENADE (MAKES ABOUT 1 CUP)

¾ cup artichoke hearts in brine or oil (about 5 large hearts), drained
15 pitted green olives (about ⅓ cup)
1 to 2 tablespoons freshly squeezed lemon juice, to taste
2 tablespoons olive oil
1 small garlic clove
Freshly ground black pepper
¼ cup chopped fresh dill

1 tablespoon olive oil
8 ounces salmon steaks
Salt and freshly ground black pepper

- Prepare the tapenade: Combine all the tapenade ingredients, except the dill, in the bowl of a food processor and process until slightly chunky. Add the dill and pulse a few times. Be careful not to puree. Adjust the seasoning and transfer to a serving bowl. Cover and refrigerate until ready to serve.
- Grill the salmon steaks: Preheat the grill. Have a clean plate ready for the cooked fish. Oil the grill rack, season the salmon with salt and pepper, then grill the fish for about 5 minutes on each side, or until cooked through. The cooking time will depend on the heat of the grill and the thicknesses of the fish.

Meal ideas

- Salad or vegetable
- Whole grain or starch (Couscous Salad with Chickpeas and Artichokes, page 272)
- Reduced-fat milk or yogurt
- Fresh fruit

Meal ideas and tips for diabetes

- Salad or nonstarchy vegetable
- Whole grain or starch (above), 1 CARB
- Reduced-fat milk or unsweetened reduced-fat yogurt, 1 CARB
- Fresh fruit, 1 CARB

4 ounces salmon: Calories: 235 cals; Protein: 23 g; Carbohydrates: 0 g; Fat: 15 g; Fiber: 0 g; Sodium: 67 mg; Vitamin D: 500 IU; Vitamin E: 4 mg; B_6: 0.7 mg; B_{12}: 3 mg; Niacin: 10 mg; Phosphorus: 272 mg; Selenium: 27 mcg; Omega-3 DHA: 1.2 g; 0 CARBS
4 tablespoons tapenade: Calories: 95 cals; Protein: 1 g; Carbohydrates: 5 g; Fat: 8 g; Fiber: 2 g; Sodium: 408 mg; 0 CARBS

(continued)

- Alternatively, to sauté the salmon steak, heat the olive oil in a medium-size skillet over medium-high heat. Season the fish with salt and pepper, then add it to the skillet. Cook for 3 to 4 minutes on each side, or until completely cooked through. Check the doneness by pulling the flesh away from the center bone; it should be opaque and flaky.
- Serve the fish topped with some of the artichoke-olive tapenade.

Baked or Fried Chicken Tenders

Protein and B vitamins foster your baby's cell, brain, nervous system, and muscle development.

CHICKEN tenders are loved by all ages, not just kiddies, and they can be healthy, even superhealthy if you coat them with ground flaxseeds instead of bread crumbs. Gluten-free? Use gluten-free panko or flaxseeds; see the note in Step 3. Apart from the standard ketchup (which your kids might prefer, or you, too), use any of the sauces or salsas in this book. These chicken tenders keep for three days refrigerated, and they can be frozen for up to one month.

MAKES 20 TO 25 CHICKEN TENDERS

1¼ pounds chicken tenders or boneless, skinless chicken breasts
½ cup all-purpose flour
2 large eggs
Salt and freshly ground black pepper
1 cup plain or seasoned bread crumbs or panko
⅓ cup finely grated Parmesan cheese
A pinch of Old Bay seasoning, Italian herbs, or dried oregano
Canola oil cooking spray if baking the tenders, or 1 to 3 tablespoons olive oil, if sautéing

- Cut the chicken tenders in half. If using boneless breasts, cut each lengthwise into three strips, then cut each strip on the diagonal into 2- to 2½-inch strips. (Don't worry too much about the size and shape.) Place the tenders in a bowl and set aside.
- Place the flour in a shallow pie dish or rimmed plate. Place the eggs and a sprinkle of salt and pepper in a bowl and beat; set aside. Combine the bread crumbs, Parmesan cheese, and seasonings in a shallow pie dish or a rimmed plate and mix well; set aside.
- Set up your workstation in a row as follows: chicken tenders, flour, egg mixture, bread crumb mixture, and two large plates. Place about half of the tenders in the flour and toss gently to coat all sides. Transfer the tenders in batches to the egg mixture and coat them with egg, then transfer them to the bread crumbs. Cover the tenders with the bread crumbs, pressing gently so they adhere, then place the breaded tenders on the plates. Repeat this procedure with the remaining tenders.

Meal ideas

- Whole grain or starch (Yummy Three-Bean Salad, page 138)
- Green salad or vegetable
- Reduced-fat milk or yogurt
- Fresh fruit

Meal ideas and tips for diabetes

- Bake the chicken tenders.
- Use the flax-coated version, if possible.
- Whole grain or starch (above), 1 CARB
- Green salad or nonstarchy vegetable

5 chicken tenders (made with bread crumbs): Calories: 318 cals; Protein: 34 g; Carbohydrates: 26 g; Fat: 8 g; Fiber: 1 g; Sodium: 333 mg; B$_{12}$: 0.6 mcg; Niacin: 20 mg; Riboflavin: 0.5 mg, Thiamine: 0.4 mg, Iron: 4 mg; Phosphorus: 363 mg; Selenium: 43 mcg; 2 CARBS

(continued)

Note: To make ground flaxseed–coated tenders, place ½ cup of ground flaxseeds in a bowl. Skip using the flour, egg, and bread crumb coatings and, instead, simply coat the chicken tenders on all sides with the flaxseeds.

- To bake, preheat the oven to 450°F. Just before baking, preheat a baking sheet for 3 minutes (this helps the tenders brown evenly). Remove it from the oven and spray it generously with canola oil cooking spray. Arrange the tenders on the prepared baking sheet, and lightly spray them with canola oil. Bake for 20 minutes, or until thoroughly cooked. For additional browning, after baking, broil on HIGH for about 5 minutes.

- To panfry, heat 1 tablespoon of olive oil in a large skillet over medium-high heat. Without crowding, place half of the tenders in the skillet and cook for 7 to 9 minutes, turning once or twice, until browned and crisp on both sides and fully cooked. Transfer to a clean plate lined with paper towels to drain. Use a big wad of paper towels to wipe out the skillet, then repeat the panfrying procedure with the remaining tenders. (If you use a small skillet, you may need to cook the tenders in three batches.) Serve immediately.

Hearty Beef Stew

Protein and B vitamins foster your baby's cell, brain, nervous system, and muscle development, and iron is for you.

BEEF stew has never tasted so good. Boiled potatoes or wide noodles are traditional sides. Add a green salad for vitamins and fiber. Slow cooker/Instant Pot instructions follow. This stew freezes well.

SERVES 8

2 pounds stewing beef, cut into ½-inch cubes

1 teaspoon salt

½ teaspoon freshly ground black pepper

3 tablespoons all-purpose flour

3 tablespoons olive oil

3 carrots, cut into ½-inch slices

1 large onion, halved and sliced

2 garlic cloves, minced

4 cups stock (any kind)

2 tablespoons tomato paste

1 tablespoon dried thyme

3 bay leaves

14 ounces mushrooms, quartered (3 cups)

1 tablespoon cornstarch

¼ cup chopped fresh parsley, for garnish (optional)

- Place the beef in a bowl, add the salt, pepper, and flour, and toss until the cubes are evenly coated with the flour. Heat 1 tablespoon of the olive oil in a large Dutch oven or large heavy-bottomed saucepan over medium-high heat. Add half of the beef and sauté, turning the meat occasionally, until most sides are nicely browned. Transfer the browned beef to a pie dish or heatproof bowl. Don't worry about any bits sticking to the pot; scrape them up as much as possible (do not rinse the pot). Add 1 tablespoon of the olive oil to the pot and brown the rest of the meat the same way. Transfer the meat to the pie dish. (Again, do not rinse the pot.)

- Add 1½ teaspoons of the olive oil to the pot and sauté the carrots, onion, and garlic for 3 minutes, then return the meat to the pot. Add enough stock, about 3 cups, to cover the meat completely. Add the tomato paste, thyme, and bay leaves, stir, and bring to a boil, then lower the heat to as low as possible and cook for 2 hours, or until the meat is fork-tender.

Meal ideas

- Whole grain or starch
- Green salad or vegetable (Greek-Style Broccoli, page 248)
- Reduced-fat milk or yogurt
- Fresh fruit

Meal ideas and tips for diabetes

- Whole grain or starch, 1 CARB
- Green salad or nonstarchy vegetable (above)
- Reduced-fat milk or unsweetened reduced-fat yogurt, 1 CARB

1⅓ cups of the beef stew: Calories: 256 cals; Protein: 30 g; Carbohydrates: 14 g; Fat: 10 g; Fiber: 2 g; Sodium: 653 mg; Vitamin K: 42 mcg; B Vitamins: B_6: 0.8 mg; B_{12}: 3 mg; Niacin: 9 mg; Riboflavin: 0.5 mg; Iron: 4 mg; Selenium: 36 mcg; Zinc: 7 mg; 1 CARB

(continued)

- When the stew is close to finished, prepare the mushrooms: In a medium-size skillet, heat the remaining 1½ teaspoons of oil over medium-high heat. Add the mushrooms and sauté until light golden. Add them and any juices to the stew.

- When the beef is tender, dissolve the cornstarch in ¼ cup of water and add to the stew. Mix well and then bring to a full boil. Turn off the heat, adjust the seasoning, and transfer to a serving dish. Garnish with the parsley and serve promptly.

Classic Pulled BBQ Pork

Protein and B vitamins optimize your baby's cell, brain, nervous system, and muscle development.

PULLED pork is easy and tasty and perfect for a slow cooker, Instant Pot, or Dutch oven. If you're short on time, use 1 cup of your favorite BBQ sauce mixed with 2 tablespoons of water instead of the homemade sauce below. Add hot sauce, if you desire, or simply ramp up the heat with a generous pinch of cayenne pepper. Serve on buns (dairy-free, if necessary) or rice, or with your favorite whole grain. This dish is traditionally served on soft white buns, which is yummy, but whole wheat buns are healthier.

SERVES 6

SAUCE

1 large onion, chopped
½ cup cider vinegar
1 teaspoon salt
½ teaspoon freshly ground
   black pepper
¼ cup tomato paste
¼ cup light brown sugar
1 tablespoon Worcestershire
   sauce
1 tablespoon Dijon mustard
1 teaspoon garlic powder
½ cup ketchup
Pinch of cayenne pepper
   (optional)

PORK

About 2 pounds boneless
   pork shoulder, rinsed and
   trimmed of all visible fat
1½ tablespoons cornstarch

- Prepare the sauce: In a medium bowl, mix together all the ingredients plus 2 tablespoons of water.
- Prepare the pork: Place the pork in a slow cooker, add the sauce, and turn until the pork is well coated. Cover and cook on LOW for about 5 hours, or until the pork is very tender and the meat gives easily when poked with a fork. (Note: The timing will depend on your slow cooker.)
- Transfer the cooked pork to a bowl and set aside to cool. Transfer the sauce to a medium-size saucepan and skim off as much fat as possible. If you have more than 1½ cups of sauce, simmer the sauce over low heat until reduced to that amount; otherwise, just bring it to a simmer. Dissolve the cornstarch in 1 tablespoon of water and add it to the sauce. Stir until the sauce thickens, then remove from the heat and set aside.

Meal ideas

- Whole grain or starch
- Green salad or vegetable (Favorite Broccoli Slaw, page 291)
- Reduced-fat milk or yogurt
- Fresh fruit

1 cup pulled pork: Calories: 347 cals; Protein: 31 g; Carbohydrates: 18 g; Fat: 15 g; Fiber: 1 g; Sodium: 829 mg; B$_6$: 1 mg; B$_{12}$: 1 mcg; Niacin: 15 mg; Riboflavin: 0.4 mg; Thiamine: 0.9 mg, Copper: 0.2 mg; Phosphorus: 336 mg; Selenium: 49 mcg; Zinc: 3 mg; 1 CARB

(continued)

- As soon as the pork is cool enough to handle, shred it, using two forks and a small knife. Add the pulled pork to the sauce in the saucepan and reheat it over low heat. Place some of the pork in each of the buns, if using, and serve promptly.

Meal ideas and tips for diabetes

- Whole grain or starch, 1 CARB
- Green salad or nonstarchy vegetable (Favorite Broccoli Slaw, page 291)
- Reduced-fat milk or unsweetened reduced-fat yogurt, 1 CARB

Berry-licious Shortcakes

Vitamins C and E and B vitamins promote your baby's cell, brain, and nervous system development and boost your immune system.

WHEN your sweet tooth beckons, reach for this shortcake and berry recipe. Gluten-free? Use gluten-free flour or oat flour. Dairy-free? Use plain unsweetened almond or soy milk instead of the whole milk. Skip the whipped cream and serve with your favorite nondairy sorbet. Vegan? Follow dairy-free tips, plus use vegan margarine or coconut oil in place of the unsalted butter. The strawberries should be allowed to sit for at least two hours before serving, for their juices to release. If you need to speed things up, sauté half of the berries with the sugar, combine with the uncooked berries, and serve. An equal amount of all-purpose flour can be substituted for the whole wheat flour. No time to whip heavy cream? Serve a scoop of ice cream or yogurt on the side.

SERVES 6

STRAWBERRY FILLING

1½ pounds fresh strawberries (about 6 cups), washed and hulled; cut half of the strawberries into quarters, or eighths if they are large

⅓ cup sugar, or to taste

SHORTCAKE

½ cup all-purpose flour

½ cup whole wheat flour

1½ teaspoons baking powder

¼ cup sugar

¾ cup sliced almonds, chopped

3 tablespoons unsalted butter, cut into pieces

½ cup milk

1 cup whipped cream, for topping (optional)

- Prepare the filling: Two hours before serving, combine the sliced strawberries and sugar in a bowl, mix and set aside. Place the whole strawberries in the bowl of a food processor and pulse until they are chopped into small pieces; do not puree. Add the chopped strawberries to the sliced strawberries, stir, cover, and refrigerate until ready to serve.

- Preheat the oven to 450°F. Line a baking sheet with parchment paper.

- Prepare the shortcake dough: Combine the flours, baking powder, sugar, and almonds in a large bowl and mix. Add the butter and, using your fingers, rub the mixture until it resembles coarse meal. Add the milk and stir until just combined; do not overmix.

Tips for diabetes

- Reduce your portion size, or skip this recipe.

1 shortcake with strawberries: Calories: 350 cals; Protein: 7 g; Carbohydrates: 39 g; Fat: 20 g; Fiber: 6 g; Sodium: 17 mg; Vitamin C: 85 mg; Vitamin E: 4 mg; Niacin: 4 mg; Riboflavin: 0.3 mg; Copper: 0.3 mg; Manganese: 1 mg; Selenium: 12 mcg; 2½ CARBS

(continued)

- Measure scant ¼-cupfuls of the short-cake dough and arrange on the baking sheet, gently forming into rounds. You should have six shortcakes. Bake for 10 minutes, or until light golden brown. Immediately remove the shortcake biscuits from the baking sheet and cool them on a plate or wire rack.

- To serve, slice each shortcake biscuit in half. Put the bottoms of the biscuits on the dessert plates, and cover each with some strawberry filling (and juices). Top with whipped cream, if desired, cover with the tops of the biscuits, and serve. Refrigerate leftovers.

Mango-Tango Lime Spritzer

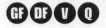

Vitamins A and C foster your baby's cell development and your immunity.

IF you love mango and lime, this drink has your name on it. As it is refreshing and loaded with vitamins, you can't find a better mocktail! Add more soda water or orange juice to thin it. Enjoy!

SERVES 2; MAKES ABOUT 3 CUPS

1 cup frozen mango pulp
2 tablespoons freshly
    squeezed lime juice,
    or to taste
½ cup orange juice
1 tablespoon sugar, agave
    nectar, or honey, or
    to taste (avoid honey
    if vegan)
1 cup club soda, or to desired
    consistency
3 ice cubes

- Place all the ingredients in the blender and mix on high speed until smooth. Adjust the sweetness and consistency. Pour into two glasses and serve. Refrigerate leftovers.

Tips for diabetes
- Reduce your portion size, or skip this recipe.

1¼ cups mango spritzer: Calories: 106 cals; Protein: 1 g; Carbohydrates: 26 g; Fat: 0 g; Fiber: 2 g; Sodium: 27 mg; Vitamin A: 1,024 IU; Vitamin C: 66 mg; 2 CARBS

Caring for Your Baby and Yourself for the Fourth Trimester

Welcome to Motherhood

Breastfeeding Your Baby

Let the beautiful, chaotic, wondrous journey of motherhood begin! Your nine months of pregnancy are finally over, and you just delivered a gorgeous baby. Now the real work of motherhood starts. If this is your first child, enjoy the fact that ignorance is bliss. If it is your second or third, or more, you know exactly how much work is involved in raising children, but you also know that the rewards far outweigh the hardships.

"Nine Months Later" is about you—yes, you. Being a new mom is not easy. We are here to help. If you want to eat healthfully while breastfeeding, read about the nutrients you need for optimal breast milk. If you need help salvaging your figure and getting back into your prepregnancy wardrobe, we can give you tips for weight loss. And, if you think you may have the "baby blues" or postpartum depression, please read on. You're not alone.

BREASTFEEDING: IDEAL NUTRITION

Breastfeeding ain't easy, but it's worth it . . . if it works for you. And, there is no shame or self-punishment if it does not. Formula feeding is a healthy alternative. To keep the spotlight on breastfeeding, research shows that it offers many health benefits for infants and mothers, as such as protection against common childhood infections and disease risk, and healthy weight gain for baby. Breastfeeding duration of at least two months was associated with reducing the risk of sudden infant death syndrome (SIDS), and breastfeeding does not need to be exclusive to confer this protection.[1] Research also shows that very early skin-to-skin contact and suckling may have physical and emotional benefits.[2] Other studies suggest that breastfeeding may reduce the risk for certain allergic diseases,[3] asthma,[4] obesity,[5] and type 2 diabetes.[6] It also may help improve an infant's cognitive development.[7] However, more research is needed to confirm these findings. In short, by consuming the proper nutrients, a nursing mother can produce nutritionally balanced breast milk that greatly enhances her baby's physical and mental development.

Every mom-and-baby breastfeeding pair is unique, and their challenges are unique, too. Certain situations, such as some of those below, may require the need for a lactation consultant and additional help along the way. In this section, we will focus only on the nutritional side of breastfeeding, not the physical mechanics or other issues.

Moms who may need extra help breastfeeding include:
- Mothers nursing multiples
- Mothers breastfeeding while pregnant (tandem nursing)
- Mothers with diabetes who nurse
- Obese or underweight nursing mothers
- Teenage nursing mothers
- Mothers nursing babies born with a cleft palate, premature babies, hospitalized babies, or any other babies with special needs
- Mothers with inverted nipples
- Mothers who have had breast surgery or have breast issues

Many moms ask whether breastfeeding will "really" help them lose weight after delivery. The short and easy answer is yes. While you're pregnant, your body automatically layers on fatty tissue to give you ample fat stores to support breastfeeding your newborn. If you chose to breastfeed, this extra padding will gradually disappear as your body adjusts to its new role as a milk factory. The fact is that moms naturally burn calories to make breast milk each time they nurse. Most nursing mothers find that even while consuming additional calories to support breastfeeding, their weight drops gradually and naturally. Losing about 1 to 2 pounds per month is the norm. Key point: Do not diet while breastfeeding, unless otherwise advised by your doctor or care team.

Some new moms wonder how breastfeeding will affect their daily meals. Will they need more calories, carbohydrates, fat, and protein? If you're eating a well-balanced diet with ample calories to satisfy your hunger, and you are getting enough liquid to stay well hydrated, especially after each nursing session, you probably don't need any major changes to your diet. One of the wonders of breast milk is that it can usually meet your baby's nutritional needs even when you're not eating "perfectly." But, just because your baby won't be harmed by your occasional dietary lapses doesn't mean that your body won't suffer. The adage applied to pregnancy also goes for breastfeeding: Your body will feed your baby first. When your nutrient intake is inadequate, your body draws on its reserves, which can eventually become depleted.

How many calories do moms need is another common question. There's no one-size-fits-all answer. In general, 2,000 to 2,500 calories per day are needed, and a minimal intake of no fewer than 1,800 calories per day. Your body is working around the clock to make breast milk for your baby, burning about 500 extra calories daily in the process. But this number may need to be adjusted based on milk volume, your rate of weight loss, extreme amounts of physical activity or exercise, and any special situations.

Instead of counting calories (unless your doctor has recommended you do so), we suggest that you follow your hunger as a guide to how much you need to eat. Many breastfeeding moms feel surges of hunger, whereas others may feel hungry all the time. Eating small meals with healthy snacks in between—the way you did during pregnancy—is a good way to keep your hunger in check and your energy level high. Here are some guidelines.

BASIC ADVICE FOR BREASTFEEDING

- Inform your OBGYN and your child's pediatrician in advance of delivery that you will be breastfeeding. Explain any dietary restrictions or special needs you may have.
- Continue taking all of your prenatal vitamins and any supplements prescribed by your doctor as long as recommended, usually for 6 months. Do not self-prescribe vitamins or supplements (synthetic or herbal), because large doses may be toxic. And remember that vitamins and supplements do not replace real food.
- Do not take any medications, prescription or over-the-counter, without your doctor's approval. Breastfeeding women should not use Retin-A or Accutane.
- Avoid all alcohol, but if you really need a drink, make sure to consume it after you've nursed, to allow a couple of hours for the alcohol to metabolize. The alcohol reaches your baby through your breast milk.
- Follow a well-balanced, varied diet that contains nutrient-dense foods. Your baby will taste the foods you consume, so if you eat healthfully, don't be surprised if your baby develops a taste for peas, carrots, spinach, squash, and peaches.
- Consume about 500 extra calories per day (or about 200 calories above your pregnancy caloric intake) for the duration of breastfeeding.

- Eliminate or severely limit caffeine to no more than 1 to 2 cups of coffee or tea per day. The caffeine passes into your breast milk. If you need energy, consume protein, go for a walk, or take a few deep breaths of fresh air.
- Drink 8 fluid ounces of water each time you breastfeed, or at least 6 to 8 cups of water per day. This, along with increased fiber, will help avoid constipation.
- Vegetarians and vegans should be able to meet all of their nutritional needs adequately, although certain supplements will be needed. As a vegetarian, you need to eat foods that contain vitamin B_{12} (such as eggs or dairy), eat foods fortified with vitamin B_{12}, and/or take supplements. If you are on a vegan or macrobiotic diet, or any other diet that does not include animal products, be sure to get enough B_{12}, calcium, iron, protein, and other nutrients that may be lacking. You may need to get advice from a registered dietitian or your doctor.
- Follow the same EPA guidelines on fish safety as you did for pregnancy. Avoid high-mercury fish, such as shark, tilefish, and mackerel, and limit canned white tuna to 6 ounces per week. See page 35 for more information.
- As your wallet and availability allow, choose organic products, free of pesticides, hormones, antibiotics, and chemicals as much as possible.
- Follow the same guidelines for sugar substitutes as during pregnancy. Basically, avoid saccharine. Safe choices include stevia, Splenda, and agave nectar. Natural sugar food sources, such as brown sugar, honey, pure maple syrup, and dried fruits, are always the best.

QUESTIONS AND ANSWERS ABOUT BREASTFEEDING

What are your daily nutritional requirements for breastfeeding?

As with pregnancy, the nutritional guidelines for breastfeeding may appear daunting on paper, but rest assured that certain nutrients in breast milk are fairly consistent, regardless of what a mother eats. A mother's body channels her nutrients into her breast milk, even if it means depleting her own stores. Remember to eat lots of lean protein. Consume calcium with every meal and snack. Consume whole-grain complex carbs with fiber and nutrients. Eat healthy fats, such as olive oil and avocados. Eat iron-rich foods. Fuel up with potassium-rich foods. And, keep in mind the basic nutrition pairs for optimal absorption: vitamin C + iron and vitamin D + calcium. The following are some of the most important nutrients for breastfeeding and how they help your baby grow.

SOME IMPORTANT NUTRIENTS FOR BREASTFEEDING WOMEN AND THEIR BABIES[8]

NUTRIENT	PREGNANCY RDI	LACTATING RDI (AGES 19 TO 50)	BABY'S DEVELOPMENT
Calcium	1,000 mg	1,000 mg	Bones, muscles, and nerve function
Choline	450 mg	550 mg	Brain development
Copper	1,000 mcg	1,300 mcg	Iron absorption
Iodine	220 mcg	290 mcg	Thyroid functioning and metabolism
Omega-3 DHA	300 mg	300 mg	Physical and cognitive development
Potassium	4,700 mg	5,100 mg	Kidney, cardiac, digestive, and muscular function
Protein	71 g	60 g	Building your baby's body
Vitamin A	770 mcg	1,300 mcg	Healthy vision, skin, cell development, and immunity
Vitamin B_{12}	2.6 mcg	2.8 mcg	Red blood cells, nerve function, and metabolism
Vitamin B_6	1.9 mg	2.0 mg	Cell formation, nervous and immune system function
Vitamin D	500 IU	200 IU	Bones
Vitamin E	15 mg	19 mg	Protects cells from damage and boosts immunity
Zinc	11 mg	12 mg	Organ development, muscles, eyes, skin, and genetic expression

What are the nutritional requirements for breastfeeding multiples?

Nursing multiples is definitely a challenge, so don't be afraid to ask for help at any point along your journey. Your pediatrician, lactation consultant, doula, or care team who have experience with multiples can offer support. The calorie math is simple for breastfeeding twins: If one baby = about 500 calories above your prepregnancy needs, two babies = about 1,000 additional calories. You may need to increase your calorie intake as your babies grow and get hungrier. Or decrease them if you supplement your nursing with formula, and later, solids. Talk to your doctor and pediatrician about any extra supplements you and your baby may need.

Are there ways to improve my milk flow?

When you're in the early days of caring for a breastfed baby, nothing can be more stressful than worrying whether you're producing enough breast milk. It can seem like every cry, hiccup, burp, or whimper from your baby is a signal he or she isn't getting enough milk. Here is some basic advice that will hopefully put your mind at ease and improve your milk flow.

Supply and demand: Your milk output is primarily based on supply and demand. Milk production is based on how many times each day your milk is drained from your breasts. The more you breastfeed or express (pump) your milk, the more milk you will make. While eating well is excellent for you (it boosts your energy and resistance to illness among other things), a "perfect" diet is not necessary to produce high quality breastmilk.

Sleep and rest: A good night's sleep or a great nap can do wonders for your milk supply. When you're burning the candle at both ends (yes, you, Supermom!), your body gets worn down. Being as rested as possible can help your body boost milk production. Stay hydrated: Research has not yet found a link between the fluids a mother drinks and her milk production. The simple guideline is drink according to thirst. To make life easy, keep a container of water where you usually breastfeed. A signal that you may need to drink more fluids is if your urine is dark yellow instead of a light, straw color.

Why is vitamin D so important for my baby?

In 2000 and 2001, studies on rickets (a softening of the bones in children caused by a lack of vitamin D) among breastfed infants in North Carolina, Texas, Georgia, and the mid-Atlantic region of the United States prompted researchers to take a closer look at whether all breastfed infants were getting adequate amounts of vitamin D. Based on their findings and other data, in 2003, the American Academy of Pediatrics recommended a daily supplement of 200 IU (5 mcg) of vitamin D for all breastfed infants and all nonbreastfed babies whose daily intake of vitamin D-fortified formula or milk is less than 500 ml. If you have any concerns, consult your child's pediatrician.[9]

Does my baby's fussiness mean that I'm consuming the wrong foods?

A fussy baby is likely not related to something you've eaten; almost all babies have fussy periods. Signs of your baby's intolerance or an allergy to a certain food can include fussiness, dry skin or eczema, congestion, bloody stool, diarrhea, vomiting, rash, and wheezing. If you think your baby has an allergy, or if you have a family history of allergies, consult your baby's pediatrician.

In general, there are no specific foods that every breastfeeding mother must avoid. Some common culprits that may cause gassiness in your baby include garlic, onions, cabbage, broccoli, cauliflower, beans, and spicy or acidic foods. It takes between two and six hours for certain foods to affect the taste and composition of your breastmilk, so if you suspect a food is affecting your baby, chart it but keep in mind this time lag.

Avoid that food for a few days or weeks, then try it again and record your baby's response. You'll find your baby's nursing groove—we promise!

What are some challenges obese women face?

Severely overweight and obese mothers often experience increased challenges when it comes to breastfeeding. In fact, studies indicate that they are more likely to experience difficulty with the mechanics of nursing, which may be one reason they are less likely to start breastfeeding in the first place, or more inclined to breastfeed for a short duration. Studies show that obese mothers also tend to take longer to produce sufficient milk, possibly because of a lower prolactin (a milk-producing hormone) response to suckling. If you are overweight and are experiencing any difficulties, please (please!) don't give up before seeking support.

Navigating Postpartum Depression

Your baby is healthy, your nursery is cozy and adorable, your partner and family love you—but there's one big problem. You are painfully depressed, anxious, and angry, and you're not sure why. Even worse, you're scared to share your disturbing feelings and thoughts with anyone. If this describes you, please know that you are not alone. Approximately one in seven new mothers worldwide (about 15 percent) suffers from postpartum depression (PPD). PPD usually begins during the first three months after birth, but it may begin anytime during the first year postpartum.

The excellent news is that PPD and its related disorders are 100 percent treatable! You might have faced depression during pregnancy, or prior to it, but when there is a flare-up following delivery or a continuation of pregnancy depression, this bout of depression is termed PPD. Even if you are already on medication for depression, you might experience breakthrough symptoms postpartum that require a change in treatment. It's important that you're under the care of a practitioner who specializes in perinatal mental health, since perinatal depression differs from depression at other times in our lives. Please note that the advice here also applies to mothers with existing depression, from mild to severe, treated with medications or not.

It can be tough to know the difference between normal mood changes after giving birth and the more severe symptoms that require treatment. As moms, new and old, we all have bad days, even bad weeks that leave us feeling down, frustrated, irritated, or helpless. A mild state of the "baby blues" is common after delivery and should be gone by two weeks postpartum. Despite our temporary slumps, with the milder baby blues, there is still a light at the end of the tunnel. But for mothers experiencing PPD, that bright new-baby-light goes off. Low self-esteem and a roller coaster of emotions torture a new mother's head, heart, and soul, leaving her behavior erratic and often self-destructive.

One mother who knows these feelings all too well is Shoshana Bennett, PhD, widely known as Dr. Shosh. Her journeys through PPD following both of her pregnancies sparked her commitment to helping women all over the globe recover from this disorder. We asked her to share her story and her expertise on the critical role of nutrition and exercise in recovery.

DR. SHOSH'S PERSONAL STORY

Immediately after I delivered our first baby in 1983, I knew there was something very wrong with me. I became anxious and obsessive—scary thoughts were spinning non-stop in my head about my baby being harmed. I didn't trust myself to be alone with her, thinking I might be the one to hurt her. I was overwhelmed and frightened. I thought my life was over—there was nothing but doom and gloom. I was a mere shell of the person I had been before the birth.

My ob-gyn at that time did what some unfortunately still do, through no fault of their own, since many ob-gyns don't know a lot about prenatal or postpartum mood/anxiety disorders. When I exclaimed, "If life's going to be like this, I don't want to be here anymore," he laughed. He told me that all new mothers feel this way, I should go home and do something nice for myself and that feeling would pass. He tried to normalize a serious disorder and dismissed it as the baby blues. *If this is normal*, I thought, *then clearly I'm an inadequate mother and I wasn't cut out to do this*. I was convinced I was a burden to my family, and my husband and baby would be better off without me. I'm quite grateful to still be here—there were a couple of very close calls when I almost took myself out.

When my daughter was two and a half years old, I remember thinking, *maybe I can be a mom!* I now realize that my chemistry was starting to return to normal. My hair regained its curl, I could see in color again instead of in shades of gray, and I was able to taste my food and enjoy it. We decided to have another baby. Everything went well during my pregnancy, just like the first time, until I delivered. I dropped into the same nightmarish state.

One year into my second life-threatening and undiagnosed postpartum depression, I learned that my condition had a name and there may even be help for it! I vowed to myself at that moment that I would do everything in my power to help other families prevent the devastating effects of this illness. It became my mission to educate all professionals working with pregnant and postpartum parents and the public.

Still coming out of the depression, I started pioneering in Northern California, founded an organization called Postpartum Assistance for Mothers, and became president of California's state organization. More recently, I served as president of our international organization, Postpartum Support International. The help I never received but desperately needed is what I've given to tens of thousands women around the globe.

Along with therapy that empowers new parents to discard the unrealistic expectations of motherhood, a basic plan of action always includes some uninterrupted hours of sleep at night, excellent nutrition, exercise, and emotional and physical support that allow them to nurture themselves. With proper help, postpartum depression is totally treatable and leads to 100 percent wellness—often better than before.

LET'S START BY DEFINING YOUR DEPRESSION

Identifying the symptoms of PPD and distinguishing them from the baby blues is an essential first step. A thyroid imbalance, which affects about 10 percent of postpartum women, can mimic the symptoms of PPD, so it should be ruled out by your doctor as a physiological cause of depression.[1] No matter what, every new mom and parent needs support, and the following list should help you determine whether what you're feeling is "normal" or whether you should seek out a professional.

Baby Blues

Symptoms begin the first week and should be gone by two to three weeks following delivery. If these mild symptoms haven't ended by then, or if they intensify, contact a psychologist or other health practitioner who specializes in perinatal mental health. This professional should give you a thorough assessment and a wellness strategy.

- Crying for no apparent reason
- Lack of concentration
- Feeling stressed out
- Difficulty sleeping at night

Postpartum Depression

PPD can appear immediately after delivery and anytime up to one year postpartum. The feelings are more intense than baby blues and they can get in the way of normal feelings and functioning. If you identify with any of the following feelings or have other symptoms getting in your way, please find a health-care practitioner who specializes in perinatal mental health.

- Sadness
- Difficulty sleeping at night
- Irritability or anger
- Feeling overwhelmed
- Fatigue and exhaustion
- Loss of interest in sex
- Lack of joy in life
- Feelings of shame, guilt, or hopelessness
- Anxiety
- Difficulty bonding with your baby
- Withdrawal from family and friends

Postpartum Psychosis

A rare but serious condition that almost always develops within the first month after delivery. If you experience any of these symptoms, get help immediately.

- Confusion or disorientation
- Thoughts about needing to hurt yourself
- Seeing or hearing things that others don't (hallucinations)
- Speech that doesn't make sense to others
- Paranoia
- Obsessing about death (including of your baby)
- Feeling that you don't need much sleep

BASIC ADVICE FOR THE BABY BLUES AND POSTPARTUM DEPRESSION

Maintaining a well-balanced diet and taking supplements postpartum is essential for both your physical and mental health. From vitamins and minerals to healthy fats and lean proteins—your diet has a huge impact on your strength, stamina, ability to produce breast milk, and solid emotional well-being.

- Take a daily multivitamin with minerals to make sure that you are getting all the essential nutrients your body and brain need. Talk to your doctor or care team about your specific needs. Additional supplements may be required to make sure your body is not lacking any vital nutrients that could affect your emotional health.
- Do not diet if you are suffering from PPD. Depriving your body of nutrients is detrimental to recovery.
- If you've lost your appetite and can't manage to eat three meals a day, nibble foods throughout the day.
- Consume lots of protein, ideally at least 60 grams per day. High-protein foods will help prevent your blood sugar level from rising; keeping it steady is important for balancing your moods.
- Eat complex carbohydrates, such as whole grains, fruits, and vegetables. These slow-releasing sugars are the type your brain likes, especially if it is struggling with depression.
- Avoid refined carbohydrates as much as possible. A box of chocolates may be fleetingly pleasurable, but the sugar high and crash that follow can send your blood sugar levels and emotions into a tailspin. Keep these foods out of the house. If you want a cookie, buy a single, delicious cookie, not a whole bag.
- Stay well hydrated with water. Aim for at least 8 to 10 glasses a day, particularly when exercising, or if you suffer from panic attacks. Dehydration can exacerbate anxiety.
- Try to avoid caffeine; it won't aggravate depression but may increase anxiety.
- Avoid alcohol, which is a depressant.
- Get exercise, ideally outdoors. Even a walk will make a difference.
- Get plenty of sleep. Naps are great, too.

QUESTIONS AND ANSWERS ABOUT POSTPARTUM DEPRESSION

Are there any special nutrients to combat depression?

Yes, there certainly are.[2] In tandem with other treatments, the foods you eat and supplements you take can have a positive effect. Here are some of the top nutrients, why they matter, and where you can find them.

- Chromium to bust sugar cravings.[3] Aim for about 45 micrograms daily. Chromium helps stabilize serotonin, a neurotransmitter that affects anger, aggression, mood, sleep, and other brain functions. A drop in serotonin levels can trigger sugar cravings. It is found in meat, poultry, broccoli, spinach, romaine lettuce, peanuts, potatoes, whole grains, and apples.

- Iron to combat fatigue:[4] Aim for at least 9 milligrams per day. Iron can be severely depleted during pregnancy and breastfeeding. Talk to your care team to see if you're getting enough (see page 342 for iron sources).

- DHA to alleviate depression:[5] Get plenty of serotonin-raising DHA omega-3 fatty acids (at least 300 milligrams of DHA) during pregnancy and postpartum from fish or supplements. DHA omega-3s are proven to help alleviate and prevent depression, in general, not just during pregnancy and postpartum. If you are breastfeeding, they are critical for your baby's brain development, too. And if you're not breastfeeding, speak with your pediatrician about adding a liquid omega-3 supplement to the infant formula. See page 37 for more information on omega-3 supplements.

- B_{12} for energy:[6] Aim for at least 2.8 milligrams per day of B_{12}, which is needed to convert amino acids into serotonin and dopamine, two important neurotransmitters linked to depression and low energy. Animal products, fortified breakfast cereals, and brewer's yeast are good sources.

- Folate for energy and mental health:[7] Raising your daily folate intake to at least 600 micrograms has been associated with increased energy and mental clarity. Studies show that 15 to 38 percent of adults with depressive disorders have low levels of B vitamins, including folate. This B vitamin is also believed to enhance the effects of antidepressant medications (see page 347 for folate sources).

- B_6 for mood balance:[8] Aim for 2.0 mg daily. This vitamin helps conduct the neurotransmitters responsible for balancing your moods. Consume B_6 from poultry, fish, eggs, whole grains, and nuts, and thiamine from whole grains, brewer's yeast, lean pork, legumes, nuts, and seeds.

- Vitamin D to ward off depression:[9] Adequate vitamin D from the sun can help alleviate feelings of depression, but it might not be enough. It's a good idea to get your Vitamin D level checked. There is an inverse relationship with vitamin D levels and depression. People with low levels of vitamin D have more depression, and those with higher D tend to have less. At least 500 mcg or 200 IU are recommended.

How can exercise can help reduce depression?

Exercise is an important part of any PPD recovery plan. One of the best reasons to exercise is that it elevates serotonin and dopamine, and it releases endorphins, or happy hormones. Ironically, during a bout of depression, when you most need those happy chemicals, getting exercise can be extremely difficult due to lack of energy and motivation. Go easy, and remember your body is still recovering. Dr. Shosh suggests doing whatever you can. If all you can do is walk from the living room to the kitchen on a given day, fine. If you can walk outside only far enough to get your mail, that's okay. It may be hard to imagine being this paralyzed by depression, but some women are. If it helps, ask a support person to be your buddy for a walk around the block. Here are some tips to help you start exercising after your doctor gives you clearance.

- Try to take a walk outside every day. Ten minutes is a good start, ideally work up to 30 minutes. Sunshine can be an added serotonin booster.
- If a walk outside sounds overwhelming, do some body stretches that can help relieve tension and stress. If you're sitting a lot, stand up every 20 minutes to get the blood flowing.
- Even if your mobility is restricted due to doctor's orders, certain breathing exercises can oxygenate your brain and help your moods.
- Stay well hydrated, particularly if you're breastfeeding.
- Take lots of breaks, and don't push yourself too hard. If a woman is experiencing a panic disorder, she should avoid overly strenuous exercise because it may cause an adrenaline surge, which could spark a panic attack.
- Yoga is an excellent stress reducer.

Does sleep affect depression?

Catch your zzz's at night and whenever you can. Easier said than done, especially if you have a baby who does not sleep through the night. Sleep deprivation can rob mothers of melatonin, a naturally occurring hormone vital to the regulation of circadian rhythms, and it can reduce serotonin. Low levels of either of these brain chemicals may cause depression, anxiety, and other negative feelings. Finding a sleep schedule that works for you and your baby is the best advice. A few hours of uninterrupted nighttime sleep a few nights a week will propel PPD recovery, and without it, recovery will be harder. Throw out the myths of motherhood, such as, "I'm the mother, so the responsibility of nighttime care is all on me." Allow your baby to bond with Daddy, Gramma, or another trusted adult during those hours so you can recover. You can provide a bottle in case your baby needs to feed while you're sleeping. Everyone benefits this way. Solicit help with child care or chores whenever you can.

If you are at the breaking point of requiring medication to sleep (or you want to avoid getting to that point) and want to try a natural option first, Dr. Shosh suggests getting a pair of low blue light glasses, available online at www.lowbluelights.com. In the spectrum of light, blue light suppresses melatonin and keeps you awake. These special lenses are designed to block out 95 percent of blue light. Wearing them 2 to 3 hours before bedtime can start the flow of natural melatonin in the brain.

Bottom line: PPD is totally treatable and in many cases preventable. It's important to recognize emotional and physical symptoms and to embrace nutrition, exercise, and regular emotional support to greatly minimize the severity of PPD and possibly even to completely avoid it. You're an amazing mom. With proper help from a health-care practitioner who specializes in perinatal mental health, you will succeed, and be on your happy way!

WEIGHT LOSS AFTER BABY
Choose the Right Time and Take It Slow

Before we begin this section, take a deep breath and repeat this new mom's weight-loss mantra: I have an amazing body and I just gave birth to a beautiful child. I accept my body just as it is. I will be patient and compassionate as I take this journey. I will not compare myself to others.

Pregnancy was work. Labor and delivery were work. Breastfeeding is work. Caring for a newborn is tons of work. And weight loss is yet more work. You need a break, mama! And only you can give yourself permission to take a break and to ask others for help when you need it. Before you overwhelm yourself with thinking about weight loss, consider the basic advice we offer below. Most important: Set a natural pace. Most women lose half of their "baby weight" by six weeks after childbirth. The rest often comes off over the next several months.

BASIC ADVICE FOR WEIGHT LOSS POSTPARTUM

- Weight loss from delivery. Take one 7- to 8-pound baby, plus about 2 pounds of blood and amniotic fluid, and you're pretty much assured a 10-pound weight loss in the hospital after you deliver. In the first week, you will probably lose another 3 to 4 pounds of water weight. So, up to 15 pounds can be lost without effort. That's the good news!
- To lose the rest will take work. But ideally wait until after your 6-week checkup before starting a diet. Get clearance from your doctor or care team to diet. Those entire first 6 weeks are a transitional period for mom and baby. It takes about that long for your baby to adapt to the rhythms of the outside world, for breastfeeding to gel, and for planning a daily routine.

- Aim for a weight loss of about 1½ pounds per week. A healthy diet combined with daily exercise will help you shed the pounds. Ideally, you should plan to return to your prepregnancy weight by 6 to 12 months after delivery.
- Get your doctor's approval to exercise. Many women wait at least 6 to 8 weeks before starting or restarting a serious exercise regimen.
- Keep at it. Everyone loses weight at a different rate, so don't be discouraged if your weight loss happens more slowly than it does for all those celeb mamas. It took 9 months to put that weight on, so give yourself at least 9 months to get it off and get your body back.
- Prioritize breastfeeding. If you are breastfeeding, wait until your baby is at least 2 months old and your milk supply has normalized before cutting calories. It's generally safe to diet while breastfeeding, as long as your total caloric intake doesn't dip below 1,800 calories per day and you keep eating a wide variety of nutritious foods. Be sure to check with your doctor and your child's pediatrician to get the green light.
- Quick weight loss can reduce your milk supply. Losing about 1½ pounds (680 grams) a week should not affect your milk supply or your health. You may want to make a note of when you start your weight loss program in case it does affect your milk supply.
- You may not be able to return to your exact prepregnancy shape. For many women, pregnancy causes lasting changes in the body. You may have a softer belly, wider hips, larger breasts, feet, or waistline, and that is normal. Make your goals about your new body realistic.
- Weigh yourself only once a week and remember that sometimes it takes a week for your efforts to catch up with the scale. You won't see a cause-and-effect relationship every week.

QUESTIONS AND ANSWERS FOR WEIGHT LOSS POSTPARTUM

As we all know, one key to successful weight loss is being psychologically at peace with yourself and your new family situation before you begin. This equilibrium is not always obvious or easy to achieve. According to Linda Wade, PhD, a clinical psychologist with a private practice in New York, a woman must connect with her "inner self" before beginning any effective weight loss plan at any stage in her life, not just postpartum. Dr. Wade sees many clients seeking to reduce their weight. Here she shares some of the advice she offers them.

How will I know when the timing is right to start dieting?

The right time to start dieting depends very much on the individual and can be determined only by you. Don't compare yourself to anyone else. We all carry our own weight, both emotional and physical. Check in with yourself and take inventory of what's going on in your life at the moment. As wonderful as the birth of a child is, there can also be losses associated with it: loss of personal time, loss of your prepregnant body image, and sometimes loss of income due to a change of employment. In general, losses tend to make a woman want to use food for comfort, so begin by understanding how you feel about your new place in life and ask yourself whether you are happy there. If you are not, think about why not and how you can adjust. Ideally, try to eliminate as much stress and conflict as possible from your life before you begin dieting. Get support from your partner, family, friends, or a diet group.

What reasonable goals can I set for myself and how can I prioritize them?

It is very important to be realistic about what can be accomplished. Small changes tend to be more lasting. An initial goal of simply maintaining your weight while you try to reduce your stress and manage your life, is an admirable goal. When you get an inner reading that things are calm enough for you to effectively change your food intake and begin exercising, 1 to 2 pounds per week is a healthy and realistic goal. Many women have an impatient side that will want to set much higher goals, but this invariably leads to failure, self-judgment, and often to giving up. Dropping a few hundred calories from your day requires a lot of physical and mental work.

Making the time to eat right, exercise, journal, and do other self-care activities is one of the biggest challenges of early motherhood. As tired as you may be, set aside 15 minutes for yourself—maybe before the baby and anyone else in the house wakes up—to make a cup of tea, to read something inspirational, to get quiet within yourself, or to journal. During this time, think through your day with this question in mind: *When can I be free to take care of myself?* Try to carve out time to exercise, take a walk with your baby, make yourself a nice salad for lunch, or nap if you are exhausted. You will know you are strong and confident enough to make positive changes to your lifestyle when you listen to and connect with yourself.

How can I control my cravings and urges to indulge when others are indulging?

There is an old saying—"hungry, angry, lonely, and tired," also known as HALT—that reminds us that if we are experiencing one or all of these feelings, we are vulnerable to overeating. Exhaustion is especially difficult—and very common in early motherhood. Again, self-knowledge will serve you well. Don't overcommit yourself to nonessential activities and ask for assistance with basic chores and shopping. Try to keep only healthy foods and snacks in your home, reach out to friends for advice or support, and share your frustration, anger, or anxieties with your partner. If you can eliminate these four feelings, your cravings and overindulgence will likely subside.

Know yourself—your strengths and weaknesses—and figure out how you can feel satisfied without feeling deprived. Once you find harmony, make a deal with yourself that you will try a small portion of appealing dishes and that you won't take seconds. Eat slowly, so you aren't finished before everyone else. Think about the number of calories in the high-sugar desserts and ask yourself if they are really worth the extra hours of exercise that will be necessary to burn them off. The answer is probably no.

What if my weight classifies me as obese and I feel defeated and depressed without even trying?

There are two issues here. One is long-term weight loss and the other is depression. While dieting, you need to discover how to live with the knowledge that you are doing the best you can to lose weight, even though from day to day the amount of weight being lost does not seem significant. But think: at the rate of one pound per week you will lose 52 pounds in one year! That's a considerable amount. Keep returning to the positive—what you have accomplished so far—and keep moving ahead. If you find that your depression is not lifting with positive self-talk, consulting a professional is the best next step. Psychotherapy and/or medication can be very helpful.

What if my partner or others are not supportive?

While dieting is inner work, it helps to have support from the outside. In fact, the ability to speak up for one's self is an expression of inner work. Letting your friends and partner know that you are following a healthy diet plan to lose weight will help you, particularly if you make decisions in front of them. You might also want to ask them not to take personally any refusal of food they offer you. If your partner wants to have certain foods in the house that are not helpful foods for you, ask him or her to find a special closet or space in the refrigerator for them. Some experts may advise that the partner forgo these foods altogether, but in general, I would not agree with this. Ultimately, we cannot place the control of what we eat on anyone or anything outside ourselves.

What is the best way to start a diet?

Journaling would be my advice. Getting into the habit of recording your daily thoughts and feelings is important inner work for any life change, including weight loss. You can write in a food journal, or you can use a separate journal for your entries. Now, to get started, sit somewhere comfortable with a notebook and a pen. Take a big, deep breath and relax. Then begin to notice your emotional body. What is that? you may ask. Well, it's the part of your body that carries a hunch or feels anxiety or tension. Just notice it. Notice what thoughts are coming. There might be judgment: *I hate this*, or *Why do I have to feel this way?* or *What's wrong with me?* There might be opinions: *I have to go on a diet today*, or *This is impossible, it will never work*. Or just feelings: *I'm feeling kind of down today*, *I'm happy because the baby finally slept through the night*. Don't judge anything you write but be curious about your thoughts and feelings. These are some of your parts coming forward. They need space and acknowledgement. After you do this for a while, you will begin to notice your "whole self" start to relax. Ultimately, you will be in a better place to take actions, such as making smart food choices and doing exercises, which will serve your entire well-being. If you don't have time to journal, even thinking about these things is helpful.

Dieting can bring up a lot of emotional baggage. How should I sort through it?

The therapeutic technique I use most in my practice is based on the Internal Family Systems Model (IFS) developed by Richard C. Schwartz, PhD. In a nutshell, the IFS is based on the understanding that there are many different parts of our mind that affect our thinking. They are almost like separate individuals subconsciously guiding our thoughts and actions. We must acknowledge our "parts" and possibly even name them. For instance, one part might be protective and managerial, another might try to keep our vulnerabilities under wraps, and a third part might try to keep any emotional pain, past or present, from surfacing by suppressing it using unhealthy means, such as alcohol abuse, binge eating, or overworking. In addition to our different parts, everyone also has a Self, a curious, compassionate, and nonjudgmental center to their entire being. The goal of this work is to be more and more led by one's Self, and to leave those other parts behind.

If one's parts are being heard and understood by one's Self, a person can approach dieting in a calm, confident, and creative way. If one or more parts are not being acknowledged, and food has become an antidote for emotional pain or conflict, trying to diet is going to be tricky and, in the end, could add to a person's emotional distress. The IFS Model is, of course, a lot more intricate than this brief description implies. If you would like to learn more about it, visit www.selfleadership.org. *Introduction to the Internal Family Systems Model* is an excellent description of the theory that can be ordered from the website.

CREATING A HEALTHY AND BALANCED DIET PLAN THAT WORKS FOR YOU

Aim for a healthy, balanced diet within your calorie limits and shun all unhealthy foods. Crash and yo-yo diets don't work and are not healthy for your recovering body. And seasoned moms will tell you, don't try to make changes all at once. A common mantra is "Nine months up, nine months down." These healthy eating tips will help you lose weight safely.

- Do not skip meals. With a new baby, many new moms forget to eat. If you do not eat, you will have less energy, and it will not help you lose weight.
- Eat 5 to 6 small meals a day with healthy snacks in between (rather than 3 larger meals). Planning out meals and snacks for the day or week is an excellent idea if you have the ability to do so. Once you have a system that works, meaning you're losing weight at an appropriate pace, stick with it as long as possible.
- Eat breakfast. Even if you do not normally eat in the mornings, get into the habit of having breakfast. It will give you energy to start your day and stop you from feeling tired and hungry later.
- Aim for a full-range of nutrients from foods, just as you did during your pregnancy. Choose foods high in vitamins, minerals, healthy fats, complex carbs, and fiber. Refer to the charts and recipes throughout this book for ideas. Keep taking your prenatal vitamin for up to 6 months postpartum.
- Slow down. When you take your time eating, you will notice that it is easier to tell that you are full. It is tempting to multitask, but if you focus on your meal you will be less likely to overeat.

- Make sure you get enough protein throughout the day.
- Drink plenty of water—aim for 10 glasses per day. Keep a water bottle near the spot where you usually feed the baby, that way you'll remember to drink when your baby does.
- Choose whole foods (also called real foods) as much as possible and try to cook at home as often as you can. Limit high-calorie or empty-calorie drinks, such as sodas (including all diet sodas), fruit juices, and other beverages with added sugar. They can keep you from losing weight.
- Choose broiled or baked rather than fried foods. Avoid sugary sauces as much as possible. A squeeze of lemon and some fresh herbs adds a boost of flavor.
- Choose high-fiber whole grains, not refined ones. Reducing your bread intake can cut a ton of calories and carbs.
- Limit sweets and foods with added sugar. Be picky about the carbs you consume.
- Cut back on takeout. Skip the junk food and fast food. Try to plan ahead and pack foods from home as much as possible. Keeping healthy snacks on hand can save you from grabbing a candy bar or other less optimal snack.
- Avoid fad diets. They can lead to mood swings and—hey, let's face it—you're already juggling a lot as a new mom recovering from pregnancy and getting your hormones to rebalance.

COUNTING CALORIES AND GAUGING YOUR ENERGY-BASED NEEDS

Everyone's calorie needs are different. The following chart outlines calorie guidelines for maintaining weight and for weight loss, depending on your age and how active you are. Generally, when you are in the weight-loss mode, you drop approximately 500 calories from your daily maintenance calories to lose 1 pound per week:

1 pound equals 3,500 calories (500 calories x 7 days = 3,500 calories)

These guidelines are just that—guidelines. Your calorie needs may be higher or lower, and might change depending on the results you get. If you find that a suggested calorie level is just too low and you are always hungry, even if you are losing weight, increase your calorie intake a bit. If you're not losing weight, you may need to cut back a bit more. In the end, you are better off losing the weight at a slower pace, while changing your eating habits, than losing pounds quickly and not being able to keep them off.

DAILY MAINTENANCE AND WEIGHT LOSS CALORIES GUIDELINES FOR WOMEN (CALORIES PER DAY)[1]

AGE	SEDENTARY MAINTAIN	SEDENTARY WEIGHT LOSS	MODERATELY ACTIVE MAINTAIN	MODERATELY ACTIVE WEIGHT LOSS	ACTIVE MAINTAIN	ACTIVE WEIGHT LOSS
14 to 18	1,800	1,300	2,000	1,500	2,400	1,900
19 to 30	2,000	1,500	2,000 to 2,200	1,500 to 1,700	2,400	1,900
31 to 50	1,800	1,300	2,000	1,500	2,200	1,700
51 +	1,600	1,200	1,800	1,300	2,000 to 2,200	1,500 to 1,700

To determine whether you are sedentary, moderately active, or active, in addition to your daily routine (additional activities might include brisk walking, jogging, biking, aerobics, or yard work), think about the amount of moderate or vigorous activity you do on most days of the week. Consider yourself active if you do more than 60 minutes; moderately active, 30 to 60 minutes; and sedentary, fewer than 30 minutes.

Many women find it difficult to initiate dietary changes and to begin exercising at the same time. You do not have to do both at the same time. Start with changing your diet while maintaining your current level of activity, whether it is sedentary or very active. Once you have your eating plan under control (which might take a few weeks), then start to add exercise to your daily routine. If you already exercise, by all means continue.

Before you begin dieting or exercising, promise yourself not to get on the scale every day. Choose one day a week to weigh yourself when you wake up. As we mentioned earlier, don't be disappointed if the scale does not reflect a decrease right away. Results can sometimes take a few weeks, but they will come. Factors, such as salt intake and your body's fluid status, can alter your weight. Also, if you are toning up and building muscle, the scale numbers may not decrease as much, even though your body is getting leaner. Take out a tape measure or use your old clothes to measure the inches you are losing on your waistline, thighs, and hips.

EXERCISE IS KEY

If exercise has always been a part of your life, you are extremely fortunate. Keep it that way. When you are ready to shed your pregnancy weight, first and foremost, get medical clearance, then gradually resume your old routines. If you don't have an old routine, and exercise is new to you, don't worry. It's never too late to start. Some new moms get so into exercise they have an even better body after pregnancy than before getting pregnant. That mom might be you!

A healthy diet combined with regular exercise is the best way to shed the pounds. Exercise will help you lose fat instead of muscle. Once you are ready to start losing weight, eat a little less and move a little more each day. Many moms feel that going to the gym and carving out that time for themselves not only helps them get in shape, but also reduces stress and gives them energy. Some say it keeps them emotionally stable in their crazy new-mom world.

We know that not everyone has access to a gym, but there are many exercises you can do at home. Ask someone to watch your little one, close your door, turn on an exercise video, and get to work. You don't need a gym to do deep squats, leg lefts, stomach crunches (make sure you get clearance from your doctor for these), to lift free weights, or to jog in place. It's really amazing how much you can do at home.

It may be tempting to push yourself into a strenuous routine for fast weight loss. But rapid weight loss is not healthy and is hard on your body. Please don't overdo it. Just a quick walk around the block with your baby in the stroller is a great way to start adding exercise to your daily routine (and maybe even relieve that nagging backache). Take the stairs whenever you can. Put your baby in a carriage and walk in the mall with a friend (a great way to exercise in the winter or on a rainy day, or if you just need some retail therapy).

Getting Started

- Medical clearance from your doctor or health-care provider is essential. Explain your exercise plan and ask if there are any exercises you should avoid. Inform your doctor if you are breastfeeding.
- Complications during pregnancy or a C-section will prolong post-delivery healing time, and abdominal exercises may need to be delayed. Check with your doctor to make sure.
- Stomach muscle separation requires special attention. Ask about exercises that are safe and beneficial to your healing process.
- Back pain can often be relieved with stretching and exercise, but start slowly, don't push yourself, and be aware of any warning signals. Stop immediately if something does not feel right.
- Start with 15 minutes a day and gradually work your way up. Keep reminding yourself that exercise is not an all-or-nothing proposition. A 10-minute walk has benefits.

- Treat yourself to some new gym clothes, especially shoes if your feet have expanded from pregnancy.
- Get as much support as you can and share your goals with your partner.

During Exercise
- Get well hydrated before exercising. Drink a glass or two of water, even if you don't feel thirsty, about an hour *before* you begin your routine. Sip water during your routine, if you need to.
- Change into comfortable clothes. Wear a sports bra with strong support.
- Factor your warm-up time and after-exercise stretches into your routine. It is vital to warm up your body before you exercise to prevent injuries, muscle sprains, and strains.
- Be aware of your body as you work out. Know when to stop. Warning signals include pain, dizziness, feeling faint, shortness of breath, palpitations (irregular heartbeats), back pain, pelvic pain, and bleeding.

After Your Routine
- Stretch to prevent muscle cramping.
- If you have the time, lie on the floor on your back with your arms and legs relaxed for 5 minutes of total relaxation. This is called the corpse pose in yoga; it is designed to relax your body and clear your mind.
- Your muscles may feel sore, which is okay, but they should not feel painful. Take a minute to distinguish between feeling sore and being in pain. If pain is what you feel, refrain from exercising for a day or two. If the pain is severe, consult your doctor immediately.
- Stand tall for the rest of the day. Suck in your tummy, straighten your back, lift the top of your head to the sky, tuck in your chin, and distribute your weight evenly on both feet.

Always remember you are beautiful and strong. Be compassionate and kind with yourself. Ask for help when you need it. Don't try to do it all alone. We wish you and your families a beautiful and healthy life ahead. Sending all of our new moms love and big hugs!

BMI Basics
Understanding Body Mass Index (BMI)

The body mass index (BMI) is a helpful tool for determining if you are at a healthy weight. It is a single number based on the ratio of your weight to your height. An ideal BMI is less than 25. Because muscle and bone are denser than fat, an athletic or muscular person may have a high BMI, but not be overweight or obese.

There are four categories of BMI:

Underweight = **less than 18.5**
Normal weight = **18.5 to 24.9**
Overweight = **25 to 29.9**
Obese = **30 or greater**

You can use the chart on page 338 to find out your BMI.

FORMULA FOR DETERMINING YOUR CURRENT BODY WEIGHT AND IDEAL BODY WEIGHT

To determine your ideal body weight (IBW):

The first 5 feet of your total height = **100 pounds**
For every inch over the first 5 feet add 5 pounds
Your IBW should be within a plus/minus 10-pound range.
For example: A woman who is 5 foot 4:
5 feet = **100 pounds**
4 inches x 5 pounds per inch = **20 pounds**
100 + 20 = **120 pounds**
Plus or minus 10-pound range: 110 to 130 pounds (average 120 pounds)

To convert pounds to kilograms, divide by 2.2
For example: 120 pounds divided by 2.2 = **55 kilograms**
Plus or minus 10-pound range: 50 to 59 kilograms

Body Mass Index Table

	Normal						Overweight					Obese										Extreme Obesity														
BMI	19	20	21	22	23	24	25	26	27	28	29	30	31	32	33	34	35	36	37	38	39	40	41	42	43	44	45	46	47	48	49	50	51	52	53	54
Height (Inches)												Body Weight (pounds)																								
58	91	96	100	105	110	115	119	124	129	134	138	143	148	153	158	162	167	172	177	181	186	191	196	201	205	210	215	220	224	229	234	239	244	248	253	258
59	94	99	104	109	114	119	124	128	133	138	143	148	153	158	163	168	173	178	183	188	193	198	203	208	212	217	222	227	232	237	242	247	252	257	262	267
60	97	102	107	112	118	123	128	133	138	143	148	153	158	163	168	174	179	184	189	194	199	204	209	215	220	225	230	235	240	245	250	255	261	266	271	276
61	100	106	111	116	122	127	132	137	143	148	153	158	164	169	174	180	185	190	195	201	206	211	217	222	227	232	238	243	248	254	259	264	269	275	280	285
62	104	109	115	120	126	131	136	142	147	153	158	164	169	175	180	186	191	196	202	207	213	218	224	229	235	240	246	251	256	262	267	273	278	284	289	295
63	107	113	118	124	130	135	141	146	152	158	163	169	175	180	186	191	197	203	208	214	220	225	231	237	242	248	254	259	265	270	278	282	287	293	299	304
64	110	116	122	128	134	140	145	151	157	163	169	174	180	186	192	197	204	209	215	221	227	232	238	244	250	256	262	267	273	279	285	291	296	302	308	314
65	114	120	126	132	138	144	150	156	162	168	174	180	186	192	198	204	210	216	222	228	234	240	246	252	258	264	270	276	282	288	294	300	306	312	318	324
66	118	124	130	136	142	148	155	161	167	173	179	186	192	198	204	210	216	223	229	235	241	247	253	260	266	272	278	284	291	297	303	309	315	322	328	334
67	121	127	134	140	146	153	159	166	172	178	185	191	198	204	211	217	223	230	236	242	249	255	261	268	274	280	287	293	299	306	312	319	325	331	338	344
68	125	131	138	144	151	158	164	171	177	184	190	197	203	210	216	223	230	236	243	249	256	262	269	276	282	289	295	302	308	315	322	328	335	341	348	354
69	128	135	142	149	155	162	169	176	182	189	196	203	209	216	223	230	236	243	250	257	263	270	277	284	291	297	304	311	318	324	331	338	345	351	358	365
70	132	139	146	153	160	167	174	181	188	195	202	209	216	222	229	236	243	250	257	264	271	278	285	292	299	306	313	320	327	334	341	348	355	362	369	376
71	136	143	150	157	165	172	179	186	193	200	208	215	222	229	236	243	250	257	265	272	279	286	293	301	308	315	322	329	338	343	351	358	365	372	379	386
72	140	147	154	162	169	177	184	191	199	206	213	221	228	235	242	250	258	265	272	279	287	294	302	309	316	324	331	338	346	353	361	368	375	383	390	397
73	144	151	159	166	174	182	189	197	204	212	219	227	235	242	250	257	265	272	280	288	295	302	310	318	325	333	340	348	355	363	371	378	386	393	401	408
74	148	155	163	171	179	186	194	202	210	218	225	233	241	249	256	264	272	280	287	295	303	311	319	326	334	342	350	358	365	373	381	389	396	404	412	420
75	152	160	168	176	184	192	200	208	216	224	232	240	248	256	264	272	279	287	295	303	311	319	327	335	343	351	359	367	375	383	391	399	407	415	423	431
76	156	164	172	180	189	197	205	213	221	230	238	246	254	263	271	279	287	295	304	312	320	328	336	344	353	361	369	377	385	394	402	410	418	426	435	443

Source: Adapted from Clinical Guidelines on the Identification, Evaluation, and Treatment of Overweight and Obesity in Adults: The Evidence Report.

Nutrition Sources

PROTEIN SOURCES
(Recommended Daily Intake for protein during pregnancy is 71 grams.)

FOOD	SERVING SIZE	PROTEIN (G)
Chicken, cooked	3 ounces	26
Turkey breast, roasted	3 ounces	26
Pork loin or chops, roasted	3 ounces	24
Beef, cooked	3 ounces	23
Shrimp, cooked	4 ounces	23
Tuna fish, canned	3 ounces	22
Ham, cured	3 ounces	19
Salmon, cooked	3 ounces	19
Cottage cheese	½ cup	16
Catfish, cooked	3 ounces	15
Tempeh	½ cup	15
Cheddar cheese	1 cup	14
Reduced-fat yogurt	1 cup	13
Egg, hard-boiled	1 egg	6
Edamame, cooked	⅓ cup	11
Tofu, extra-firm	4 ounces	11
Roasted peanuts	¼ cup	10
Lentils, cooked	½ cup	9
Deli ham	2 ounces	9
Peanut butter	2 tablespoons	8
Milk, reduced-fat 2%	1 cup	8
Kidney beans	½ cup	7

FOOD	SERVING SIZE	PROTEIN (G)
Chickpeas, cooked	½ cup	7
Mozzarella string cheese	1 cheese string	7
Vegetarian baked beans	½ cup	6
Turkey loaf (breast meat)	4 slices	6
Jarlsberg cheese	1 slice	6
Muenster cheese	1 slice	6
Kraft Singles cheese	1 slice	4
Frozen yogurt	½ cup	4

VEGAN PROTEIN SOURCES

(Recommended Daily Intake for protein during pregnancy is 71 grams.)

FOOD	SERVING SIZE	PROTEIN (G)
Soy nuts (dried and roasted)	¼ cup	11
Edamame, cooked	½ cup	11
Seitan	3 ounces	15
Tempeh	½ cup	14
Soy protein bar (average)	1 bar	14
Tofu	4 ounces	11
Kashi Go Lean cereal	1¼ cups	12
Soy burger (average)	1 burger	14
Peanuts, raw	¼ cup	10
Pumpkin seeds	¼ cup	10
Lentils, cooked	½ cup	9
Kashi Go Lean Crisp cereal	¾ cup	9
Hemp seeds	3 tablespoons	9
Peanut butter	2 tablespoons	8
Veggie dog (average)	1 veggie dog	8
Canned bean soup	1 cup	8
Spirulina, dry	2 tablespoons	8
Soy nut butter	2 tablespoons	7
Kidney beans, cooked	½ cup	7
Chickpeas, cooked	½ cup	7

FOOD	SERVING SIZE	PROTEIN (G)
Vegan baked beans	½ cup	6
Hummus	½ cup	6
Soy sausage link (average)	1 sausage link	6
Sprouted bread	1 slice	5
Chia seeds, dry	2 tablespoons	5
Almond milk, protein enriched	1 cup	5
Soy yogurt	1 cup	9
Nutritional yeast	2 tablespoons	4
Soy milk with added A and D	1 cup	7
Green peas, boiled	½ cup	4
Quinoa, cooked	½ cup	4
Spinach, cooked	½ cup	3
Artichokes, cooked	1 artichoke	3

OMEGA-3 SOURCES: DHA AND EPA

(Recommended Daily Intake for pregnancy for DHA and EPA during pregnancy is 300 mg or 3 grams; see page 13 for more information. Amounts of EPA and DHA in fish and fish oils and the amount of fish consumption required to provide about 1 gram of EPA and DHA per day)[1]

FISH SOURCES (3-OUNCE SERVING SIZE) AND CAPSULES	DHA AND EPA CONTENT IN MILLIGRAMS[a]	REQUIRED NUMBER OF SERVINGS FOR ABOUT 1 GRAM OF DHA AND EPA[b]
Tuna, light, canned in water, drained	0.26	12
Tuna, white, canned in water, drained	0.73	4
Sardines	0.98–1.70	2–3 (good source)
Salmon, chum	0.68	4.5
Salmon, sockeye	0.68	4.5
Salmon, pink	1.09	2.5 (good source)
Salmon, chinook	1.48	2 (good source)
Salmon, Atlantic, farmed	1.09–1.83	1.5–2.5 (good source)
Salmon, Atlantic, wild	0.9–1.56	2–3.5 (good source)
Mackerel	0.34–1.57	2–8.5 (good source)
Herring, Pacific	1.81	1.5 (good source)
Herring, Atlantic	1.71	2 (good source)
Trout, rainbow, farmed	0.98	3 (good source)

FISH SOURCES (3-OUNCE SERVING SIZE) AND CAPSULES	DHA AND EPA CONTENT IN MILLIGRAMS[A]	REQUIRED NUMBER OF SERVINGS FOR ABOUT 1 GRAM OF DHA AND EPA[B]
Trout, rainbow, wild	0.84	3.5
Halibut	0.4–1.0	3–7.5
Cod, Pacific	0.13	23
Cod, Atlantic	0.24	12.5
Haddock	0.2	15
Catfish, farmed	0.15	20
Catfish, wild	0.2	15
Flounder/sole	0.42	7
Oyster, Pacific (meat only)	1.17	2.5
Oyster, Eastern (meat only)	0.47	6.5
Oyster, farmed (meat only)	0.37	8
Lobster (meat only)	0.07–0.41	7.5–42.5
Crab, Alaskan king (meat only)	0.35	8.5
Shrimp, mixed	0.27	11
Clam (meat only)	0.24	12.5
Scallops (meat only)	0.17	17.5
Cod liver oil capsule[c]	0.19	5
Omega-3 fatty acid concentrate capsule	0.50	2 (good source)

Note: The intakes of fish given above are very rough estimates because oil content can vary markedly (>300%) with species, season, diet, and packaging and cooking methods.

[a] The EPA and DHA content of fish is per 3-ounce serving (edible portion).

[b] The amount required to provide about 1 gram of EPA and DHA per day is measured in ounces of fish per day, or grams per gram of oil per day.

[c] This intake of cod liver oil would provide approximately the recommended daily allowance of vitamins A and D.

IRON SOURCES
(Recommended Daily Intake for iron during pregnancy is 27 mg.)

FOOD	SERVING SIZE	IRON (MG)
Cream of Wheat, cooked with water	¾ cup	8.9
Blackstrap molasses	2 tablespoons	7.0
All-bran cereal	½ cup	4.5
Soybeans, cooked	½ cup	4.4
Spirulina	2 tablespoons	3.9

FOOD	SERVING SIZE	IRON (MG)
Oysters, canned	2 ounces	3.7
Spinach, cooked	½ cup	3.2
Lentils, cooked	½ cup	3.2
Pumpkin seeds	¼ cup	3.0
Baked potato with skin	1 potato	2.7
Split peas, cooked	½ cup	2.5
Beef (short loin)	3 ounces	2.3
Chickpeas, cooked	½ cup	2.3
Tempeh	½ cup	2.2
Edamame, cooked	½ cup	2.2
Pinto beans, cooked	1.2 cup	2.2
Hearts of palm, canned	½ cup	2.2
Flour tortillas	2 tortillas	2.1
Lima beans, cooked	½ cup	2.0
Black beans, cooked	½ cup	1.8
Tempeh	3 ounces	1.8
Ground beef patty	3 ounces	1.7
Tofu	4 ounces	1.7
Whole wheat bread	2 slices	1.6
Almonds, dry roasted	¼ cup	1.5
Kidney beans, canned	½ cup	1.5
Quick-cooked oatmeal	1 cup	1.5
Lamb loin	3 ounces	1.5
Prune juice	4 ounces	1.5
Quinoa, cooked	½ cup	1.4
Romaine lettuce	2 cups	1.2
Sunflower seeds	¼ cup	1.2
Turkey breast	3 ounces	1.1
Dried figs	¼ cup	1.1
Dried apricot halves	5 halves	1.0
Wheat germ	2 tablespoons	1.0
Avocado	½ avocado	1.0

DAIRY CALCIUM SOURCES
(Recommended Daily Intake for calcium during pregnancy is 1,000 mg.)

FOOD	SERVING SIZE	CALCIUM (MG)
Swiss cheese	2 ounces	545
Yogurt, nonfat plain	1 cup	488
Yogurt, reduced-fat plain	1 cup	448
Monterey Jack cheese	2 ounces	423
Mozzarella cheese, part-skim, low-moisture	2 ounces	414
Cheddar cheese	2 ounces	409
Processed cheese	2 ounces	325
Fontina cheese	2 ounces	312
Milk, nonfat	8 ounces	301
Milk, reduced-fat 1%	8 ounces	300
Milk, reduced-fat 2%	8 ounces	298
Milk, whole (3.3%)	8 ounces	290
Milk, nonfat dry	⅓ cup	283
Pasteurized feta cheese	2 ounces	280
Pasteurized goat cheese	1 ounce	253
Ricotta cheese, part-skim	¼ cup	167
Buttermilk, reduced-fat	½ cup	142
Parmesan cheese	2 tablespoons	138
Frozen yogurt, vanilla	½ cup	138
Ice cream, vanilla	½ cup	87
Cottage cheese	½ cup	78

NONDAIRY CALCIUM SOURCES
(Recommended Daily Intake for calcium during pregnancy is 1,000 mg.)

SOURCE	SERVING SIZE	CALCIUM (MG)
Calcium-fortified orange juice	8 ounces	350
Blackstrap molasses	2 tablespoons	344
Soy beverage, enriched	8 ounces	300
Calcium-fortified bread	2 slices	160
All-bran cereal	½ cup	150

SOURCE	SERVING SIZE	CALCIUM (MG)
Spinach, cooked	½ cup	122
Canned salmon (bone-in)	2 ounces	121
Turnip greens, cooked	½ cup	99
Tempeh	½ cup	92
Almonds, dry roasted	¼ cup	92
Corn tortillas	2 tortillas	91
Soybeans, cooked	½ cup	88
Almond butter	2 tablespoons	86
Molasses	2 tablespoons	82
Flour tortillas	2 tortillas	80
Bok choy, cooked	½ cup	79
Tofu (not fortified)	4 ounces	75
Dried figs	¼ cup	72
Vegetarian baked beans	½ cup	64
Plain bagel	1 bagel	53
Mustard greens, cooked	½ cup	52
Okra, cooked	½ cup	50
Kale, cooked	½ cup	47
Acorn squash, baked	½ cup	45
Butternut squash, baked	½ cup	42
Fresh orange, medium	1 orange	42
Pinto beans, cooked	½ cup	41
Chickpeas, cooked	½ cup	40
Collard greens, cooked	½ cup	40

VITAMIN A SOURCES
(Recommended Daily Intake for vitamin A during pregnancy is 2,300 IU.)

SOURCE	SERVING SIZE	VITAMIN A (IU)
VEGETABLES		
Spinach, cooked	½ cup	9,433
Sweet potato, cooked	½ cup	9,343
Kale, cooked	½ cup	8,854

SOURCE	SERVING SIZE	VITAMIN A (IU)
Butternut squash, chopped or pureed, cooked	½ cup	7,441
Collard greens, cooked	½ cup	7,220
Romaine lettuce, sliced	1½ cups	6,140
Pumpkin, chopped or pureed, cooked	½ cup	4,938
Kale, raw	2 cups	2,667
Red bell pepper	½	1,863
Baby carrots	8 baby carrots	1,132
Asparagus, cooked	½ cup	504
Brussels sprouts, cooked	½ cup	332
Broccoli, cooked	½ cup	283
FRUITS		
Cantaloupe, diced	¾ cup	4,058
Mango	½ mango	1,120
Tangerines	2 tangerines	1,199
Apricots, dried	5 dried apricots	631
OTHER SOURCES		
Tuna, bluefin, cooked	2.5 ounces	1,786
Herring, pickled	2.5 ounces	610
Eggs, cooked	2 eggs	520
Pasteurized goat cheese, semi-soft	1 ounce	415
Ricotta cheese	¼ cup	236

VITAMIN C SOURCES

(Recommended Daily Intake for vitamin C during pregnancy is 85 mg.)

SOURCE	SERVING SIZE	VITAMIN C (MG)
VEGETABLES		
Red bell pepper, raw	½ pepper	76
V8 low-sodium or tomato juice	1 cup	72
Broccoli florets	½ cup	41
Snow peas, cooked	½ cup	38
Brussels sprouts, cooked	½ cup	37
Cauliflower, cooked	½ cup	27

SOURCE	SERVING SIZE	VITAMIN C (MG)
Kale, cooked	½ cup	26
Cabbage, raw	1 cup	20
Mustard greens, cooked	½ cup	18
Baked potato	1 potato	17
Bok choy, cooked	½ cup	16
Turnip greens, cooked	½ cup	15
FRUITS		
Guava	1 guava	126
Orange or grapefruit juice	1 cup	124
Grapefruit, pink or red	½ grapefruit	94
Kiwi	1 kiwi	91
Orange	1 orange	70
Lychee	½ cup	68
Papaya, diced	¾ cup	64
Cantaloupe, diced	¾ cup	44
Strawberries	½ cup	42
Mango	½	37
Pineapple, diced	1 cup	37
Clementine	1 clementine	36
Soursop	½ cup	23

FOLATE SOURCES

(Recommended Daily Intake for folate (folic acid) during pregnancy is 600 mcg.)

SOURCE	SERVING SIZE	FOLATE (MCG)
All-bran cereal	½ cup	400
Edamame, frozen, prepared	½ cup	241
Lentils, cooked	½ cup	179
Romaine lettuce	2 cups	152
Chickpeas, cooked	½ cup	141
Pasta, enriched, dry	2 ounces	134
Asparagus, cooked	½ cup	131
Black beans, cooked	½ cup	128

SOURCE	SERVING SIZE	FOLATE (MCG)
Spinach, cooked	½ cup	131
Artichoke, boiled, drained	1 artichoke	107
Brewer's yeast	1 teaspoon	104
Baby spinach, raw	2 cups	106
Sunflower seeds	¼ cup	76
Orange juice	1 cup	74
Beets, cooked	½ cup	74
Kidney beans, canned	½ cup	64
Avocado, medium	½ avocado	56
Wheat germ	2 tablespoons	51
Tomato juice	1 cup	49
Calcium-fortified white bread	2 slices	48
Brussels sprouts, cooked	½ cup	47
Peanuts, roasted	¼ cup	45
Orange, medium	1 orange	39
Broccoli, cooked	½ cup	39

FIBER SOURCES
(Recommended Daily Intake for fiber during pregnancy is 28 g.)

SOURCE	SERVING SIZE	FIBER (G)
General Mills Fiber One cereal	½ cup	14
All-bran cereal	½ cup	10
Chia seeds, dry	2 tablespoons	9
Raspberries	1 cup	8
Lentils, cooked	½ cup	8
Black beans, cooked	½ cup	7
Chickpeas, cooked	½ cup	5
Potato with skin	1 potato	5
Kidney beans, canned	½ cup	5
Green peas, cooked	⅓ cup	4
Kellogg's Raisin Bran cereal	½ cup	4
Quick-cooked oatmeal (prepared with water)	1 cup	4

SOURCE	SERVING SIZE	FIBER (G)
Blueberries	1 cup	4
Apple with skin, medium	1 apple	4
Whole wheat bread	2 slices	3
Strawberries	1 cup	3
Orange, medium	1 orange	3
Wheat germ	¼ cup	3
Dried dates	5 dates	3
Broccoli, cooked	½ cup	2
Whole wheat crackers	5 crackers	2
Brussels sprouts, cooked	½ cup	2

Low-Carb Recipes for
Diabetes During Pregnancy
(20 or less carbs per serving)

Month 1 Recipes

High-Folate Spinach Bean Dip = 15

Swiss Chard or Spinach with Soy Sauce = 7

Baked Salmon and Broccoli Rabe with
  Scallion-Ginger Sauce = 12

Awesome Chicken Burgers = 2

Make It Again Meat Loaf = 13

Month 2 Recipes

Ginger-Mint Soother for Morning Sickness = 0

Quick Romaine and Avocado Salad = 12

Pr-Egg-O Salad = 6

Kale with Cranberries and Walnuts = 17

Salmon with Artichoke-Olive Tapenade = 5

Grilled Chicken with Red or White
  Homemade BBQ Sauce Marinade = 0

Month 3 Recipes

Easy Veggie Frittata = 7

Creamy Asparagus Artichoke Soup = 20

Hot and Sweet Veggie Salad = 13

Just Plain Good Guacamole = 12

Yummy Three-Bean Salad = 19

Salmon with Toasted Almonds, Capers,
  and Herbs = 5

Family-Friendly Chicken Curry = 15

Month 4 Recipes

Glorious Edamame Dip = 7

Spinach and Cheese Omelet for One = 3

My Big Fat Greek Salad = 13

Lemony Slaw = 6

Easy Garlicky Spinach = 4

Maple Glazed Carrots = 20

Zucchini Noodles with Spicy Shrimp = 9

Sheet Pan Roasted Chicken Dinner = 16

Indian-Spiced Salmon with Cucumber-Tomato
  Salsa = 2

Chili-Rubbed Pork Chops = 0

Best-Ever Flank Steak with Salsa Verde = 1

Month 5 Recipes

Great Green Broccoli-Spinach Soup = 18

Cucumber-Tomato Yogurt Salad = 8

Tomato-Mozzarella Salad = 7

Roasted Asparagus = 4

Crab Cakes with Homemade Tartar Sauce = 8

Grilled Chicken Kebabs = 14

Month 6 Recipes

Creamy Cauliflower Soup = 18

Awesome Homemade Salad Dressings = 0

Chicken Salad with Dried Apricots and Almonds = 11

Month 6 Recipes *continued*

Classic Creamed Spinach = 11

Light and Healthy Vegetable Ragout = 18

Twenty-Minute Tomato Sauce = 8

Easy-Bake Meatballs = 7

Baked Salmon with Mustard-Dill Sauce = 0

Grilled or Broiled Lamb Chops = 0

Month 7 Recipes

Easy Cheese-y Toast = 14

Tomato, Hearts of Palm, and Asparagus Salad = 10

Snappy Mediterranean-Style Chicken Salad = 20

Grilled or Roasted Vegetables = 10

Greek-Style Broccoli = 6

Tilapia Mediterranean Style = 8

Lemon-Herb Grilled Chicken = 0

Month 8 Recipes

Ham and Egg Cups = 3

Beef, Barley, and Vegetable Soup = 19

Beets with Goat Cheese and Greens = 15

Roasted Brussels Sprouts = 7

Lemony Cauliflower-Broccoli Rice = 12

Slow-Cooked Ginger-Garlic Chicken = 13

Mustard-Tarragon Pork Tenderloin = 0

Steak on the Grill = 0

Month 9 Recipes

Gazpacho (Without the Gas) = 12

Healthy Hummus = 17

Okra and Tomatoes Greek Style = 12

Panfried Chicken with Terrific Tzatziki = 3

Hearty Beef Stew = 14

Classic Pulled BBQ Pork = 18

Menus for Pregnancy

The following seven 2,000-calorie menus are meant as a guideline for ideas on how to build healthy meals and snacks. Please ask your doctor and/or care team what the ideal daily calorie intake is for you at your various stages of pregnancy. Mix and match. Change ingredients and dishes according to your needs, tastes, and ingredient availability.

DAY ONE

Breakfast

1 cup fortified whole-grain breakfast cereal

1 cup reduced-fat milk

1 slice whole wheat bread, toasted

1 tablespoon peanut or nut butter

½ cup calcium-fortified orange juice

Lunch

1 whole wheat pita pocket

½ cup hummus or bean dip (Healthy Hummus, page 290, or Glorious Edamame Dip, page 161)

5 cherry tomatoes, 4 cucumber slices, and 1 cup mixed greens with 1 tablespoon light salad dressing (see Awesome Homemade Salad Dressings, page 214)

1 peach or your favorite fruit

Snack

1 high-protein bar

1 cup reduced-fat plain or flavored yogurt

Dinner

4 ounces store-bought roasted chicken breast

1 medium-size baked potato

2 tablespoons sour cream

½ cup broccoli florets (Greek-Style Broccoli, page 248)

½ cup coleslaw (Lemony Slaw, page 164)

1 cup reduced-fat milk

½ cup frozen vanilla yogurt

DAY ONE

Calories: 1,956 cals	Fiber: 29 g
Fat: 49 g	Iron: 35 mg
Carbohydrates: 294 g	Calcium: 2,671 mg
Protein: 99 g	Folic acid: 877 mcg

DAY TWO

Breakfast

- 1 or 2 eggs, cooked (Spinach and Cheese Omelet for One, page 159)
- 2 slices whole wheat bread
- ¾ cup cantaloupe or your favorite fruit
- 1 cup calcium-fortified orange juice

Lunch

- 1 sandwich made with 3 ounces leftover roasted chicken on whole wheat bread with lettuce and tomato slices or chicken salad (Chicken Salad with Dried Apricots and Almonds, page 216, or Snappy Mediterranean-Style Chicken Salad, page 245)
- 8 baby carrots and 5 celery sticks with 2 tablespoons ranch dressing
- 1 cup reduced-fat milk

Snack

- 1 apple or banana
- 1 tablespoon peanut or nut butter

Dinner

- 1½ cups spaghetti with meat sauce (Favorite Spaghetti and Meat Sauce, page 198)
- 1 tablespoon Parmesan cheese
- 2 cups romaine lettuce with 2 tablespoons light dressing (Quick Romaine and Avocado Salad, page 109)
- 1 cup reduced-fat vanilla yogurt with 3 tablespoons granola (Yummy Granola Parfait, page 239)

DAY TWO

Calories: 1,999 cals	Fiber: 28 g
Fat: 53 g	Iron: 16 mg
Carbohydrates: 274 g	Calcium: 1,537 mg
Protein: 110 g	Folic acid: 563 mcg

DAY THREE

Breakfast

- 1 medium-size whole wheat bagel, toasted
- 2 tablespoons cream cheese or your favorite cheese
- 1 cup fresh papaya or your favorite fruit
- 1 cup reduced-fat milk

Lunch

- 1½ cups bean soup (Easy Black Bean Soup, page 107)
- 5 whole wheat crackers with 2 ounces Cheddar cheese
- 1 orange or your favorite fruit
- 1 cup reduced-fat milk

Snack

- ¼ cup hummus (Healthy Hummus, page 290)
- ½ whole wheat pita pocket

Dinner

- 4 ounces meat loaf (Make It Again Meat Loaf, page 95)
- 1 cup brown rice or whole grain
- 8 asparagus spears (Roasted Asparagus, page 189)
- 2 cups mixed green salad with 2 tablespoons light French dressing
- ½ cup frozen vanilla yogurt with ½ cup fresh strawberries or berries

DAY THREE

Calories: 2,074 cals	Fiber: 36 g
Fat: 66 g	Iron: 16 mg
Carbohydrates: 294 g	Calcium: 1,672 mg
Protein: 99 g	Folic acid: 521 mcg

DAY FOUR

Breakfast

1 pack instant or regular oatmeal

1 cup reduced-fat milk

1 banana or your favorite fruit

Lunch

1 serving grilled chicken Caesar salad (from a restaurant or takeout)

1 cup reduced-fat vanilla or fruit yogurt

Snack

1 plain brown rice cake

½ cup mandarin oranges or your favorite fruit

Dinner

2 slices vegetarian pizza

¾ cup sautéed zucchini or a green vegetable

½ cup raspberry or your favorite fruit sorbet

DAY FOUR

Calories: 1,984 cals	Fiber: 19 g
Fat: 77 g	Iron: 13 mg
Carbohydrates: 238 g	Calcium: 1,540 mg
Protein: 95 g	Folic acid: 298 mcg

DAY FIVE

Breakfast

1 oat bran muffin (Gingery Cran-Bran Muffins, page 79)

1 tablespoon peanut or nut butter

1 fruit smoothie with yogurt (Pineapple-Banana-Calcium Smoothie, page 207)

Lunch

1 salad bar salad (2 cups romaine lettuce, 1 hard-boiled egg, ½ cup cottage cheese, 1 tomato, 5 cucumber slices, and 2 tablespoons light salad dressing)

1 whole wheat dinner roll

½ cup fresh pineapple slices or your favorite fruit

Snack

1 cup vanilla yogurt

¼ cup granola (Perfect Homemade Granola, page 105)

½ cup blueberries or your favorite fruit

Dinner

4 ounces grilled or broiled pork chops (Chili-Rubbed Pork Chops, page 174)

1 cup sweet potato or sweet potato casserole (Southern-Style Sweet Potato Casserole, page 250)

¾ cup green beans

1 cup reduced-fat milk

½ cup unsweetened applesauce (Chunky Apple and Apricot Sauce, page 280)

DAY FIVE

Calories: 1,994 cals	Fiber: 31 g
Fat: 55 g	Iron: 14 mg
Carbohydrates: 275 g	Calcium: 1,118 mg
Protein: 109 g	Folic acid: 506 mcg

DAY SIX

Breakfast

2 whole wheat or enriched waffles (Weekend Pecan Waffles, page 208)

2 tablespoons maple syrup

½ cup blueberries or berries

1 cup reduced-fat milk

Lunch

1 grilled cheese sandwich on whole wheat bread with 2 slices of cheese

1 cup reduced-fat milk

1 oatmeal cookie with raisins

1 banana or your favorite fruit

Snack

1 fruit smoothie with yogurt (Berry-Peach-Flax Smoothie, page 287)

Dinner

4 ounces salmon, grilled, sautéed, or roasted (Indian-Spiced Salmon with Cucumber-Tomato Salsa, page 172)

2 cups mixed greens with 2 tablespoons light salad dressing

1 cup whole wheat couscous (Couscous Salad with Chickpeas and Artichokes, page 272)

½ cup broccoli florets

¾ cup mango sorbet

DAY SIX

Calories: 2,010 cals	Fiber: 25 g
Fat: 43 g	Iron: 14 mg
Carbohydrates: 324 g	Calcium: 1,518 mg
Protein: 87 g	Folic acid: 405 mcg

DAY SEVEN

Breakfast

2 slices French toast (French Toast Banana Sandwich, page 104)

1 cup calcium-fortified orange juice

Lunch

½ cup tuna salad sandwich on whole wheat bread with romaine lettuce and tomatoes (Tasty Tuna Salad Sandwich, page 187)

1 dill pickle

1 cup reduced-fat milk

1 apple or your favorite fruit

Snack

⅓ cup dried apricots

1 high-protein bar

Dinner

4 ounces flank steak, or other lean beef steak, grilled (Best-Ever Flank Steak with Salsa Verde, page 175)

1 cup Loaded Sesame Noodles, page 292)

½ cup asparagus (Roasted Asparagus, page 189)

½ cup frozen vanilla yogurt

DAY SEVEN

Calories: 1,980 cals	Fiber: 28 g
Fat: 55 g	Iron: 16 mg
Carbohydrates: 283 g	Calcium: 1,079 mg
Protein: 99 g	Folic acid: 399 mcg

Menus for Vegetarian and Vegan Pregnancies

The following seven 2,000-calorie menus for vegetarians and vegans are meant as a guideline for ideas on how to build healthy meals and snacks. Please ask your doctor and/or care team what the ideal daily calorie intake is for you at your various stages of pregnancy. If you have any special nutrition needs, please focus on those foods when you build your menus. Mix and match. Change ingredients and dishes according to your needs, tastes, and ingredient availability.

DAY ONE VEGETARIAN

Breakfast

- 2 enriched whole wheat waffles (Weekend Pecan Waffles, page 208)
- 2 tablespoons maple syrup or blackstrap molasses
- 1 cup calcium-fortified orange juice
- 1 banana or your favorite fruit

Snack

- 1 cup smoothie (Mango-Chia Smoothie, page 157)

Lunch

- 1 quesadilla with cheese and vegetables (Black Bean, Mushroom, and Spinach Quesadillas, page 293)
- 3 tablespoons salsa
- 2 cups mixed greens with ½ avocado (or ⅓ cup guacamole, Just Plain Good Guacamole, page 135)
- 2 tablespoons salad dressing (see Awesome Homemade Salad Dressings, page 214)
- 1 apple or your favorite fruit
- 1 cup enriched reduced-fat dairy or nondairy milk

Snack

- 6 ounces dairy or nondairy yogurt
- ⅓ cup granola (Perfect Homemade Granola, page 105)
- ½ cup berries or your favorite fruit

Dinner

- One serving vegetable lasagne (Best-Ever Vegetarian Lasagne, page 296)
- 8 asparagus spears or broccoli (Roasted Asparagus, page 189, or Favorite Broccoli Slaw, page 291)
- 1 whole wheat roll
- 1 teaspoon butter or olive oil
- ½ cup reduced-fat dairy or nondairy frozen yogurt

DAY ONE VEGETARIAN

Calories: 2,010 cals	Fiber: 39 g
Fat: 65 g	Iron: 18 mg
Carbohydrates: 313 g	Calcium: 1,157 mg
Protein: 51 g	Folic acid: 421 mcg

DAY TWO VEGETARIAN

Breakfast

- 2 eggs, cooked (Spinach and Cheese Omelet for One, page 159 or Easy Veggie Frittata, page 133)
- 2 slices whole wheat bread, toasted
- 2 teaspoons butter or olive oil
- 1 cup calcium-fortified orange juice or green drink (Supergreen Drink, page 129)

Snack

- 1 high-protein bar
- 6 ounces reduced-fat dairy or nondairy fruit yogurt

Lunch

- ¾ cup bean salad (Yummy Three-Bean Salad, page 138)
- 2 cups mixed greens with 5 cherry tomatoes and 5 cucumber slices
- 2 tablespoons salad dressing (see Awesome Homemade Salad Dressings, page 214)
- ½ cup cottage cheese
- 5 whole wheat crackers, or 1 slice whole-grain bread
- 1 cup enriched reduced-fat dairy or nondairy milk

Dinner

- 1½ cups whole wheat spaghetti with ½ cup tomato sauce and 3 ounces sautéed tofu (Spaghetti with Herbed Tofu Balls, page 273)
- ½ cup broccoli florets or green vegetable (Tomato, Hearts of Palm, and Asparagus Salad, page 244)
- ½ cup mango or your favorite fruit sorbet

DAY TWO VEGETARIAN

Calories: 2,103 cals	Fiber: 35 g
Fat: 65 g	Iron: 17 mg
Carbohydrates: 306 g	Calcium: 1,632 mg
Protein: 93 g	Folic acid: 419 mcg

DAY THREE VEGETARIAN

Breakfast

- 2 slices French toast (French Toast Banana Sandwich, page 104)
- 1 cup calcium-fortified orange juice or green drink (Supergreen Drink, page 129)
- 6 ounces reduced-fat dairy or nondairy fruit yogurt

Snack

- 1 banana or your favorite fruit
- 2 tablespoons peanut or nut butter
- 2 brown rice cakes

Lunch

- 1 cup squash or carrot soup (Butternut Squash Soup, page 106)
- ½ cup egg salad (Pr-Egg-O Salad, page 110)
- 2 slices whole wheat bread
- 1 cup enriched dairy or nondairy milk
- ½ cup (4 ounces) mandarin orange slices in light syrup or fresh fruit

Dinner

- 1 serving tofu cakes (Old Bay Tofu Cakes with Cocktail Sauce, page 116)
- ½ cup tabbouleh salad (Best-Ever Tabbouleh Salad, page 111)
- ½ cup green vegetable
- 1 cup mixed greens
- 1 tablespoon salad dressing (see Awesome Homemade Salad Dressings, page 214)
- ½ cup raspberry or your favorite fruit sorbet

DAY THREE VEGETARIAN

Calories: 2,060 cals	Fiber: 23 g
Fat: 62 g	Iron: 13 mg
Carbohydrates: 324 g	Calcium: 1,382 mg
Protein: 66 g	Folic acid: 363 mcg

DAY FOUR VEGAN

Breakfast

1 cup fortified vegan whole-grain breakfast cereal

1 cup enriched nondairy plant-based milk

1 banana or your favorite fruit

1 cup vegan calcium-fortified orange juice

Snack

1 medium-size vegan whole wheat bagel or vegan whole-grain roll

2 slices vegan cheese or spread or ⅓ cup bean dip (High-Folate Spinach Bean Dip, page 81)

¼ cup soy nuts or edamame

Lunch

1 vegan burger

1 vegan whole wheat bun

Salad Bar Salad made with 2 cups romaine lettuce, 5 cherry tomatoes, ¼ cup shredded carrots (Quick Romaine and Avocado Salad, page 109)

2 tablespoons vegan salad dressing (see Awesome Homemade Salad Dressings, page 214)

6 ounces nondairy fruit yogurt

Dinner

3 ounces sautéed tofu with ½ cup bok choy and sesame seeds

1 cup brown rice or your favorite whole grain

2 cups salad with vegan dressing (see Awesome Homemade Salad Dressings, page 214)

2 vegan oatmeal cookies (No-Bake Nutty Energy Balls, page 97)

½ cup nondairy pudding or yogurt

DAY FOUR VEGAN

Calories: 2,048 cals	Fiber: 49 g
Fat: 56 g	Iron: 43 mg
Carbohydrates: 324 g	Calcium: 1,192 mg
Protein: 85 g	Folic acid: 911 mcg

DAY FIVE VEGAN

Breakfast

1 cup vegan oatmeal

1 tablespoon molasses

¼ cup nuts or seeds

1 cup enriched nondairy milk

½ cup berries or your favorite fruit

Snack

1 medium-size vegan whole wheat bagel

2 slices vegan turkey or bean spread (Healthy Hummus, page 290)

1 high-protein vegan granola bar

Lunch

1 vegan burrito (Protein-Packed Burritos, page 255)

2 cups mixed greens, ½ cut seasoned croutons, ¼ cup shredded carrots

2 tablespoons vegan salad dressing (see Awesome Homemade Salad Dressings, page 214)

1 cup tomato juice

1 banana or your favorite fruit

Dinner

3 ounces tofu sautéed with vegetables (Hot and Sweet Veggie Salad, page 137)

½ cup cooked spinach (Swiss Chard with Soy Sauce, page 90, prepared with spinach)

1 cup whole wheat couscous with chopped parsley and sunflower seeds

1 vegan ice-cream sandwich

½ cup blueberries or your favorite fruit

DAY FIVE VEGAN

Calories: 2,063 cals	Fiber: 39 g
Fat: 67 g	Iron: 23 mg
Carbohydrates: 300 g	Calcium: 1,010 mg
Protein: 78 g	Folic acid: 490 mcg

DAY SIX VEGAN

Breakfast

1 vegan avocado toast (Just Plain Yummy Avocado Toast, page 80)

½ cup strawberries or your favorite fruit

1 cup nondairy yogurt

Snack

½ cup hummus (Healthy Hummus, page 290)

1 whole wheat pita pocket

8 baby carrots or your favorite veggies

Lunch

1½ cups vegan lentil soup (Lentil Soup with Brown Rice and Spinach, page 82)

1 slice vegan sprouted spelt bread

1 vegetable and bean vegan tamale

1 cup enriched nondairy milk

1 apple or your favorite fruit

Dinner

1 cup vegan vegetable ragout (Light and Healthy Vegetable Ragout, page 218)

1½ cups vegan whole wheat pasta

2 cups mixed greens with ⅓ cup roasted walnuts and 2 tablespoons dried cranberries

2 tablespoons balsamic salad dressing (see Awesome Homemade Salad Dressings, page 214)

½ cup peach or your favorite vegan sorbet

½ cup blueberries or berries

DAY SIX VEGAN

Calories: 2,028 cals	Fiber: 48 g
Fat: 39 g	Iron: 23 mg
Carbohydrates: 378 g	Calcium: 1,071 mg
Protein: 61 g	Folic acid: 615 mcg

DAY SEVEN VEGAN

Breakfast

1 cup fortified vegan whole-grain breakfast cereal

1 cup enriched nondairy milk

½ cup blueberries or your favorite fruit

1 slice whole vegan wheat bread, toasted

1 tablespoon almond or nut butter

Snack

½ cup vegan bean dip (Glorious Edamame Dip, page 161)

10 vegan whole wheat crackers, or 1 slice vegan whole-grain bread

¼ cup mixed nuts

1 cup vegan green drink (Supergreen Drink, page 129)

Lunch

1½ cups vegan miso soup with tofu and greens or bean soup

7 pieces vegan vegetable maki (takeout) with 1 teaspoon soy sauce, pickled ginger, and wasabi

½ cup vegan seaweed salad or cabbage slaw (Lemony Slaw, page 164)

1 orange or your favorite fruit

1 cup enriched nondairy milk or yogurt

Dinner

1 cup vegan chili (Three-Bean Chili, page 91)

1 cup brown rice or your favorite whole grain

2 cups green salad (Asian-Inspired Spinach Salad, page 186)

½ cup vegan frozen nondairy ice cream or vegan sorbet

½ cup fresh raspberries or your favorite fruit (Refreshing Fruit Salad, page 130)

DAY SEVEN VEGAN

Calories: 2,010 cals	Fiber: 56 g
Fat: 68 g	Iron: 44 mg
Carbohydrates: 315 g	Calcium: 1,191 mg
Protein: 61 g	Folic acid: 1,028 mcg

Menus for Diabetes During Pregnancy

The following menus for diabetes during pregnancy are meant as a guideline for ideas on how to build healthy meals and snacks. Please ask your doctor and/or care team about your ideal daily carbohydrate intake for meals and snacks and your blood glucose levels post meals and fasting. Please also inquire about your daily calorie intake needs and any other special nutrition needs at your various stages of pregnancy. Mix and match the menus. Pull out foods from the menu meal plans to eat as snacks. Change ingredients and dishes according to your needs, tastes, and ingredient availability. Load up on colorful vegetables and fruits. Remember that peas, corn, potatoes, and winter squash are all starchy veggies and contain more carbs. Aim for lots of protein and fiber in your snacks and meals. See "Low-Carb Recipes for Diabetes During Pregnancy (20 or less carbs per serving)" for more ideas. We hope all this helps!

15-GRAM CARB SNACK IDEAS

1 plain rice cake = 7
2 tablespoons unsalted peanut or nut butter = 7

2 plain rice cakes = 14
½ cup plain cottage cheese = 3
A sprinkle of chia seeds = 0

½ large apple or banana, or other fruit = 15 or celery sticks = 0
2 tablespoons unsalted peanut or nut butter = 7

2 cups air-popped popcorn = 16
A light spray of olive oil = 0
A sprinkle of nutritional yeast flakes (high B-vitamin seasoning) = 0
2 mozzarella cheese sticks = 0

1 hard-boiled egg = 0
1 slice sprouted grain bread = 15
1 tablespoon mayonnaise = 0

2 Crisp Light Wasa crackers or similar crackers = 10 or 7 whole wheat crackers = 14
2 slices Cheddar cheese = 2 or ½ cup plain cottage cheese = 3 or 2 slices provolone = 2

⅓ cup prepared hummus = 15 (Healthy Hummus = 17, page 290)
Veggie sticks of cucumbers, carrots, celery, daikon, red radishes, red, yellow, or green bell peppers, or your favorite vegetables = 3

½ cup plain reduced-fat unsweetened Greek yogurt or nondairy yogurt = 10
½ cup raspberries or a single portion of your favorite fruit = 7
¼ cup chopped walnuts or your favorite nuts or seeds = 4
Sprinkle of chia seeds or ground flaxseeds = 0

½ cup grapes (about 15 grapes) = 13
1 cheese stick = 0

½ cup guacamole = 12 (Just Plain Good
Guacamole, page 135)

Romaine lettuce leaves and other veggies for
dipping = 3

1 cheese stick = 0

5 pita chips = 10

1 cup nonstarchy vegetable soup (Gazpacho
[Without the Gas] = 12, page 289)

1 cheese stick = 0

5 pita chips = 10

⅓ cup bean dip = 16 (High-Folate Spinach
Bean Dip = 15, page 81)

Veggie sticks of cucumbers, carrots, celery, daikon,
red radishes, red, yellow, or green bell peppers,
or your favorite vegetables = 3

1 cheese stick = 0

15- TO 30-GRAM CARB BREAKFAST AND BRUNCH IDEAS

Eggs and Ham or Sausages 17 carbs and
27 grams protein

2 eggs, cooked = 0 (Spinach and Cheese
Omelet for One = 3, page 159, or Ham and
Egg Cups = 3, page 262)

2 slices all-natural ham or 2 breakfast links = 1

1 slice whole-grain bread = 15

1 tablespoon cream cheese = 1

½ cup cucumber slices = 0

Oatmeal with Nuts and Seeds 23 carbs and
18 grams protein

¾ cup regular oatmeal, plain, prepared with water
and cinnamon = 21

2 tablespoons sunflower or pumpkin seeds = 2

¼ cup chopped walnuts, or other nuts = 1

1 cooked egg = 0

Avocado Toast with Hard-boiled Egg 23 carbs and
16 grams protein

1 slice whole wheat toast = 15 (Just Plain Yummy
Avocado Toast = 32, page 80)

½ avocado = 6

2 tablespoons sunflower or pumpkin seeds = 2

1 hard-boiled egg = 0

Cinnamon Toast with Eggs and Cheese 15 carbs and
17 grams protein

1 slice cinnamon whole wheat toast with a sprinkle
of cinnamon and stevia = 15

1 cheese stick = 0

1 cooked egg = 0

1 tablespoon mayonnaise = 0

Bagel and Cottage Cheese 27 carbs and 25 grams
protein

½ whole wheat bagel = 18

½ cup cottage cheese = 3

1 cooked egg = 0

½ cup sliced cucumbers = 2

½ cup low-sodium tomato juice = 4

45- TO 60-GRAM CARB LUNCH IDEAS

Special Note: To reduce the total amount of carbs, consume the dairy (milk and yogurt) and/or fruit suggestions as a snack. Most of the dairy and fruit portions listed contain 15 grams of carbs.

Classic Chicken Caesar Salad 43 carbs and 42 grams protein
1 store-bought packaged Caesar salad = 6 (Everyone's Favorite Caesar Salad = 24, page 84)
3 ounces cooked chicken = 0
1 whole wheat roll = 15
1 cup reduced-fat dairy or nondairy milk or 6 ounces reduced-fat plain yogurt = 12
½ cup fresh berries, or other fruit = 10

Egg Salad Plate 49 carbs and 33 grams protein
¾ cup egg salad = 2 (Pr-Egg-O Salad = 6, page 110)
1 cheese stick = 0
1 whole wheat roll = 15
2 cups sliced romaine = 3 (Quick Romaine and Avocado Salad = 12, page 109)
2 tablespoons Italian salad dressing = 3
½ cup cucumber slices = 2
¾ cup honeydew melon = 12
1 cup reduced-fat dairy or nondairy milk or 6 ounces reduced-fat plain yogurt = 12

Panera's Soup and Salad 50 carbs and 20 grams protein
1 cup Panera broccoli cheddar soup = 16 (Creamy Cauliflower Soup = 18, page 211)
1 Panera Greek salad, half portion = 7 (My Big Fat Greek Salad = 13, page 163)
½ medium apple, or other fruit = 15
1 cup reduced-fat dairy or nondairy milk or 6 ounces reduced-fat plain yogurt = 12

Chicken Salad 48 carbs and 31 grams protein
¾ cup chicken salad made with 3 ounces cooked chicken = 11 (Chicken Salad with Dried Apricots and Almonds = 11, page 216 or Snappy Mediterranean-Style Chicken Salad = 20, page 245)
1 whole wheat roll = 15
2 cups sliced romaine = 3
¼ cup pumpkin seeds = 4
2 tablespoons salad dressing = 3 (see Awesome Homemade Salad Dressings = 0, page 214)
1 cup reduced-fat dairy or nondairy milk or 6 ounces reduced-fat plain yogurt = 12

Pasta with Shrimp 51 carbs and 27 grams protein
1 cup whole wheat pasta = 21
3 ounces cooked shrimp = 0
2 cups baby spinach = 2
2 tablespoons salad dressing = 3
½ avocado = 6
1 cup reduced-fat dairy or nondairy milk or 6 ounces reduced-fat plain yogurt = 12
⅓ cup blueberries = 7

45- TO 60-GRAM CARB DINNER IDEAS

Special Note: To reduce the total amount of carbs in the following menus, eat the dairy and fruit suggestions as a snack. Most dairy and fruit portion listed equal 15 grams of carbs each.

Meat Lovers Steak Night 24 carbs and 32 grams protein

3 ounces grilled steak = 0 (Best-Ever Flank Steak with Salsa Verde = 1, page 175)

2 cups baby spinach = 2

5 cherry tomatoes = 2

½ avocado = 6

2 tablespoons ranch salad dressing = 2

1 cup reduced-fat dairy or nondairy milk or 6 ounces reduced-fat plain yogurt = 12

Rotisserie Chicken with Rice 41 carbs and 30 grams protein

3 ounces store-bought rotisserie chicken = 0

⅓ cup cooked brown rice or whole grain = 15

1 cup cooked broccoli = 6

1 cup coleslaw = 8 (Lemony Slaw = 6, page 164)

1 cup reduced-fat dairy or nondairy milk or 6 ounces reduced-fat plain yogurt = 12

Salmon and Couscous 41 carbs and 33 grams protein

3 ounces cooked salmon = 0 (Salmon with Artichoke-Olive Tapenade = 5, page 298 or Salmon with Toasted Almonds, Capers, and Fresh Herbs = 5, page 144)

2 tablespoons tartar sauce = 4 (Tartar Sauce = 2, page 193)

⅓ cup cooked couscous = 13

½ cup green beans = 5

2 cups baby kale = 2

2 tablespoons French salad dressing = 5

1 cup reduced-fat dairy or nondairy milk or 6 ounces reduced-fat plain yogurt = 12

Pasta and Shrimp Dinner 62 carbs and 36 grams protein

3 ounces cooked shrimp = 0 (Zucchini Noodles with Spicy Shrimp = 9, page 169)

½ cup cooked whole wheat pasta = 21 (ideally whole grain)

½ cup store-bought tomato-basil pasta sauce = 14 (Twenty-Minute Tomato Sauce = 8, page 221)

½ cup zucchini = 2

1 cup reduced-fat dairy or nondairy milk or 6 ounces reduced-fat plain yogurt = 12

½ banana = 13

Veggie Burgers with Quinoa 62 carbs and 24 grams protein

1 Amy's Veggie Burger (no bun) = 16 (Groovy Veggie Burger (with a whole wheat bun) = 55, page 142)

⅓ cup cooked quinoa = 13

2 cups baby kale salad = 2

5 cherry tomatoes = 3

2 tablespoons sunflower seeds = 2

2 tablespoons ranch salad dressing = 2

1 cup reduced-fat dairy or nondairy milk or 6 ounces reduced-fat plain yogurt = 12

½ cup strawberries = 12

Conversions for Easy Cooking

VOLUME CONVERSIONS

AMERICAN	METRIC (MILLILITERS)	FLUID OUNCES
¼ teaspoon	1.25	
½ teaspoon	2.5	
1 teaspoon	5	
½ tablespoon (1½ teaspoons)	7.5	
1 tablespoon (3 teaspoons)	15	
2 tablespoons	30	1
¼ cup (4 tablespoons)	60	2
⅓ cup (5⅓ tablespoons)	75	2⅔
½ cup (8 tablespoons)	125	4
⅔ cup (10 tablespoons)	150	5
¾ cup (12 tablespoons)	175	6
1 cup (16 tablespoons; ½ pint)	250	8
1¼ cups	300	10
1½ cups	350	12
2 cups (1 pint)	500	16
3 cups	750	24
4 cups (1 quart, 2 pints)	1,000 (1 liter)	32
5 cups	1,250	40
16 cups (4 quarts, 1 gallon)	4,000	128

DRY WEIGHT CONVERSIONS

AMERICAN	METRIC (GRAMS AND KILOGRAMS)
¼ ounce	7 grams
½ ounce	15 grams
1 ounce	30 grams
2 ounces	60 grams
3 ounces	90 grams
4 ounces	115 grams
5 ounces	150 grams
6 ounces	175 grams
7 ounces	200 grams
8 ounces	225 grams
9 ounces	250 grams
10 ounces	300 grams
11 ounces	325 grams
12 ounces	350 grams
13 ounces	375 grams
14 ounces	400 grams
15 ounces	425 grams
16 ounces (1 pound)	450 grams
1 pound 2 ounces	500 grams
1 pound 8 ounces	750 grams
2 pounds	900 grams
2 pounds 2 ounces	1,000 grams (1 kilogram)
3 pounds	1.4 kilograms
4 pounds	1.8 kilograms
4 pounds 8 ounces	2 kilograms
5 pounds	2.4 kilograms

OVEN TEMPERATURE CONVERSIONS

DESCRIPTION	DEGREES FAHRENHEIT	DEGREES CENTIGRADE
Very Low	250 to 275	121 to 133
Low	300 to 325	149 to 163
Moderate	350 to 375	177 to 190
Hot	400 to 425	204 to 218
Very Hot	450 to 475	232 to 246
Extremely Hot	500 to 525	260 to 274

Notes

INTRODUCTION

1. Cliantha Padayachee and Jeff S. Coombes, "Exercise Guidelines for Gestational Diabetes Mellitus," *World Journal of Diabetes* 6, no. 8 (July 2015): 1033–1044, https://www.wjgnet.com/1948-9358/full/v6/i8/1033.htm.

2. E. R. Magro-Malosso et al., "Exercise During Pregnancy and Risk of Gestational Hypertensive Disorders: A Systematic Review and Meta-analysis, *Acta Obstetricia et Gynecologica Scandanavica* 96, no. 8 (August 2017): 921–931, https://obgyn.onlinelibrary.wiley.com/doi/abs/10.1111/aogs.13151.

YOUR NUTRITIONAL NEEDS, PLUS A WHOLE LOT MORE

1. Institute of Medicine and National Research Council of the National Academies, Committee to Reexamine IOM Pregnancy Weight Guidelines Food and Nutrition Board on Children Youth, and Families; Kathleen M. Rasmussen and Ann L. Yaktine, eds., *Weight Gain During Pregnancy, Reexamining the Guidelines* (Washington, DC: National Academies Press, 2009), PDF download http:///12584/weight-gain-during-pregnancy-reexamining-the-guidelines.

2. Institute of Medicine, "Physical Activity Coefficients (PA Values) for Use in EER Equations," in *Dietary Reference Intakes: The Essential Guide to Nutrient Requirements* (Washington, DC: National Academies Press, 2006).

3. Institute of Medicine and National Research Council of the National Academies, *Weight Gain During Pregnancy, Reexamining the Guidelines*, "Table S-1: New Recommendation for Total Rate of Weight Gain During Pregnancy, by Prepregnancy BMI," 2.

4. American College of Obstetricians and Gynecologists, "Food, Pregnancy, and Health," pamphlet (1986), Resource Center, 409 12th Street SW, Washington, DC, 20024.

5. Carol J. Lammi-Keefe, Sarah C. Couch, and Elliot H. Philipson, eds., *Handbook of Nutrition and Pregnancy* (Totowa, NJ: Humana Press, 2008), 8.

6. Institute of Medicine and National Research Council of the National Academies, *Weight Gain During Pregnancy, Reexamining the Guidelines*, "Chart: Dietary Reference Intakes for

Pregnancy, Table b-1a Equations to Estimate Energy Requirement for Pregnant Women by Trimester," 316.

7. H. H. Butchko et al., "Aspartame: Review of Safety," *Regulatory Toxicology and Pharmacology* 35, no. 2 part 2 (April 2002): S1–S93, https://www.ncbi.nlm.nih.gov/pubmed?term=12180494.

8. M. A. Pereira, "Sugar-Sweetened and Artificially-Sweetened Beverages in Relation to Obesity Risk," *Advances in Nutrition* 5, no. 6 (November 2014): 797–808, https://www.ncbi.nlm.nih.gov/pubmed?term=25398745.

9. Juliana F. W. Cohen et al., "Maternal *Trans* Fatty Acid Intake and Fetal Growth," *American Journal of Clinical Nutrition* 94, no. 5 (November 2011): 1241–1247, https://academic.oup.com/ajcn/article/94/5/1241⁄4597860.

10. James A. Greenberg, Stacey J. Bell, and Wendy van Ausdal, "Omega-3 Fatty Acid Supplementation During Pregnancy," *Reviews in Obstetrics and Gynecology* 1, no. 4 (Fall 2008): 162–169, https://www.ncbi.nlm.nih.gov/pmc/articles/PMC2621042/.

11. Martha Neuringer, Gregory J. Anderson, and William E. Connor, "The Essentiality of N-3 Fatty Acids for the Development and Function of the Retina and Brain," *Annual Review of Nutrition* 8 (July 1988): 517–541, cited in British Associate Parliamentary Food and Health Forum, *The Links Between Diet and Behavior: The Influence of Nutrition on Mental Health* (January 2008), 9.

12. M. A. Klebanoff et al., "Fish Consumption, Erythrocyte Fatty Acids, and Preterm Birth," *Obstetrics & Gynecology* 117, no. 7 (May 2011): 1071–1077, https://www.ncbi.nlm.nih.gov/pubmed?term=21508745.

13. V. Leventakou et al., "Fish Intake During Pregnancy, Fetal Growth, and Gestational Length in 19 European Birth Cohort Studies," *American Journal of Clinical Nutrition* 99, no. 3 (March 2014): 506–516, https://www.ncbi.nlm.nih.gov/pubmed?term=24335057; Lammi-Keefe, Couch, and Philipson, eds., 96.

14. Lammi-Keefe, Couch, and Philipson, *Handbook of Nutrition and Pregnancy*, 357–383.

15. M. P. Freeman et al., "Evidence Basis for Treatment and Future Research in Psychiatry," *Journal of Clinical Psychiatry* 67 (2006): 1954–1967, cited in British Associate Parliamentary Food and Health Forum, *The Links Between Diet and Behavior: The Influence of Nutrition on Mental Health* (January 2008): 26.

16. Gerard Hornstra, "Essential Fatty Acids in Mothers and Their Neonates," *American Journal of Clinical Nutrition* 71, no. 5 (May 2000): 1262S–1269S, https://doi.org/10.1093/ajcn/71.5.1262s.

17. J. Villar et al., "Strategies to Prevent and Treat Preeclampsia: Evidence from Randomized Controlled Trials," *Seminars in Nephrology* 24, no. 6 (November 2004): 607–615, https://www.ncbi.nlm.nih.gov/pubmed?term=15529296.

18. J. F. Williams and V. C. Smith, Committee on Substance Abuse. Fetal Alcohol Spectrum Disorders, *Pediatrics* 136, no. 5 (November 2015): e1395–1406, https://www.ncbi.nlm.nih.gov/pubmed?term=26482673.

19. S. Hartmann et al., "Exposure to Retinoic Acids in Non-pregnant Women Following High Vitamin A Intake with a Liver Meal." *International Journal for Vitamin and Nutrition Research* 75, no. 3 (May 2005): 187–194, https://econtent.hogrefe.com/doi/10.1024/0300-9831.75.3.187.

20. R. Blomhoff and J. Alexander, "Vitamin A and Toxicity. Should Pregnant Women and Small Children Reduce Their Intake of Liver Products and Vitamin A?," *Tidsskr Nor Laegeforen* 113, no. 24 (October 1993): 113:3037-9, https://www.ncbi.nlm.nih.gov/pubmed?term=8259577; H. Van den Berg H., K. F. Hulshof, and J. P. Deslypere, "Evaluation of the Effect of the Use of Vitamin Supplements on Vitamin A Intake Among (Potentially) Pregnant Women in Relation to the Consumption of Liver and Liver Products," *European Journal of Obstetrics, Gynecology, & Reproductive Biology* 66, no. 1 (May 1996): 17–21, https://www.ncbi.nlm.nih.gov/pubmed?term=8735753.

21. "Folic Acid," Pregnancy and Newborn Health Education Center March of Dimes, 2008, http://www.marchofdimes.com/pnhec/173_769.asp.

22. American Dietetic Association, "Position of the American Dietetic Association: Nutrition and Lifestyle for a Healthy Pregnancy Outcome," *Journal of the American Dietetic Association* (2008): 555.

23. K. D. Wenstrom et al., "Role of Amniotic Fluid Homocysteine Level and of Fetal 5, 10-Methylenetetrahydrafolate Reductase Genotype in the Etiology of Neural Tube Defects," *American Journal of Medical Genetics* 90, no. 1 (January 2000): 12–16, https://www.ncbi.nlm.nih.gov/pubmed?term=10602111.

24. For more general information on MTHFR, see https://rarediseases.info.nih.gov/diseases/10953/mthfr-gene-mutation.

25. A. Shrim et al., "Pregnancy Outcome Following Use of Large Doses of Vitamin B$_6$ in the First Trimester," *Journal of Obstetrics & Gynaecology* 26, no. 8 (November 2006): 749–751, https://www.ncbi.nlm.nih.gov/pubmed?term=17130022.

26. Institute of Medicine and National Research Council of the National Academies, *Weight Gain During Pregnancy, Reexamining the Guidelines*.

27. Institute of Medicine, *Dietary Reference Intakes: The Essential Guide to Nutrient Requirements*, "Table 1: Dietary Reference Intakes for Water by Life Stage Group (National Academies Press, Washington, DC, 2006): 156–157, PDF available at https://www.nal.usda.gov/sites/default/files/fnic_uploads//DRIEssentialGuideNutReq.pdf.

28. G. B. Piccoli et al., "Vegan-Vegetarian Diets in Pregnancy: Danger or Panacea? A Systematic Narrative Review," *British Journal of Obstetrics and Gynaecology* 122, no. 5 (April 2015): 623–633, https://www.ncbi.nlm.nih.gov/pubmed?term=25600902.

29. Marie V. Krasue and L. Kathleen Mahan, *Food, Nutrition and Diet Therapy*, 6th ed. (Philadelphia, PA: W. B. Saunders, 1979).

30. Lammi-Keefe, Couch, and Philipson, eds., *Handbook of Nutrition and Pregnancy*, 218.

31. Ibid., 219.

32. "Food Safety for Pregnant Women," Food and Drug Administration, accessed August 19, 2018, https://www.fda.gov/food/foodborneillnesscontaminants/peopleatrisk/ucm312704.htm;

Additional Food Safety Resource: https://www.foodsafety.gov; Gateway to Government Food Safety Information, including all recalls and alerts: https://www.cdc.gov/foodsafety/, 1-800-232-4636 (24-hour recorded information).

33. "Toxoplasmosis," Centers for Disease Control and Prevention, accessed August 19, 2018, https://www.cdc.gov/parasites/toxoplasmosis/gen_info/faqs.html.

34. "E. coli (Escherichia coli)," Centers for Disease Control and Prevention, accessed August 19, 2018, https://www.cdc.gov/ecoli/index.html.

35. "Salmonella, Information for Healthcare Professionals and Laboratories Centers for Disease Control and Prevention," accessed August 19, 2018, https://www.cdc.gov/salmonella.

36. "Salmonella and Eggs," Centers for Disease Control and Prevention, accessed August 19, 2018, https://www.cdc.gov/Features/SalmonellaEggs/.

37. "Listeria Listeriosis," Centers for Disease Control and Prevention, accessed August 19, 2018, https://www.cdc.gov/listeria/index.html.

38. "Dirty Dozen, EWG's 2018 Shopper's Guide to Pesticides in Produce," Environmental Working Group, accessed August 19, 2018, https://www.ewg.org/foodnews/dirty-dozen.php.

39. "Clean 15," Environmental Working Group, accessed August 19, 2018, https://www.ewg.org/foodnews/clean-fifteen.php.

40. Stephanie Spear, "Why You Should Drink Organic Coffee," ECO Watch, posted August 14, 2014, accessed August 19, 2018, https://www.ecowatch.com/why-you-should-drink-organic-coffee-1881940567.html.

41. United States Environmental Protection Agency, "2017 EPA-FDA Advice About Eating Fish and Shellfish," accessed August 19, 2018, https://www.epa.gov/fish-tech/2017-epa-fda-advice-about-eating-fish-and-shellfish.

42. "Keep Food Safe," Centers for Disease Control and Prevention, accessed August 19, 2018, https://www.cdc.gov/foodsafety/keep-food-safe.html.

43. Dr. Mercola, "How to Recognize Plastics That Are Hazardous to You," April 11, 2013, accessed August 19, 2018, https://articles.mercola.com/sites/articles/archive/2013/04/11/plastic-use.aspx.

44. A. Shrim et al., "Pregnancy Outcome," 749–751.

45. E. Viljoen et al., "A Systematic Review and Meta-analysis of the Effect and Safety of Ginger in the Treatment of Pregnancy-Associated Nausea and Vomiting," *Nutrition Journal* 13 (March 2014): 20, https://nutritionj.biomedcentral.com/articles/10.1186/1475-2891-13-20.

46. R. Gaillard, "Maternal Obesity During Pregnancy and Cardiovascular Development and Disease in the Offspring," *European Journal of Epidemiology* 30, no. 11 (November 2015): 1141–1152, https://link.springer.com/article/10.1007%2Fs10654-015-0085-7.

47. K. Blomberg, "Maternal Obesity, Mode of Delivery, and Neonatal Outcome," *Obstetrics & Gynecology* 122, no. 1 (July 2013): 50–55, https://www.ncbi.nlm.nih.gov/pubmed?term=23743457.

48. L. Schummers et al., "Risk of Adverse Pregnancy Outcomes by Prepregnancy Body Mass Index: A Population-Based Study to Inform Prepregnancy Weight Loss Counseling,"

Obstetrics & Gynecology 125, no. 1 (January 2015): 133–143, https://www.ncbi.nlm.nih.gov /pubmed?term=25560115.

49. L. Duley, D. Henderson-Smart, and S. Meher, "Altered Dietary Salt for Preventing Pre-eclampsia, and Its Complications," *Cochrane Database System* (revised October 2005): CD005548, https://www.ncbi.nlm.nih.gov/pubmed?term=16235411.

50. J. A. Hutcheon, S. Lisonkova, and K. S. Joseph, "Epidemiology of Pre-eclampsia and the Other Hypertensive Disorders of Pregnancy," *Best Practice and Research Clinical Obstetrics and Gynaecology* 25, no. 4 (August 2011): 391–403, https://www.ncbi.nlm.nih.gov /pubmed?term=21333604.

51. C. V. Ananth, K. M. Keyes, and R. J. Wapner, "Pre-eclampsia Rates in the United States, 1980–2010: Age-Period-Cohort Analysis," *British Medical Journal* 347 (November 2013): f6564, https://www.ncbi.nlm.nih.gov/pubmed?term=24201165.

52. C. Briceno-Preez, L. Briceno-Sanabria, and P. Vigil–De Gracia, "Prediction and Prevention of Preeclampsia," *Hypertension in Pregnancy* 28, no. 2 (May 2009): 138–155, https://www .ncbi.nlm.nih.gov/pubmed?term=19437225.

53. "Tobacco Use and Pregnancy," Centers for Disease Control and Prevention Reproductive Health, accessed August 18, 2018, https://www.cdc.gov/reproductivehealth/maternalinfant health/tobaccousepregnancy/index.htm.

54. B. L. Rooney, M. A. Mathiason, and C. W. Schauberger, "Predictors of Obesity in Childhood, Adolescence, and Adulthood in a Birth Cohort," *Maternal and Child Health Journal* 15, no. 8 (November 2011): 1166–1175, https://www.ncbi.nlm.nih.gov/pubmed?term=20927643; M. R. Torloni et al., "Prepregnancy BMI and the Risk of Gestational Diabetes: A Systematic Review of the Literature with Meta-analysis," *Obesity Reviews* 10, no. 2 (March 2009): 194–203, https://www.ncbi.nlm.nih.gov/pubmed?term=19055539.

55. L. Schummers et al., "Risk of Adverse Pregnancy Outcomes," 133–143.

56. B. E. Metzger et al., "Hyperglycemia and Adverse Pregnancy Outcomes," HAPO Study Cooperative Research Group, *New England Journal of Medicine* 358 (2008): 1991–2002.

57. The ADA and the American College of Obstetricians and Gynecologists (ACOG) recommend the following upper limits for glucose levels, with insulin therapy initiated if they are exceeded, but acknowledge that these thresholds have been extrapolated from recommendations proposed for women with preexisting diabetes. Little guidance is available as to what proportion of measurements exceeding these thresholds should trigger intervention, and some suggest insulin for two or more elevated values in a two-week interval while others await more consistent elevations, particularly if it is judged that further nutritional counseling may be effective.

ADA and ACOG glucose targets are:

Fasting blood glucose concentration: <95 mg/dL (5.3 mmol/L)
One-hour postprandial blood glucose concentration: <140 mg/dL (7.8 mmol/L)
Two-hour postprandial glucose concentration: <120 mg/dL (6.7 mmol/L)

American Diabetes Association, "Management of Diabetes in Pregnancy: Standards of Medical Care in Diabetes," *Diabetes Care* 41 (supplement 1) (January 2018): S137–S143, http://care.diabetesjournals .org/content/41/Supplement_1/S137.

58. R. Artal and T. Tomlinson, "Exercise: The Logical Intervention for Diabetes in Pregnancy," in *Diabetes in Pregnancy*, ed. O. Langer (Beijing: People's Medical Publishing House, 2015): 189.

59. W. K. Nicholson et al., "Therapeutic Management, Delivery, and Postpartum Risk Assessment and Screening in Gestational Diabetes," *Evidence Report/Technological Assess (Full Report)* 162 (March 2008): 1–96, https://www.ncbi.nlm.nih.gov/pmc/articles/PMC4781072/; D. S. Feig et al., "Risk of development of diabetes mellitus after diagnosis of gestational diabetes," *CMAJ* 179(3) (Jul 2008): 229-34, http://www.cmaj.ca/content/179/3/229.

60. American College of Obstetricians and Gynecologists, "Frequently Asked Questions, Exercise During Pregnancy," FAQ 119, July 2017, https://www.acog.org/Patients/FAQs/Exercise-During-Pregnancy.

PRECONCEPTION: OPTIMIZING YOUR BODY FOR PREGNANCY

1. Xiaoping Weng, Roxana Odouli, and De-Kun Li, "Maternal Caffeine Consumption During Pregnancy and the Risk of Miscarriage: A Prospective Cohort Study," *American Journal of Obstetrics and Gynecology* 198, no. 3 (March 2008): 279.e1–299.e8.

2. "Caffeine Content for Coffee, Tea, Soda, and More," Nutrition and Healthy Eating, Mayo Clinic, accessed August 19, 2018, https://www.mayoclinic.org/healthy-lifestyle/nutrition-and-healthy-eating/in-depth/caffeine/art-20049372; "Caffeine Chart," Center for Science in the Public Interest, accessed August 19, 2018, https://cspinet.org/eating-healthy/ingredients-of-concern/caffeine-chart.

LIFE AFTER DELIVERY: BREASTFEEDING YOUR BABY

1. J. M. D. Thompson et al., "Duration of Breastfeeding and Risk of SIDS: An Individual Participant Data Meta-analysis," *Pediatrics* 5 (2017): 140, https://www.ncbi.nlm.nih.gov/pubmed?term=29084835.

2. L. Gray, L. Watt and E. M. Blass, "Skin-to-Skin Contact Is Analgesic in Healthy Newborns," *Pediatrics* 105, no. 1 (January 2000): e14, https://www.ncbi.nlm.nih.gov/pubmed?term=10617751.

3. Arne Høst et al., "Dietary Prevention of Allergic Diseases in Infants and Small Children," *Pediatric Allergy & Immunology* 19, no. 1 (February 2008): 1–4, https://www.ncbi.nlm.nih.gov/pubmed?term=18199086.

4. Leslie Elliott et al., "Prospective Study of Breast-Feeding in Relation to Wheeze, Atopy, and Bronchial Hyperresponsiveness in the Avon Longitudinal Study of Parents and Children (ALSPAC)," *Journal of Allergy and Clinical Immunology* 122, no. 1 (July 2008): 49-54e1-3, https://www.jacionline.org/article/S0091-6749(08)00618-0/fulltext.

5. T. Harder et al., "Duration of Breastfeeding and Risk of Overweight: A Meta-analysis," *American Journal of Epidemiology* 162, no. 5 (September 2005), 397–403, https://www.ncbi.nlm.nih.gov/pubmed?term=16076830.

6. S. Ip et al., "A Summary of the Agency for Healthcare Research and Quality's Evidence Report on Breastfeeding in Developed Countries," *Breastfeeding Medicine* Supplement 1 (October 2009): S17–S30, https://www.ncbi.nlm.nih.gov/pubmed?term=19827919.

7. C. G. Victora et al., "Association Between Breastfeeding and Intelligence, Educational Attainment, and Income at 30 Years of Age: A Prospective Birth Cohort Study from Brazil," *Lancet Global Health* (2015); 3:e199, https://www.ncbi.nlm.nih.gov/pubmed?term=26869575; A. Sacker, M. A. Quigley, and Y. J. Kelly, "Breastfeeding and Developmental Delay: Findings from the Millennium Cohort Study," *Pediatrics* 118 (September 2006): e682, https://www.ncbi.nlm.nih.gov/pubmed?term=16950960; B. L. Horta, C. Loret de Mola, and C. G. Victora, "Breastfeeding and Intelligence: A Systematic Review and Meta-analysis," *Acta Paediatrica* 104 (July 2015): 14, https://onlinelibrary.wiley.com/doi/abs/10.1111/apa.13139.

8. Institute of Medicine and National Research Council of the National Academies, *Weight Gain During Pregnancy, Reexamining the Guidelines.*

9. Lawrence M. Gartner and Frank R. Greer, "Prevention of Rickets and Vitamin D Deficiency: New Guidelines for Vitamin D Intake," *Pediatrics* 111, no. 4 (April 2003): 908–910.

BLUES AFTER BIRTH: NAVIGATING POSTPARTUM DEPRESSION

1. Maria Le Donne et al., "Postpartum Mood Disorders and Thyroid Autoimmunity," *Frontiers in Endocrinology* 8 (May 2017): 98, https://www.frontiersin.org/articles/10.3389/fendo.2017.00091/full.

2. B. M. Leung and B. J. Kaplan, "Perinatal Depression: Prevalence, Risks, and the Nutrition Link—A Review of the Literature," *Journal of the American Diet Association* 109, no. 9 (September 2009): 1566–1575, https://www.ncbi.nlm.nih.gov/pubmed/19699836; S. Etebary et al., "Postpartum Depression and the Role of Serum Trace Elements," *Iranian Journal of Psychiatry* 5, no. 2 (Spring 2010): 40–46, https://www.ncbi.nlm.nih.gov/pubmed/22952489.

3. Stephen D. Anton et al., "Effects of Chromium Picolinate on Food Intake and Satiety," *Diabetes Technology & Therapeutics* 10, no. 5 (October 2008): 405–412, https://www.ncbi.nlm.nih.gov/pmc/articles/PMC2753428/; Richard Malter, "Preventing Postpartum Depression: A Case Report," *Journal of Orthomolecular Medicine*, 16, no. 4 (2001): 213–217, https://pdfs.semanticscholar.org/9ab7/2cf087b2fa81f633ca8a5b5ca17be0531549.pdf; R. B. Singh et al., "Micronutrient Formulations for Prevention of Complications of Pregnancy," *Frontiers in Bioscience, Scholar Edition* 10 (January 2018): 175–184, https://pdfs.semanticscholar.org/d921/8ac0bc421cd045437687a0a557a457531010.pdf.

4. Carol J. Lammi-Keefe, Sarah C. Couch, and Elliot H. Philipson, eds., *Handbook of Nutrition and Pregnancy* (Totowa, NJ: Humana Press, 2008), 96; Andreanne Wassef, Quoc Dinh, and Martin St-Andre, "Anaemia and Depletion of Iron Stores as Risk Factors for Postpartum Depression: A Literature Review," *Journal of Psychosomatic Obstetrics & Gynecology* (October 2017), https://doi.org/10.1080/0167482X.2018.1427725; Manish Dama et al., "Iron Deficiency and Risk of Maternal Depression in Pregnancy: An Observational Study," *Journal of Obstetrics and Gynaecology Canada* 40, no. 6 (June 2018): 698–703, https://doi.org/10.1016/j.jogc.2017.09.027; B. M. Leung and B. J. Kaplan, "Perinatal Depression: Prevalence, Risks, and the Nutrition Link—A Review of the Literature," *Journal of the American Dietetic Association* 109, no. 9 (September 2009): 1566–1575, https://www.ncbi.nlm.nih.gov/pubmed/19699836.

5. Lammi-Keefe, Couch, and Philipson, eds., *Handbook of Nutrition and Pregnancy*, 357–383; Mei-Chi Hsu, Chia-Yi Tung, and Hsing-E Chen, "Omega-3 Polyunsaturated Fatty Acid Supplementation in Prevention and Treatment of Maternal Depression: Putative Mechanism and Recommendation," *Journal of Affective Disorders* 238 (October 2018): 47–61, https://doi.org/10.1016/j.jad.2018.05.018; Michelle P. Judge et al., "Pilot Trial Evaluating Maternal Docosahexaenoic Acid Consumption During Pregnancy: Decreased Postpartum Depressive Symptomatology," *International Journal of Nursing Sciences* 4, no. 1 (December 2014): 339–345, https://www.sciencedirect.com/science/article/pii/S2352013214000982; M. Freeman et al., "An Open Trial of omega-3 Fatty Acids for Depression in Pregnancy," *Acta Neuropsychiatrica* 18, no. 1 (2006): 21–24; M. Makrides and R. Gibson, "Long-Chain Polyunsaturated Fatty Acid Requirement During Pregnancy and Lactation," *American Journal of Clinical Nutrition* 71 (2000): 307–311; Joseph. R. Hibbeln, "Seafood Consumption, the DHA Content of Mothers' Milk and Prevalence Rates of Postpartum Depression: A Cross-national, Ecological Analysis," *Journal of Affective Disorders* 69, no. 1-3 (May 2002): 15–29, https://www.sciencedirect.com/science/article/pii/S0165032701003743.

6. A. Coppen and C. Bolander-Gouaille, "Treatment of Depression: Time to Consider Folic Acid and Vitamin B$_{12}$," *Journal of Psychopharmacology* 19, no. 1 (January 2005): 59–65, https://www.ncbi.nlm.nih.gov/pubmed/15671130; Mary F. F. Chong et al., "Relationship of Maternal Folate and Vitamin B$_{12}$ status During Pregnancy with Perinatal Depression: The GUSTO Study," *Journal of Psychiatric Research* 55 (August 2014): 110–116; Yoshihiro Miyake et al., "Dietary Folate and Vitamins B$_{12}$, B$_6$ and B$_2$ Intake and the Risk for Postpartum Depression in Japan: The Osaka Maternal and Child Health Study," *Journal of Affective Disorders* 96, no. 1-2 (November 2006): 133–138, https://www.sciencedirect.com/science/article/pii/S0165032706002564.

7. Miyake et al., "Dietary Folate and Vitamins B$_{12}$, B$_6$ and B$_2$," 133–138; Chong et al., "Relationship of Maternal Folate," 110–116.

8. Miyake et al., "Dietary Folate and Vitamins B$_{12}$, B$_6$ and B$_2$," 133–138.

9. Sue Penckofer et al., "Vitamin D and Depression: Where Is All the Sunshine?" *Issues Mental Health Nursing* 31, no. 6 (June 2010): 385–393, https://www.ncbi.nlm.nih.gov/pmc/articles/PMC2908269/; Fariba Aghajafari et al., "Vitamin D Deficiency and Antenatal And Postpartum Depression: A Systematic Review, *Nutrients* 10, no. 4 (February 2018): 478,

http://www.mdpi.com/2072-6643/10/4/478; Katharine M. Lange et al., Department of Psychology, Southern Oregon University and Department of Experimental Psychology, University of Regensburg, Germany, "Vitamin D and Depression," *Vitamins and Food Proteins Agro Food Industry High Tech* 27, no. 2 (March/April 2016), http://www.teknoscienze.com/getpdf.php?filename=Contents/Riviste/PDF/VITAMINS-FOOD%20PROTEINS_2016_low.pdf&beginpage=31&endpage=34&filetitle=Vitamin%20D%20and%20depression.

WEIGHT LOSS AFTER BABY: CHOOSE THE RIGHT TIME AND TAKE IT SLOW

1. Jack F. Hollis et al., "Weight Loss During the Intensive Intervention Phase of the Weight-Loss Maintenance Trial," *American Journal of Preventative Medicine* 35, no. 2 (2008): 118–126. For a more exact reading of your calorie needs, go to http://www.caloriecontrol.org/calcalcs.html and plug in your height, weight, age, and activity level, and you will get your estimated daily maintenance calorie needs.

NUTRITIONAL SOURCES

1. Penny M. Kris-Etherton, William S. Harris, and Lawrence J. Appel for the Nutrition Committee, "Fish Consumption, Fish Oil, Omega-3 Fatty Acids, and Cardiovascular Disease," *Circulation* 106 (November 2002): 2747–2757.

Thanks

CATHERINE JONES

Wow! Third edition! I'm thrilled, blessed, and extremely grateful to everyone who made it happen. This book has always been a true labor of love. My coauthor since the first edition, Rose Ann Hudson, RD, LD, is a remarkable woman. She combines deep knowledge of perinatal nutrition with a warm and compassionate approach to her patients, and life in general. I'm so proud of our awesome collaborators: Elna Narula, RN, CDE; Shoshana Bennett, PhD; and Linda Wade, PhD. All are experts in their fields with decades of experience. I am thankful that Dr. Knight's beautiful words and her infinite wisdom are immortalized in these pages. She will forever be my hero.

Claire Schulz, my acquiring editor at Da Capo Press, brought her sensitivity and smarts to this edition and embraced my new approach of chapters divided by months. I'm indebted to Dan Ambrosio, senior editor, and his skilled team for their insights and wisdom—a serious group of talent including Renée Sedliar and Miriam Riad in the editorial office, and Anna Hall and Lauren Ollerhead in publicity and marketing. Cisca Schreefel, my brilliant editorial production manager, worked with copyeditor Iris Bass, proofreader Katie Malm, and indexer Elizabeth Parson, to push this edition across the finish line. I owe a big thanks to interior designer, Trish Wilkinson, and cover designer, Kerry Rubenstein, for their beautiful work. Big hug of appreciation to all of my recipe testers for this edition and all the previous ones. I am grateful to my literary agents, Lisa and Sally Ekus, who have been by my side for decades.

My family is my anchor and sanity. My two incredible children, Aleksandra and Hale, bring me more joy, pride, and love than they will ever know. My husband, Paul, has given me the strength and freedom to reach for the stars. His intelligence, humor, and love are bottomless. My parents and siblings, Jack, Paul, Mark, and Elizabeth, have always been my bedrock of support. My mother is a gem, a smart beautiful woman who raised us all with grace and patience. My late father always believed in me and gave me courage to chase my dreams. I miss you, dad.

To all moms, dads, and others who read and cook from this book, thank you! Whether this is your first baby and you're embarking on your wondrous journey of parenthood, or you are already riding the sometimes crazy, always gorgeous road, you are the reason we wrote this book. Keep your sense of humor. Tell your little ones you love them and are proud of them every day. Hug often. Exhale. *There is no perfect.* You're amazing!

ROSE ANN HUDSON

I would like to thank my parents, the late and beloved Thomas and Lilian Angotti, who have always given me the love, guidance, and support I needed to achieve my goals. They have my deepest gratitude. Other members of my family have given a part of themselves to this project and I thank them: my wonderful husband, Mark, and beautiful daughters, Emily and Rachel, who gave me love and encouragement throughout. My sisters, Angela Angotti Morris and Antoinette Angotti, who have always been there for me. And, my eldest sister, Alma Angotti, who helped me organize my thoughts for this book on paper.

I would like to thank all of my colleagues for sharing their expertise and words of encouragement through the revision of this book: Martha Betts, RD, CNM; Julie Thorsen, RD; Elyse Kouri, RD; Ruth Osborne, RD; Maria Novak, RD; Brandi Suarez, RD; Katy Azzam, RD; Taylor Horne, RD; and Hannah Hallgrath, RD. They are an outstanding group of professional women making an impact on patients' health and nutrition every day. Finally, I would like to thank Catherine Jones for her hard work and tremendous dedication. It has been my great pleasure to work with Catherine, and I am confident that this new edition will help pregnant women for many years to come.

About the Authors

CATHERINE JONES

Catherine is an award-winning author of four books and the founder and CEO of Werbie, a health-tech company providing solutions for women with diabetes. The company's first product, GlucoseMama, is a complete system to improve the management of gestational diabetes. Catherine's two high-risk pregnancies with complications and her love of cooking inspired her to write the first edition of *Eating for Pregnancy* in 2003. She is passionate about helping moms and their families eat well and cook at home. She is a graduate of Connecticut College and La Varenne Culinary School in France. She was born in India and has lived around the globe as the daughter and spouse of Foreign Service officers. She has two children (her son is a vegan) and a precocious labradoodle from Poland named Miko. Contact Catherine at catherinejonescooks@gmail.com.

ROSE ANN HUDSON, RD, LD

Rose Ann is a registered dietitian and licensed dietitian specializing in perinatal nutrition. She has been on the staff of Inova Fairfax Hospital, in the obstetrics department, for more than twenty years. She served on the staff of Columbia Hospital for Women in Washington, DC for thirteen years, and has a private practice specializing in high-risk pregnancies for more than twenty-five years. Seeing thousands of patients every year, she is an expert on the nutritional needs of both low-risk and high-risk pregnancies. She lives with her husband in Rockville, Maryland. She has two daughters who have many of the same nutrition and baby passions. Her daughter Emily is a writer, vegan, and enjoys cooking and experimenting with healthy recipes. Rachel is a labor and delivery registered nurse.

DR. TERESA KNIGHT, OB-GYN, FACOG

Special Note: We are all deeply saddened that Dr. Knight lost her battle with cancer in October 2018. She was an incredible physician with unparalleled compassion. We will always remember and love her. Teresa was a board-certified obstetrician/gynecologist and a Fellow of the American College of Obstetrics and Gynecology. She was the founder of Women's Health Specialists of Saint Louis. In addition to her medical practice, she was an advisor to health-tech companies. Teresa received recognition for her contribution to the development of a traveling health clinic for perinatal services for homeless women. She was the medical director for the Family Planning Clinic of Franklin County. She has also worked in Tanzania, providing women's health training for medical providers. Teresa appeared regularly on local TV program and other media in her hometown of St. Louis, Missouri. She is survived by her husband, Bradford Smith, and her two children, Vincent and Elisa.

About the Contributors

ELNA NARULA, RN, CDE

Elna is a registered nurse and certified diabetes educator with a diverse background in maternal-child health, diabetes, high risk pregnancies, and clinical research. She has taught thousands of women and health-care professionals about diabetes in pregnancy for the past twenty-five years in an array of clinical settings, in both individualized and group sessions, giving presentations at community events and national conferences, and developing educational and marketing materials for healthcare and diabetes technology companies. Elna has trained patients and health-care professionals on insulin pumps and other medical devices. She is particularly interested in providing the best in available diabetes tools and resources to those living with gestational, type 1, and type 2 diabetes. Her passion for this springs from having a daughter with type 1 diabetes. Together they have worked in advocacy roles for many years promoting diabetes research and technology in the quest for a cure, which also led to her working on a number of type 1 diabetes clinical trials. At present she is working on a clinical trial for an autoimmune disease. Elna particularly enjoys teaching gestational diabetes classes because she believes it has a tremendous ripple effect of crystallizing lifelong healthy habits that can offset future metabolic and diabetes conditions for both mom and baby, as well as her entire family in the years ahead.

LINDA WADE, PHD

Linda is a clinical psychologist in private practice in Westchester County, New York. She is certified in Internal Family Systems, Focusing and Imago Relationship Therapy. She has over thirty years of experience, both professionally and personally, tackling the challenges of extra weight. She lives with her husband, and has a grown son and two grandchildren.

SHOSHANA BENNETT, PHD

Shoshana is the author of *Children of the Depressed, Postpartum Depression for Dummies,* and *Pregnant on Prozac,* and is coauthor of *Beyond the Blues: Understanding and Treating Prenatal and Postpartum Depression & Anxiety.* She is the creator of the app *PPD Gone!* and is an executive producer of the documentary *Dark Side of the Full Moon.* She cofounded the Postpartum Action Institute, committed to promoting parental health. After two life-threatening bouts of postpartum illness, Shoshana helped pioneer the field of maternal mental health. She founded Postpartum Assistance for Mothers in 1987, became president of California's state organization Postpartum Health Alliance, and then served as president of Postpartum Support International. Shoshana has helped tens of thousands of moms and dads around the world through private consultations, conferences, webinars, and support groups. Contact Shoshana at www.DrShosh.com.

General Index

calories *(continued)*
  daily needs for, 6–8
  estimated energy requirement, 7
  inadequate, 6
  during pregnancy, 10, 50
  for multiples, 50
  for teens, 47
  weight-loss guidelines, 333–334
carbohydrates
  CARBS, 11, 64
  complex, choosing, 11
  consuming daily, 64
  counting, 53, 64
  for fetal development, 11
  gluten-free, 25
  for PPD, 323
cats, and toxoplasmosis, 28–30
celiac disease, 25
cell development, 12, 13, 16–22, 71–71
Changes in mom's body month-by-month
  bloating, 76, 100, 126, 154, 178, 204, 234, 258, 284
  blood volume, 284
  Braxton Hicks contractions, 178, 204, 234, 258, 284
  breast changes, 76, 100, 126, 154, 204, 234, 258, 284
  cervix dilation, 284
  constipation, 76, 100, 126, 154, 178, 204, 234, 258, 284
  dizziness, 100, 126, 154, 178, 204, 234, 284
  fatigue, 76, 100, 126, 154, 234, 284
  food aversions and cravings, 100, 126, 154
  frequent urination, 76, 100, 126, 154, 178, 203, 234, 258, 284
  gas, 76, 100, 126, 154, 178, 203, 234, 258, 284
  headaches, 178, 204, 234, 284
  heartburn, 178, 204, 234, 258, 284
  heightened smell, 100, 126, 154, 204

  hemorrhoids, 178, 204, 234, 258, 284
  indigestion, 178, 204, 234, 258, 284
  leg cramps, 178, 204, 234, 258, 284
  lightening, 284
  lightheadedness, 100, 126, 154, 178, 204, 234, 284
  mood swings, 100
  morning sickness, 76, 100, 126
  mucus plug, 284
  nasal congestion/nose bleeds, 154
  nausea, 76, 100, 126
  nesting syndrome, 284
  placenta brain, 100
  shortness of breath, 258, 284
  sleep issues, 258, 284
  spotting/bleeding, 76, 100, 126
  stretch marks, 257, 284
  swelling, 178, 204, 258
  vaginal discharge, 100, 126, 154
  water break, 284
chia seeds, 44
chicken, cooking to well-done stage, 38
cholesterol, 16
choline, 22, 315
chromium, 15, 22, 324
coffee, 69, 70
complete meal ideas, 65
complex carbohydrates, 11
constipation, 23, 43–44
continuous glucose monitors, 54
cooking odors, 41
copper, 15, 22, 315
corpse pose, 336
counting calories for weight loss, 333
counting carbohydrates, 53, 64
couscous, cooking instructions and tips, 112
crash diets, 332
cravings, 43, 324, 330
Crohn's disease, 21, 45
C-sections, 51, 335

D
dairy-free recipe symbol, 65
dairy products, 25, 344
dehydration, 24, 60, 323
dental care, 47
depression. *See also* postpartum depression
  consulting a professional about, 330
  exercise for, 325
  sleep and, 325–326
  vitamin D for, 19, 324
DHA (docosahexaenoic acid), 13, 38, 324, 341–342
diabetes and gestational diabetes mellitus (GDM)
  about, 51
  blood glucose target levels, 54
  complications, 51
  defined, 51
  dietary guidelines, 52–53
  entering pregnancy with, 68
  exercise and, 55–56, 69
  finger pricking, 52
  low-carb recipes for, 351–352
  meal planning, 42
  menus for, 361–364
  pregnancy after 35, 48
  pregestational, 51
  progression to type 2, 58
  questions and answers about, 53–58
  reducing risk of, 68
  risk factors for, 54
  type 1, 51, 57
  type 2, 57, 58
diabetes educators, 53
diarrhea, 31, 32
diets and dieting
  best way to start, 331
  consulting doctor about, 327
  deciding when to begin, 329
  emotional baggage and, 331–332
  getting support for, 330–331
  healthy eating tips, 332–333
  in teens, 48
dinners, for diabetes during pregnancy, 52
dinners, low-carb ideas for, 364
dizziness, 47, 59

DNA, 19–20doctors
confirming pregnancy with, 2
consulting, about dieting, 327
consulting, about exercise, 69, 328, 335
before you conceive, 67
dopamine, 324, 325
drugs, 2, 48
due date calculations, 72

E
eating disorder, 69
eclampsia, 46
E. coli, 30–31
eggs, raw, 32–33, 160
emotional baggage, 331–332
emotional support, 326
endorphins, 325
energy needs during pregnancy, 10
EPA (eicosapentaenoic acid), 13, 38, 341–342
erythritol, 12
essential oils, 41
estimated energy requirements, 7, 10
exercise
benefits of, 3, 58–59, 325
consulting doctor about, 69, 328, 335
controlling blood sugar with, 55–56, 59
as a daily habit, 68
with diabetes, 53, 55, 61
to ease constipation, 44
at home, 335–336
with PIH, 61
for PPD, 232
precautions for certain women, 69
for pregnant women over 35, 49
reducing depression with, 325
safety tips, 53
warning signs to stop, 59–61, 336
for weight loss, 334–336
exhaustion, 330
eye development, 13, 18

F
fad diets, 333
fast food, 333
fatigue, 3, 41, 47, 324
fats, healthy, 12–13, 52, 64. *See also* omega-3 fatty acids
fertilization, 75
fetal age, 72
fetal alcohol exposure (FAE), 18
fetal alcohol syndrome (FAS), 18
fetal brain development, 10, 12
Fetal development
month-by-month
bone, 125, 153, 177, 203, 233, 257, 283
brain, 75, 99, 125, 153, 177, 203, 233, 257, 283
cell, 75, 99, 125, 153, 177, 203, 233, 257, 283
ear/hearing, 125, 153, 177, 203, 233, 257, 283
eye/vision, 99, 125, 153, 177, 203, 233, 257, 283
fat stores, 233, 257, 283
head-down position, 257, 283
heart, 99, 125, 153, 177, 203, 233, 257, 283
hiccups, 177, 203, 233, 283
immune system, 257, 283
kicks, 177, 203, 233, 283
lung, 153, 177, 203, 233, 257, 283
muscle, 125, 153, 177, 203, 233, 257, 283
nervous system, 177, 203, 233, 257, 283
neural tube, 75, 99, 125
organ, 75, 99, 125, 153, 177, 203, 233, 257, 283
placenta, 75, 99, 125
sensory, 153, 177, 203, 233, 257, 283
sexual organ, 125, 153, 177, 203, 233, 283
tooth, 125, 153, 177, 203, 233, 283
vernix caseosa, 177, 203, 233, 257, 283
fever, 32, 34
fiber, 23, 44, 52, 348–349

fiber, supplemental, 44
finger pricking, 54, 57
first trimester
calorie requirements, 7
constipation during, 43
heartburn in, 41
month 1 (weeks 1–4), 75–77
month 2 (weeks 5–8), 99–101
month 3 (weeks 9–13), 125–127
progesterone levels in, 3
fish
DHA and EPA content in, 341–342
fish sandwiches, safety of, 37
fish sticks, safety of, 37
high in mercury, risks from, 3, 35–37, 314
low in mercury, 36
omega-3 fatty acids in, 13
raw, avoiding, 36
safe choices in, 13
USDA and EPA guidelines on, 36, 314
fish oil supplements, 37–38
Floradix iron supplements, 44
fluoride, 22flours, gluten-free, 25
fluids. *See* water
flu-like symptoms, 30, 34
folic acid/folate, 20, 60, 64, 324, 347–348
folic acid supplements, 40, 67
food allergies, 24–26
food aversions, 43
food-borne illnesses
E. coli, 30–31
listeriosis, 33–35
salmonella, 31–33
Salmonella enteriditis (SE), 32–33, 160
Toxoplasmosis, 28
food cravings, 43
food journals, 331
food poisoning, 56
food safety tips
cooking food to "well-done" stage, 38
E. coli, 30–31
listeriosis, 33–35
methylmercury, 35–37

food safety tips *(continued)*
    safe plastics, 39
    salmonella, 31–33
    Salmonella enteriditis (SE), 32–33
    toxoplasmosis, 28–30
fourth trimester, 309
fresh air, 41
fruits, 35, 52–53, 85
fussiness, 316–317

G
gas, 42
gas-producing foods, 42
gastric bypass surgery, 45
genetic material, 20, 70
gestational age, 72
gestational diabetes. *See* diabetes
gestational hypertension, 3, 45, 46, 48
ginger supplements, 40
gingivitis, 47
glucagon, 58
glucometer, 54
glucose, 51
gluten-free diets, 25
gluten-free recipe symbol, 65
grain-based flours, 265
grains, 112–113
greens, cleaning and storing, 85
gum disease, 47

H
HALT (hungry, angry, lonely, and tired), 330
head circumference, 13
headaches, 45, 60
heart health, 16, 17, 21
heart rates, 60
heartburn, 41–42
hemorrhoids, 23, 43–44
high blood pressure, 45–46, 48
high blood sugar levels, 51
high-risk pregnancies, 44
hormones, pregnancy-related, 50–51, 55
hot tubs, 3
hyperemesis gravidarum, 40
hypertension, 3, 45–46, 61
hyperthermia, 60
hypoglycemia, 51, 57–58

I
immune system development, 13, 17
immunity, 16, 18, 19
implantation, 75
increased blood volume, 9
indigestion, 41–42
infertility, 45, 69
insulin, 15, 51, 53, 57, 58
insulin resistance, 51
Internal Family Systems Model (IFS), 331
iodine, 15, 22, 27, 315
iodized salt, 27
iron
    anemia, 15, 27
    combatting fatigue with, 324
    constipation, 43–44
    daily recommended intake, 15, 27, 342
    health benefits, 15–16
    heme, 16, 27
    hemoglobin, 15
    maximizing absorption of, 16, 27, 47
    nonheme, 16, 27
    plant-based sources of, 27
    for PPD, 324
    requirements for vegetarians and vegans, 27
    sources of, 342–343
    stores, 15
iron-deficiency anemia, 15, 43, 46–47
iron supplements, 27, 44, 47

J
journaling, 331
junk food, 333

K
Kegels, 61–62
kidney functioning, 17
king mackerel, 36

L
labor, 14
lactation. *See* breastfeeding
lactose intolerance, 14, 25
lancets, 54, 57
lancing devices, 54, 57

laxatives, 43
leg cramps, 61
listeriosis, 33–35
litter boxes, 30
liver, minimizing consumption of, 18
low birth weight, 47–48
low blood sugar, 51, 57–58
low blue light glasses, 326
low-carb recipe symbols, 65
low-carb recipes for diabetes during pregnancy, 351–352
lunches, for diabetes during pregnancy, 52
lunches, low-carb, 363
lymph node swelling, 30

M
macronutrients, 10–13
macrosomia, 54
magnesium, 16, 22, 61
manganese, 16, 22
massages, 3
meals, skipping, 332
meals, small, 11, 40, 42, 332
meat, undercooked or raw, 30, 31, 32
medications and prescriptions, 2, 42, 313
melatonin, 325, 326
mental clarity, 324
menus
    for diabetes during pregnancy, 361–364
    for pregnancy for one week, ideas for, 353–356
    suggested, on recipe pages, 65
    for vegetarian and vegan pregnancies, 357–360
mercury, about, 36
metabolism, 15–19, 21–22
methylmercury, 3, 35–37
milk production, 315–316, 328
minerals, 14–18, 64. *See also specific minerals*
miscarriages, 20, 45, 48, 68, 118
molybdenum, 16, 22
monounsaturated fats, 12
month 1 (weeks 1–4), 75–77
month 2 (weeks 5–8), 99–101
month 3 (weeks 9–13), 125–127

U

underweight women, 67–68
unsaturated fats, 12
UTI, 24
uterus, 9–10

V

vaping, 48, 68
vegan diets
  algae oil supplements for, 38
  and breastfeeding, 314
  general information, 25–26
  macronutrient, mineral, and
    vitamin needs, 26–28
  menus for, 359–360
  pantry staples for, 29
vegan recipe symbols, 65
vegetables, 35, 52–53, 85
vegetarian diets
  algae oil supplements for, 38
  and breastfeeding, 314
  general information, 25–26
  iron supplements for, 44
  macronutrient, mineral, and
    vitamin needs, 26–28
  menus for, 357–358
  optimizing nutrients in, 26
vitamin A, 12, 18, 23, 315,
  345–346
vitamin B_1, 21, 23, 315
vitamin B_2, 21, 23
vitamin B_3, 21, 23
vitamin B_4, 22
vitamin B_6
  for breastfeeding, 315
  daily recommended intake,
    21, 23
  good sources of, 21, 40, 324
  health benefits, 21
  for mood balance, 324
  for morning sickness, 40
  for PPD, 324
vitamin B_{12}
  for breastfeeding, 315
  daily recommended intake,
    20–21, 23
  good sources of, 20, 324
  health benefits, 20
  for low energy and
    depression, 324
  plant-based sources of, 28

for PPD, 324
supplements, 27
for vegetarians and vegans,
  28, 314
vitamin C
  daily recommended intake,
    19, 23, 346
  excessive, note about, 19
  good sources of, 19, 346–347
  health benefits, 19
  and iron absorption, 16, 27,
    47
  rebound scurvy, 19
vitamin D
  for breastfed infants, 315–316
  combining with calcium, 14
  daily recommended intake,
    19, 23
  good sources of, 19
  health benefits, 19
  for PPD, 324
  from sunlight, 19, 324
  supplements, 26
  toxic levels, 19
  warding off depression with,
    324
vitamin E, 19, 23, 315
vitamin K, 19, 23
vitamins. *See also* prenatal
    vitamins; *specific vitamins*
  consuming daily, 23, 64
vomiting, 32, 39–41, 47

W

Wade, Linda, 328
walking, 41, 59, 60, 325
water
  and constipation, 44
  daily intake, 23
  before exercising, 336
  importance of, 23–24
  between meals and snacks, 40
  for PPD, 323, 325
  unsafe, alternatives to, 56
  while breastfeeding, 314
  while dieting, 333
weight, healthy, 67
weight gain
  average, during pregnancy, 9
  composition of, during
    pregnancy, 9

with diabetes, 54
excessive, 9, 54
excessive during pregnancy, 46
inadequate, effect on fetus,
  6, 9
obesity, 45
for pregnant teens, 48
recommended rate for, 8
for women with triplets, 50
for women with twins, 50
weight loss postpartum. *See also*
  diets and dieting
  basic advice for, 327–328
  and breastfeeding, 312
  calorie guidelines, 333–334
  creating a diet plan, 332
  HALT, 330
  questions and answers,
    328–332
  setting goals for, 329
  weight loss mantra, 327
well-done temperature guide, 38
wound healing, 18–19, 22
wristband, for morning sickness,
  41

X

X-rays, 3, 47
xylitol, 12

Y

yoga, 3, 55, 325, 336
yogurt, for lactose intolerant
  moms, 25
yo-yo diets, 332

Z

zinc
  for breastfeeding, 315
  daily recommended intake,
    18, 23, 27
  good sources of, 18
  health benefits, 18
  requirements for vegetarians
    and vegans, 27
  vegetarian and vegan sources
    of, 27–28

Recipe Index